A Case-Based Guide to Neuromuscular Pathology

Lan Zhou • Dennis K. Burns • Chunyu Cai
Editors

A Case-Based Guide to Neuromuscular Pathology

Springer

Editors
Lan Zhou
Departments of Neurology
and Pathology
Boston University Medical Center
Boston, MA
USA

Chunyu Cai
Department of Pathology
University of Texas Southwestern
Medical Center
Dallas, TX
USA

Dennis K. Burns
Department of Pathology
Neuropathology Section
University of Texas Southwestern
Medical Center
Dallas, TX
USA

ISBN 978-3-030-25681-4 ISBN 978-3-030-25682-1 (eBook)
https://doi.org/10.1007/978-3-030-25682-1

This Springer imprint is published by the registered company Springer Nature Switzerland AG
The registered company address is: Gewerbestrasse 11, 6330 Cham, Switzerland

To my family members, husband Ming, and daughters Grace and Rebecca, for their love, encouragement, and support.

Lan Zhou, MD, PhD

To my wife Carol, my daughter Kelly, and my son Evan, for their enduring love and support.

Dennis K. Burns, MD

To Jade.

Chunyu Cai, MD, PhD

Preface

We present this book, *A Case-Based Guide to Neuromuscular Pathology*, to neurologists, pathologists, and other practitioners who take care of patients with neuromuscular diseases.

Biopsy of skeletal muscle and peripheral nerve with histopathological interpretation is frequently requested by neurologists to evaluate patients with myopathies and neuropathies as a part of the clinical workup and management. Muscle biopsy plays an important role in the diagnosis and classification of inflammatory myopathies, metabolic myopathies, congenital myopathies, muscular dystrophies, and toxic myopathies. Nerve biopsy is essential for diagnosing vasculitic neuropathy, amyloid neuropathy, infectious neuropathies, and neuropathies caused by malignant cellular infiltration of nerves. Although muscle and nerve biopsies are less frequently performed in the era of molecular testing, biopsies are still useful in many cases, as the sensitivity of many genetic tests in identifying pathological mutations in hereditary myopathies and neuropathies is not high. Moreover, biopsies can be extremely valuable in the initial characterization of some myopathies and neuropathies and can be used to direct subsequent genetic testing for specific hereditary myopathies and neuropathies. In addition, skin biopsy for the evaluation of intraepidermal nerve fiber density has emerged as the gold standard for diagnosing small fiber neuropathy and has been increasingly utilized by neuromuscular specialists.

This book covers the entire spectrum of neuromuscular pathology including skeletal muscle, peripheral nerve, and skin biopsies with biopsy interpretation. It comprises three parts. Part 1 uses three introductory chapters to review muscle, nerve, and skin biopsy indications and procedures, biopsy specimen handling and processing, utility of individual stains, normal muscle and nerve histology, and common muscle and nerve pathology. The 28 myopathy case chapters in Part 2 and 11 neuropathy case chapters in Part 3, collected from our practice over many years, illustrate the clinical and pathological features of these entities, demonstrate the indications and utilities of biopsies, discuss clinical and pathological differential diagnosis, update the individual disease management, and summarize pertinent clinical and pathology pearls for each case.

This book is intended to help neurologists understand the utility of muscle, nerve, and skin biopsies, correctly order these biopsies, become more familiar with neuromuscular pathology, perform clinical and pathological correlations, and make sound clinical decisions for management of patients with neuromuscular diseases based on biopsy findings. The book will help neurology residents and neuromuscular fellows answer questions related to the muscle and nerve pathology in their in-service and board exams. It is our hope that this book will also benefit neuromuscular pathologists and trainees as they correlate morphological alterations in muscle and nerve biopsies with clinical presentations and communicate their findings to clinical colleagues caring for patients with neuromuscular disorders.

We are enormously grateful to the authors of this book, who are experienced neuromuscular specialists and neuropathologists with sophisticated knowledge and expertise in neuromuscular medicine and pathology. We thank Springer for publishing this book, and thank Michael Wilt and other members in Springer for their excellent editorial support.

Boston, MA, USA — Lan Zhou
Dallas, TX, USA — Dennis K. Burns
Dallas, TX, USA — Chunyu Cai

Contents

Contributors

Rahul Abhyankar, MD Department of Neurology & Neurotherapeutics, University of Texas Southwestern Medical Center, Dallas, TX, USA

Dennis K. Burns, MD Departments of Pathology, Neuropathology Section, University of Texas Southwestern Medical Center, Dallas, TX, USA

Chunyu Cai, MD, PhD Department of Pathology, University of Texas Southwestern Medical Center, Dallas, TX, USA

Ryan Castoro, DO, MS Department of Physical Medicine and Rehabilitation, Vanderbilt University Medical Center, Nashville, TN, USA

Diana P. Castro, MD Department of Neurology and Neurotherapeutics, University of Texas Southwestern Medical Center, Children's Medical Center of Dallas, Dallas, TX, USA

Shan Chen, MD, PhD Peripheral Neuropathy Center, Rutgers University, Robert Wood Johnson Medical School, New Brunswick, NJ, USA

Jeffrey L. Elliott, MD Department of Neurology and Neurotherapeutics, University of Texas Southwestern Medical Center, Dallas, TX, USA

Partha S. Ghosh, MD Department of Neurology, Boston Children's Hospital, Boston, MA, USA

Elisabeth Golden, MD Department of Neurology and Neurotherapeutics, University of Texas Southwestern Medical Center, Dallas, TX, USA

Michelle Kaku, MD Department of Neurology, Boston University Medical Center, Boston, MA, USA

Shaida Khan, DO Department of Neurology and Neurotherapeutics, University of Texas Southwestern Medical Center, Dallas, TX, USA

Patrick Kwon, MD Department of Neurology, New York University Langone–Brooklyn, New York, NY, USA

Jun Li, MD, PhD Department of Neurology, Wayne State University School of Medicine and Detroit Medical Center, Detroit, MI, USA

Hart G. W. Lidov, MD, PhD Department of Pathology, Boston Children's Hospital, Boston, MA, USA

Lingchao Meng, MD Neuromuscular Division, Department of Neurology, Peking University First Hospital, Beijing, China

Susan Morgello, MD Departments of Neurology, Neuroscience, and Pathology, Icahn School of Medicine at Mount Sinai, New York, NY, USA

Rajeev Motiwala, MD Department of Neurology, New York University, New York, NY, USA

Sharon P. Nations Department of Neurology & Neurotherapeutics, University of Texas Southwestern Medical Center, Dallas, TX, USA

Dustin Jacob Paul, DO, MA Department of Neurology and Neurotherapeutics, University of Texas Southwestern Medical Center, Dallas, TX, USA

Susan C. Shin, MD Department of Neurology, Icahn School of Medicine at Mount Sinai, New York, NY, USA

Kara Stavros, MD Department of Neurology, Warren Alpert Medical School of Brown University, Rhode Island Hospital, Providence, RI, USA

Laura K. Stein, MD Department of Neurology, Ichan School of Medicine at Mount Sinai, New York, NY, USA

Jaya R. Trivedi, MD Department of Neurology & Neurotherapeutics, University of Texas Southwestern Medical Center, Dallas, TX, USA

Yun Yuan, MD Neuromuscular Division, Department of Neurology, Peking University First Hospital, Beijing, China

Lan Zhou, MD, PhD Departments of Neurology and Pathology, Boston University Medical Center, Boston, MA, USA

Part I
Introduction to Neuromuscular Pathology Evaluation

Chapter 1
Skeletal Muscle Biopsy Evaluation

Dennis K. Burns

Introduction

First introduced into clinical practice in the middle decades of the nineteenth century, muscle biopsies have played an integral role in the diagnosis and treatment of patients with neuromuscular diseases for well over a century. The interpretation of morphological changes in skeletal muscles, supplemented by enzyme histochemical and immunohistochemical stains are now regularly integrated with molecular analyses to provide physicians with an unprecedented understanding of the pathogenesis and phenotypic complexities of neuromuscular diseases. Although advances in molecular diagnoses have eliminated the need for muscle biopsies in some disorders, in many conditions, biopsies continue to provide information not readily obtainable by other methods.

Muscle Biopsy Acquisition

There are three important aspects of muscle biopsy acquisition: selecting the proper muscle, obtaining an adequate amount of tissue, and minimizing artifacts.

The importance of selecting the right muscle for biopsy cannot be overemphasized. Skeletal muscles are not equally affected by a given disease process. While the majority of myopathies predominantly affect proximal limb muscles, a few preferentially involve distal limb, trunk, or facial muscles. In order to maximize the diagnostic yield of a muscle biopsy, it is important to carefully select the biopsy site. Selection of the biopsy site can be challenging and should be done in close consultation with the

D. K. Burns (✉)
Department of Pathology, Neuropathology Section, University of Texas Southwestern Medical Center, Dallas, TX, USA
e-mail: dennis.burns@utsouthwestern.edu

L. Zhou et al. (eds.), *A Case-Based Guide to Neuromuscular Pathology*,
https://doi.org/10.1007/978-3-030-25682-1_1

treating physician. The site of the biopsy should be based on the pattern of muscle weakness, electromyography (EMG) abnormalities, and/or muscle imaging findings [1, 2]. In patients with chronic muscle injury, one should choose a muscle for biopsy that is weak but not profoundly atrophic. If a muscle is markedly atrophic, the biopsy may show "end-stage" changes with extensive fibro-fatty tissue replacement and few residual myofibers, precluding determination of the cause of the muscle injury. In patients with more acute or subacute muscle injury, in contrast, one may choose to biopsy a more severely affected muscle to better capture the muscle pathology. Since the majority of myopathies affect predominantly proximal limb muscles, deltoid, biceps, and quadriceps muscles are most commonly chosen, and these muscles have sufficient norms established for comparing myofiber size and fiber type percentages [3, 4]. If a myopathy predominantly affects distal limb muscles, the tibialis anterior or gastrocnemius muscle may be selected for biopsy. One should not choose a muscle which had recent injection or needle EMG examination, in order to avoid areas of nonspecific muscle injury caused by the needle [5]. Since muscle involvement in myopathies is typically symmetrical, needle EMG of limb muscles is usually done on one side and the biopsy is taken from corresponding contralateral muscle. It is worth mentioning that EMG can be normal in a mild myopathy, and some myopathies may have focal or asymmetrical limb muscle involvement. In these settings, skeletal muscle MRI or ultrasound is sometimes useful in targeting an affected muscle for biopsy.

As discussed in detail in the next few paragraphs, skeletal muscle can be obtained via open biopsy approach [2] or percutaneously, the latter employing a Bergstrom-type cutting needle [1, 6–8]. As an aside, "thin" needles of the type employed in fine needle aspiration biopsies seldom yield adequate material for meaningful interpretation of muscle morphology, and are almost never satisfactory for detailed enzyme histochemical and immunohistochemical studies. For these reason, we recommend that they not be used to obtain muscle biopsies in clinical work. Percutaneous biopsy has the advantage of being less invasive, while open biopsy has the advantage of providing larger specimens [1, 2]. Both procedures are quite safe in the hands of experienced operators. Open biopsy is usually done in an operating room with the patient sedated and under the care of an anesthesiologist, while percutaneous needle biopsies are often performed in outpatient clinic settings. Local anesthesia is given before a skin incision is made, taking care to not infiltrate the muscle tissue selected for biopsy with the anesthetic agent. The incision, typically around 3–4 cm in length, should be made in an area that avoids myotendinous junction whenever possible. Bleeding is usually minimal and can be controlled by firm pressure or ligation without the need for cautery. Muscle biopsy tissue should never be cauterized, inasmuch as the electrocautery destroys muscle morphology and enzyme activity. Detailed muscle biopsy procedures have been described by others [1, 2].

Initial Processing and Sectioning of Skeletal Muscle Biopsies

Procedures for processing skeletal muscle biopsies are well-established and, while not overly complex, differ significantly from procedures employed in handling most tissues submitted to surgical pathology laboratories. If muscle biopsies are not to be processed in the laboratory that initially receives the specimen, it is essential that the physician obtaining the biopsy and laboratory personnel at the institution where the biopsy is obtained communicate in advance with the laboratory that will ultimately process the specimen to ensure that tissue preservation is optimum.

For optimum evaluation, skeletal muscle biopsies should include both unfixed and fixed tissue. Properly frozen, unfixed tissue, in particular, plays a critical role in the assessment of morphological abnormalities in skeletal muscle. Fresh muscle should be transported immediately to the laboratory for freezing and subsequent processing. During transportation to the laboratory, the fresh tissue should be wrapped in gauze that has been slightly moistened in saline and placed in a waterproof container surrounded by crushed wet ice, in order to prevent drying artifact and loss of enzyme activity. The amount of saline should be sufficient to simply keep the tissue moist; excess saline can introduce freezing artifact, as well as promote a loss of enzyme activity in the muscle. Ideally, muscle biopsies should be transported to the laboratory for freezing within 60 minutes of the procedure, although satisfactory morphology can be obtained in tissue frozen within a few hours of the biopsy, as long as the specimen is kept cool. For specimens being transported overnight, it is advisable to freeze the specimen in the referring laboratory, and then transport the specimen on dry ice to the reference laboratory for processing.

As soon as the specimen arrives in the laboratory, the muscle segment should be carefully oriented so that its fibers are in cross section. In the case of larger segments, orientation can often be accomplished with the naked eye, while smaller specimens, including those obtained via a percutaneous needle biopsy, are best oriented with the aid of a dissecting microscope (Fig. 1.1a). The oriented sample is placed on an appropriately-labeled cork segment and immobilized with a small amount of either gum tragacanth or a small amount of Optimal Cutting Temperature (OCT) mounting medium at the base of the tissue. It is important that the tissue be placed *on top of the mounting medium* rather than covered by the medium, so that subsequent freezing of the tissue can occur as rapidly as possible (Fig. 1.1b).

Once oriented and immobilized on the cork, the fresh muscle is ready for freezing. The basic tools for freezing are relatively simple, and include a suspended metal beaker, an insulated container for liquid nitrogen and a supply of isopentane (Fig. 1.2a). The oriented skeletal muscle segment is frozen by placing it into a metal beaker of isopentane that has been cooled in liquid nitrogen to approximately −160° C. The isopentane will be sufficiently chilled when a delicate white rind begins to form on the inner surface of the beaker. The specimen should be completely immersed and gently stirred in the chilled isopentane in order to facilitate rapid, uniform freezing of the tissue (Fig. 1.2b). For smaller specimens, freezing is usually complete within 30 seconds, while larger specimens may require immersion for up to 50 seconds. Once the tissue has been frozen, it can be transferred directly to the cryostat for sectioning or, alternatively, stored in a sealed plastic bag at −70 to −80 °C. If long term storage is anticipated, placing a few ice crystals into the plastic bag can minimize "freezer burn" during storage.

In order to prepare frozen sections, the cork holding the specimen should be immobilized on a standard cryostat chuck using OCT embedding medium.

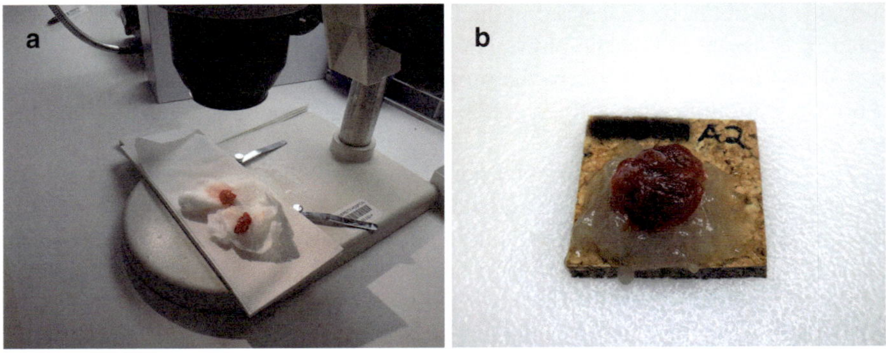

Fig. 1.1 Orientation of the muscle biopsy. (**a**) Larger specimens can sometimes be oriented with the naked eye, but in many cases, the use of a dissecting microscope can ensure that cross sections of the fresh frozen specimen are obtained. (**b**) A properly oriented muscle segment. The fresh tissue has been mounted on the surface of a small mound of gum tragacanth. Note that the specimen is not fully embedded in the mounting medium. This ensures that a maximum amount of the specimen's surface area is exposed to the chilled isopentane (2-methlybutane) during the subsequent freezing process

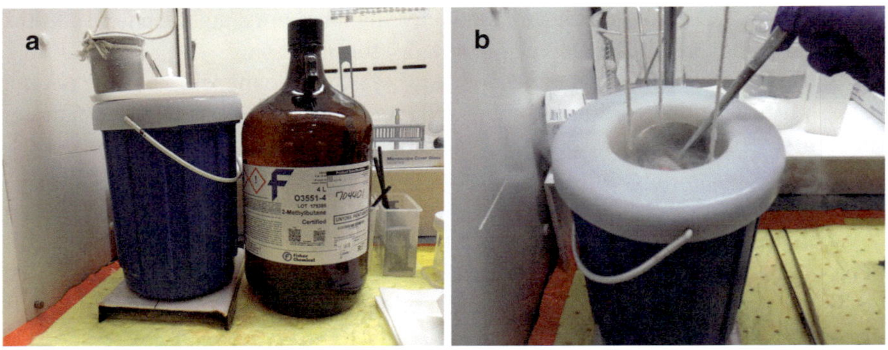

Fig. 1.2 Freezing the muscle biopsy. (**a**) The basic material for properly freezing muscle biopsies consists of an insulated, wide-mouthed container for liquid nitrogen, a metal beaker that can be suspended into the liquid nitrogen and a supply of isopentane. (**b**) To freeze the biopsy, the metal beaker is filled with isopentane and partially immersed into the liquid nitrogen, taking care to not allow the liquid nitrogen to come into direct contact with the isopentane. A white rind will form on the inner surface of the metal beaker when the isopentane has been cooled to an appropriate temperature for freezing the specimen. The oriented, mounted muscle segment is then completely immersed in the chilled isopentane and gently stirred for about 50 seconds. Once frozen, the specimen can be transferred to the cryostat for sectioning or, alternatively, stored in a sealed plastic bag at −70 to −80° C for later processing

Sections should be cut in a cryostat maintained at a temperature of −20 to −25° C. Biopsies that have been stored at −70 to −80 °C should be allowed to warm to cryostat temperatures in order to avoid shattering the tissue during sectioning. Sections of tissue destined for routine staining, including enzyme histochemical staining, should be cut at thicknesses of 10 μm, while those used for immunohistochemical staining should be cut a thicknesses of 6 μm. In our laboratory, sections are picked up directly onto commercially prepared positively-charged glass slides (*Superfrost™ Plus*), although sections can also be placed on standard glass coverslips for staining if desired. If the cryostat sections are not to be stained immediately, the slides are placed in a folder and kept in a 4 °C refrigerator until ready for use. Ideally, cryostat muscle sections should be stained within 24 hours of the time that the sections are cut.

Although skeletal muscle morphology at the light microscopic level is best demonstrated in cryostat sections of properly frozen muscle, fixed muscle can also provide useful diagnostic information in a number of important muscle disorders. In the case of open biopsies, muscle destined for fixation should be clamped *in situ* using either a single use, disposable Becton Dickinson Rayport® polypropylene clamp or a reusable Price muscle biopsy clamp. The clamped muscle segment is gently excised from the surrounding skeletal muscle, placed into 10% neutral buffered formalin, and transported to the laboratory. Once in the laboratory, the fixed muscle segment is excised from the clamp. Representative longitudinally oriented sections measuring no more than 1 mm in thickness are transferred to 3% buffered glutaraldehyde for resin embedding and, in selected cases, subsequent electron microscopy. The remainder of the skeletal muscle segment is divided into cross and longitudinal sections and placed into standard histological cassettes for paraffin histology, discussed below. Muscle tissue obtained via percutaneous needle biopsy is also suitable for fixation. Muscle fragments obtained via needle biopsy can be placed directly into fixative—either 10% neutral buffered formalin or 3% buffered glutaraldehyde—and transported to the laboratory.

Routine Histological Stains

Proper evaluation of muscle biopsies requires the use of a number of different stains on frozen and, in some laboratories, fixed tissue, some of which are familiar to general surgical pathologists and some of which are used exclusively in the evaluation of frozen skeletal muscle. In our laboratory, frozen and paraffin sections of skeletal muscle biopsies are routinely evaluated with a panel of non-enzymatic histological stains and enzyme histochemical stains as listed below:

- <u>Non-enzymatic stains (frozen sections)</u>
  - Hematoxylin and eosin (H&E)
  - Modified Gomori trichrome
  - Oil Red O
  - Non-aqueous periodic acid Schiff (PAS) with and without diastase digestion (usually reserved for cases with suspected glycogen storage abnormalities)
  - Crystal violet
  - Congo red
- <u>Enzyme histochemical stains (frozen sections)</u>
  - Myosin adenosine triphosphatases (ATPases) at pH 4.3, 4.6 and 9.4
  - Nonspecific esterase
  - Acid phosphatase

  - Alkaline phosphatase
  - NADH-tetrazolium reductase
  - Succinate dehydrogenase (SDH)
  - Cytochrome-c oxidase (COX)
  - Sequential COX-SDH
  - Myophosphorylase
  - Phosphofructokinase
  - Myoadenylate deaminase
- Non-enzymatic stains (paraffin sections)
  - H&E
  - Masson trichrome
  - Congo red
  - Morin stain (reserved for cases of suspected aluminum adjuvant-associated myopathies)

Most of the staining of frozen (cryostat) sections is performed by placing the mounted sections in new 5-slide capacity plastic slide mailers. Coplin jars are used for the same purpose in some institutions, but if used, must be scrupulously cleaned between staining runs to avoid cross contamination. The use of new slide mailers minimizes the risk of such cross contamination. Individual stains and their uses are described in the following paragraphs. Technical information about individual staining procedures is available in published protocols included in the references at the end of this chapter [1, 9–18].

Normal skeletal muscle is composed of a mixture of three different types muscle cells, each of which has a fairly predictable staining profile in the panel of stains listed above. Type 1 myofibers, also known as "slow twitch" fibers, generate most of their energy via oxidative metabolism, and, as such, have abundant mitochondria and lipid, and less glycogen. Type 1 fibers are relatively resistant to fatigue, and are adapted to prolonged, endurance-type activities. Type 2 myofibers, or "fast twitch" fibers, generate more of their energy via glycolysis and contain more abundant glycogen and have less lipid and fewer mitochondria than their type I counterparts. Type 2 myofibers can be further subdivided into type 2a (fast twitch mixed oxidative/glycolytic) fibers and type 2b (fast twitch glycolytic) fibers. Type 2a fibers can change into type 2b fibers and vice versa, depending upon an individual's exercise habits. Whether of myofiber is a type 1 or a type 2 fiber, however, is determined by the lower motor neuron that innervates it and remains constant if its innervation remains intact. The metabolic profile of a given myofiber influences its staining properties, as discussed in the following paragraphs.

Non-enzymatic Stains (Frozen Sections)

The ***hematoxylin and eosin (H&E) stain*** is arguably the single most useful stain used in the evaluation of frozen sections of skeletal muscle biopsies. H&E stained cryostat sections provide information about the presence and pattern of myofiber atrophy (e.g., group atrophy in neurogenic disorders, selective perifascicular atrophy in classical dermatomyositis), myofiber degeneration and necrosis, regenerative change, vacuoles, inflammatory infiltrates and chronic structural changes of the type seen in many muscular dystrophies. Blood vessels and structural vascular abnormalities (e.g. vasculitis) are also well demonstrated in H&E sections. In normal muscle (Fig. 1.3a), individual myofibers have a polygonal configuration in cross section, with diameters ranging from approximately 30–70 mμ in adult women and 40–80 mμ in adult men [19]. Myofiber nuclei stain blue in H&E sections. Normal myofiber nuclei are small, and typically lie at the periphery of the fiber in transverse sections. Contractile proteins give the sarcoplasm a light pink appearance. Delicate basophilic stippling is visible in well preserved specimens at higher magnification, imparted by the presence of mitochondria and "sarcotubular" components (sarcoplasmic reticulum and T-tubules) in the intermyofibrillar network. Type 1 myofibers stain a bit more darkly than type 2 fibers in H&E stains, although fiber typing is best done with other stains (see below). When muscle fibers regenerate following myofiber injury, the sarcoplasm often stains light blue, owing to the presence increased cytoplasmic ribonucleoprotein associated with protein synthesis. Enlarged nuclei with discernible nucleoli are another characteristic of regenerating myofibers. These changes are illustrated later under the heading "Interpretation of the Biopsy." Increased numbers of internalized nuclei can be seen in a number of myopathic disorders (discussed below) but are also common near myotendinous insertion sites, and in this location should not be interpreted as evidence of myofiber injury.

The ***Gomori trichrome stain*** is familiar to most pathologists as a useful stain for demonstrating collagen, which stains with a light green color in frozen sections. In frozen sections of skeletal muscle, the modified Gomori trichrome stain developed by Engel and Cunningham [9] plays an even more important role in highlighting a variety of normal and abnormal structures within the sarcoplasm of muscle fibers. Normal mitochondria and sarcotubular elements, which are visible as punctate blue structures in H&E sections, stain red in the Gomori trichrome stain owing to the affinity of sarcoplasmic membranous structures for the Chromotrope 2R dye used in the procedure (Fig. 1.3b). Abnormal collections of mitochondria produce characteristic "ragged red" change in type I myofibers in many patients with mitochondrial disorders (discussed below under "Interpretation of the Biopsy"). Tubular aggregates, discussed below in the paragraphs dealing with biopsy interpretation, are also highlighted in the Gomori trichrome stain. Additional structures that are reliably highlighted in the trichrome stain include nemaline rods and cytoplasmic bodies (both derived from sarcomeric Z-bands), and the membranous debris present in sarcoplasmic vacuoles in patients with inclusion body myositis. Figures 1.18–1.20, which will be discussed later, contain examples of some of the abnormal structures that are highlighted in Gomori trichrome-stained cryostat sections. The appearance of collagen in Gomori trichrome-stained cryostat sections is illustrated in Fig. 1.21, which will also be discussed later.

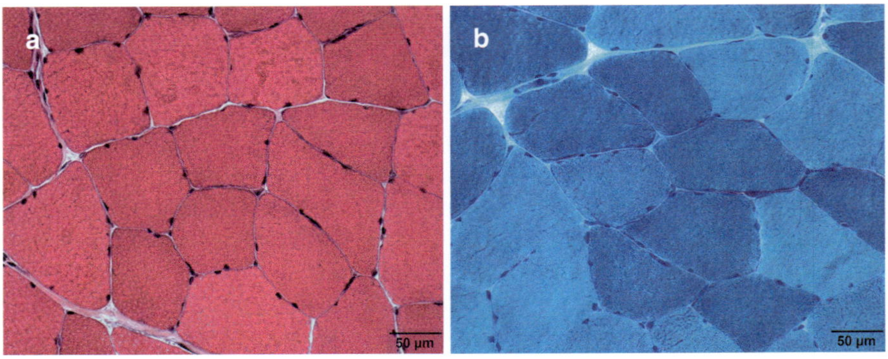

Fig. 1.3 Normal muscle (H&E and Gomori trichrome stains) . (**a**) Normal skeletal muscle, H&E. In a properly prepared skeletal muscle segment, the myofibers have a fairly uniform, polygonal appearance in cross section. The sarcoplasm of normal muscle fibers stains pink H&E stains, due to the presence of contractile proteins (myofibrils). In normal muscle myofiber nuclei characteristically lie just beneath the sarcoplasm except in the vicinity of myotendinous insertion sites, where internalized nuclei are fairly common. (**b**) Normal skeletal muscle, Gomori trichrome. The Gomori trichrome stain is an indispensable stain in the evaluation of frozen muscle biopsies. The contractile proteins stain green in the Gomori trichrome stain, while the membrane-rich elements that lie between the myofibrils (mitochondria, sarcoplasmic reticulum and T-tubules) stain red-purple, imparting a delicate stippled appearance to the sarcoplasm. Type 1 myofibers have larger numbers of mitochondria than type 2 fibers and stain more darkly in the Gomori trichrome stain

The ***Oil Red O stain*** is one of several stains available for demonstrating sarcoplasmic neutral lipid in frozen sections. Neutral lipid is present in normal skeletal muscle, particularly in type I (slow twitch) fibers. Normal sarcoplasmic lipid appears as fine red dots in the Oil Red O stain (Fig. 1.4a), and abnormal lipid stores appear as correspondingly larger red droplets (Fig. 1.4b). "Bleeding" of stained lipid over the section can occur when the muscle biopsy contains a significant amount of adipose tissue, and care must be taken to not misinterpret this phenomenon as abnormal sarcoplasmic lipid accumulation. After staining, sections are covered with glycerol or a comparable aqueous medium and coverslipped.

Periodic Acid-Schiff (PAS) stains have been used for decades to demonstrate carbohydrates in tissues, including glycogen and other molecules with carbohydrate components (e.g., glycoproteins and glycolipids). PAS stains are especially important in the evaluation of biopsies from patients with suspected glycogen storage diseases. Carbohydrate-rich structures, including glycogen, stain magenta in the PAS stain (Fig. 1.4c, d). Incubation of the tissue with diastase before staining will remove particulate glycogen, but will leave other carbohydrate-bearing structures (e.g. basement membranes) intact. The PAS reactivity basement membranes and of abnormal filamentous forms of glycogen of the type that accumulate in type IV glycogenosis and polyglucosan body disease is not affected by diastase digestion. It is worth noting that fixation of tissue in aqueous fixatives prior to staining often removes delicate particulate glycogen from the tissues, preventing adequate demonstration of abnormal glycogen stores.

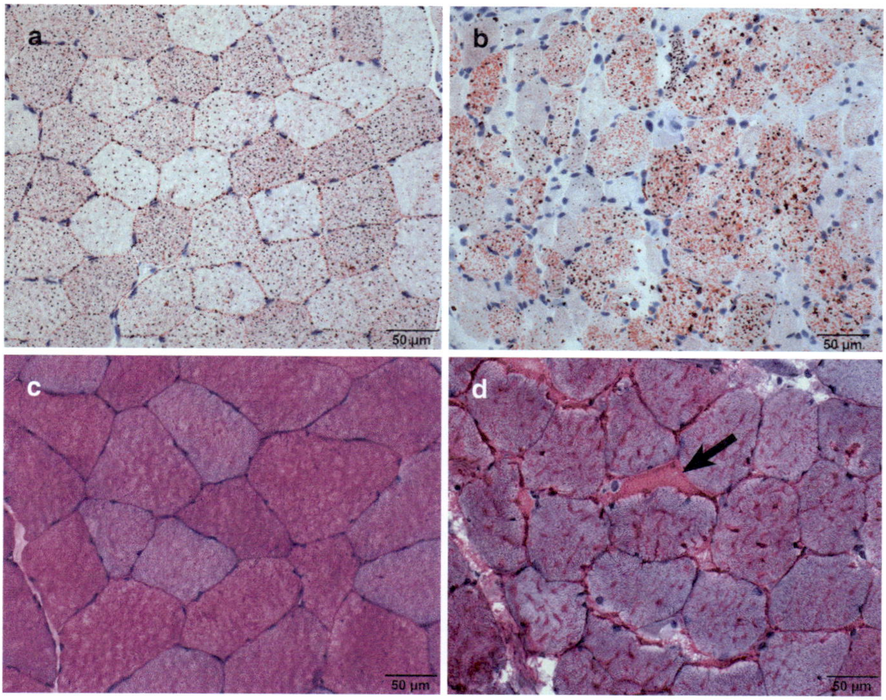

Fig. 1.4 Oil red O and PAS-stains of frozen muscle. (**a**) Normal muscle, oil red O. The oil red O stain is a very useful stain for demonstrating neutral lipids in frozen muscle, which appear as delicate red sarcoplasmic droplets. The lipid content of type 1 myofibers is higher than that of type 2 fibers. (**b**) Lipid storage myopathy, oil red O. Abnormal sarcoplasmic lipid accumulation can be seen in a wide range of conditions, including primary lipid storage myopathies, as illustrated here. Increased amounts of lipid are also seen in mitochondrial disorders and as a nonspecific reaction to myofiber injury. The abnormal lipid deposits appear as larger droplets than those seen in normal muscle. In extreme cases, these large droplets can occupy most of the cross sectional area of the affected myofiber. (**c**) Normal muscle, PAS. The PAS stain is the standard stain for demonstrating glycogen and basement membrane material. Because type 2 myofibers have a higher concentration of glycogen than type 1 fibers, they stain more intensely in the PAS stain. Incubation of the tissue section with diastase (amylase) will remove particulate glycogen, but will not affect the staining of basement membranes. (**d**) Glycogen storage disease, PAS. Abnormal glycogen deposits (arrow) stain with a magenta color in the PAS stain. In this biopsy from a patient with McArdle disease (muscle phosphorylase deficiency), particulate glycogen accumulates in subsarcolemmal regions. Pre-treatment with diastase will remove such deposits. In some conditions, exemplified by glycogen storage disease type IV and polyglucosan body disease, the abnormal glycogen deposits are composed of filamentous rather than particulate glycogen and will persist in the tissue after diastase digestion

The ***Congo Red stain*** is an essential stain for demonstrating amyloid deposits. The term "amyloid" does not refer to a specific protein, but rather to a heterogeneous group of proteins that have in common a tendency to aggregate into a β-pleated sheet configuration. Amyloid deposits can be encountered in skeletal muscle in patients with sporadic systemic amyloidosis, most commonly associated with plasma cell dyscrasias and abnormal immunoglobulin light chain (particularly lambda light chain) production. Less commonly, amyloid deposits can be seen in hereditary forms of amyloidosis associated with abnormal deposits of transthyretin and, less commonly, a

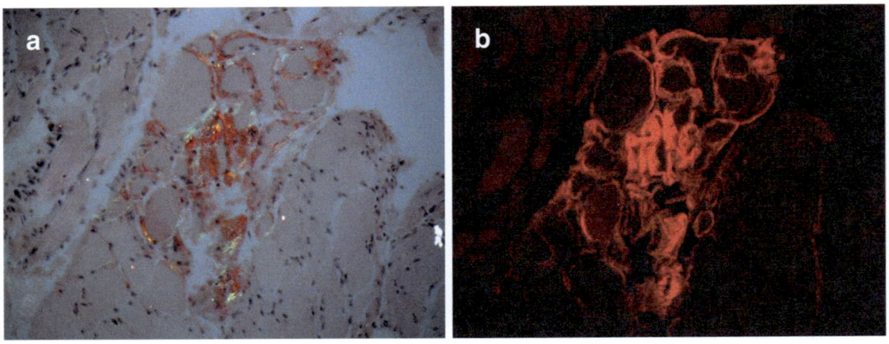

Fig. 1.5 Amyloid deposits, Congo red stain. (**a**) Amyloidosis, Congo red under polarized light. The classic method for the demonstration of amyloid deposits at the light microscopic level is the Congo red stain. When viewed under polarized light, the pink-staining amyloid has a characteristic "apple green" birefringence. (**b**) Amyloidosis, Congo red with epifluorescence illumination. When Congo red-stained sections are viewed under epifluorescence illumination with Texas red filtration, amyloid deposits have a bright red appearance. This technique is a more sensitive method for detecting amyloid deposits than polarized light microscopy, but is somewhat less specific

number of other proteins. Interestingly, amyloid deposition is also seen in two forms of autosomal recessive limb girdle muscular dystrophy – LGMD 2B (dysferlinopathy) [20] and LGMD 2 L (anoctamin-5 deficiency) [21]. In all of the preceding conditions, the amyloid is deposited extracellularly – most commonly within vessels walls and around individual myofibers. Intracellular amyloid deposits also occur in some conditions, notably variants of inclusion body myositis (IBM). In this disorder, the intracellular amyloid deposits are composed of β-amyloid, the type of amyloid encountered in the central nervous system in Alzheimer's disease and amyloid angiopathy.

Amyloid deposits appear as homogeneous, eosinophilic deposits in in H&E stained sections, and have a salmon-pink color in Congo red stains. Under polarized light, the amyloid deposits contain areas of characteristic "apple green" birefringence (Fig. 1.5a). Fluorescence microscopy with Texas Red filtration is an even more sensitive technique for detection of amyloid deposits [22]. Under fluorescence illumination with Texas Red filtration, amyloid deposits appear bright red (Fig. 1.5b).

Enzyme Histochemical Stains (Frozen Sections)

Staining for ***myosin adenosine triphosphatase (ATPase)*** activity has long been the most reliable method for distinguishing slow twitch (type 1) myofibers from fast twitch (type 2) fibers. The staining procedure involves the cleavage of a phosphate group from ATP in a frozen muscle section in a solution of aqueous calcium chloride, producing an insoluble calcium phosphate precipitate at the site of the reaction. The tissue is then incubated in a solution of cobaltous chloride, during which the calcium in the calcium phosphate is replaced by cobalt (Co^{2+}). The section is then briefly incubated in a solution of ammonium sulfide, which generates a black cobaltous sulfide reaction product in the muscle fiber [1, 10, 11]. Incubation of the section in an alkaline barbital solution (pH 9.4 in our laboratory) results in the selective activation of myosin ATPase in type 2 fibers, causing them to stain darkly, while type 1 fibers remain pale. Pre-incubation of tissue sections in a barbital buffer at pH 4.3 produces a reciprocal staining pattern – that is, darkly staining type 1 fibers and pale type 2 fibers. In addition, in the ATPase 4.3 preparation, a small subpopulation of intermediate-staining type 2c fibers is often visible. Finally, pre-incubation of the tissue section at pH 4.6 produces a pattern in which type 1 fibers stain darkly, type 2a (fast twitch oxidative) fibers are pale, and type 2b (fast twitch glycolytic) fibers stain with intermediate intensity (Fig. 1.6a–c). The use of standard mounting medium in the preparation of slides stained for ATPase activity will result in fading of the reaction product over time. Staining intensity can be preserved by cover-slipping the ATPase-stained sections with Canada balsam. In normally innervated muscle, the distribution of type 1 and type 2 fibers is random, as illustrated in Fig. 1.6a–c. A loss of randomness in the distribution of myofibers is called "fiber

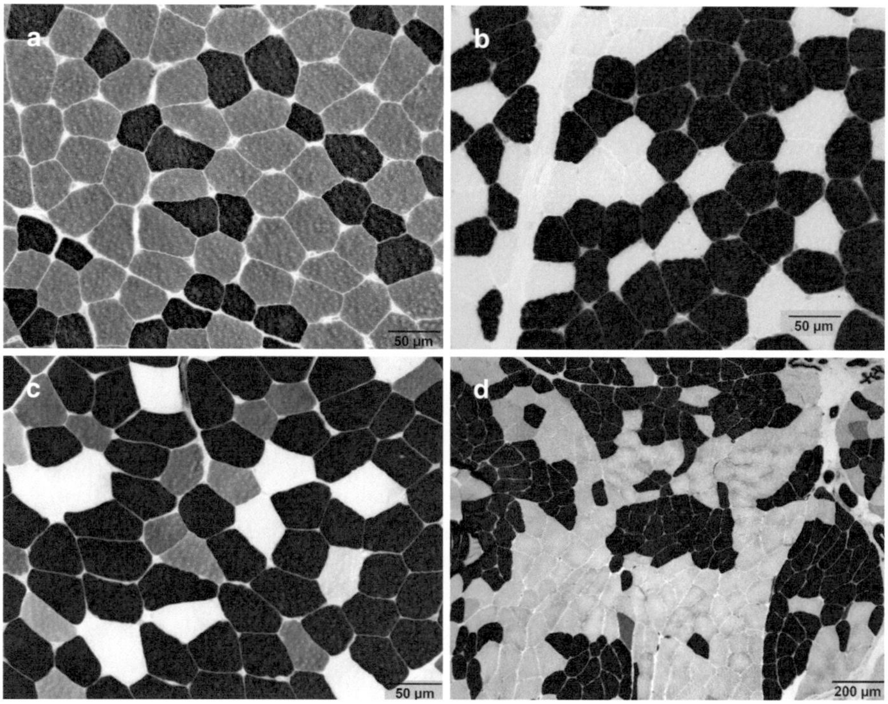

Fig. 1.6 ATPase stains. (**a**) Normal muscle, ATPase 9.4. Cryostat sections stained for myosin ATPase activity are the most reliable way to distinguish slow-twitch (type 1) from fast-twitch (type 2) subpopulations. In this section of deltoid muscle stained for ATPase activity at pH 9.4, type 2 fibers are dark, while type 1 fibers are pale. (**b**) Normal muscle, ATPase 4.3. Staining a section of the same muscle for ATPase activity at pH 4.3 reveals a reverse staining pattern, with the more numerous type 1 fibers staining darkly. (**c**) Normal muscle, ATPase 4.6. Staining of normal skeletal muscle at pH 4.6 typically reveals three levels of staining intensity: type 1 fibers are dark, type 2A (mixed oxidative-glycolytic) fibers are pale, and type 2B (fast twitch glycolytic) fibers stain with intermediate intensity. (**d**) In normal skeletal muscle, the different myofiber subtypes intermingle in a random distribution. If a muscle is denervated and then re-innervated, axonal sprouts from regenerating motor axons innervate contiguous myofibers, resulting in the formation of groups of contiguous myofibers with the same histochemical staining profile ("fiber type grouping")

type grouping" and indicates reinnervation of previously denervated muscle (Fig. 1.6d). The ATPase stain is extremely helpful in characterizing conditions associated with various patterns of type-specific myofiber atrophy or hypertrophy, and in the identification of patients with myopathy with thick filament loss ("critical illness") myopathy. Some of these patterns are illustrated later under "Interpretation of the Biopsy" in Fig. 1.12.

The ***nonspecific esterase stain*** relies on the hydrolysis of an exogenous alpha-naphthyl acetate substrate by endogenous esterase to yield naphthol, which in turn forms an insoluble azo dye when incubated with basic fuchsin, which appears brick red under the microscope [12]. The stain highlights normal neuromuscular junctions due to the presence of acetylcholinesterase in those structures, providing a reliable internal control (Fig. 1.7a). Recently denervated myofibers are highlighted in the esterase stain, owing to increased cytoplasmic esterase activity (Fig. 1.7b). The esterase stain also highlights macrophages and, in some cases, sarcoplasmic vacuoles associated with abnormal lysosomal activity, although these are usually demonstrated even more clearly in sections stained for acid phosphatase activity (discussed below). Type 1 fibers generally stain a bit more darkly than type 2 fibers in the esterase stain.

The ***acid phosphatase stain*** is based on the hydrolysis of naphthol AS-B1 phosphate by endogenous acid phosphatase to form naphthol, which, like the naphthol generated in the esterase stain, forms an insoluble azo dye in the presence of basic fuchsin [1, 11]. The red reaction product highlights macrophages (Fig. 1.7c) and other structures that have lysosomal activity, such as degenerating myofibers and pathological sarcoplasmic inclusions associated with abnormal lysosomal activity (Fig. 1.7d). The stain is generally a more sensitive marker of lysosomal activity than the nonspecific esterase stain.

The ***alkaline phosphatase stain*** is another "hydrolytic" stain that relies on the hydrolysis of an alpha-naphthyl acid phosphate substrate by endogenous alkaline phosphatase to generate naphthol, which reacts, in turn, with a diazo salt (fast blue RR salt) to form a black reaction product at sites of alkaline phosphatase activity. Glycerol or a comparable aqueous mounting medium should be used to coverslip the section, as alcohols or xylene dissolve the reaction product [13]. The alkaline phosphatase reaction generates gas that can produce distracting bubbles if the section is coverslipped prematurely. To minimize this, it is advisable to wait at least 45 minutes before placing the coverslip over the stained section. The stain highlights the sarcoplasm of regenerating myofibers (Fig. 1.7e), as well as occasional myofibers in infantile denervation of the type seen in spinal muscular atrophy type 1 (Werdnig-Hoffmann disease); normal muscle fibers lack alkaline phosphatase activity. Increased alkaline phosphatase reactivity can also be seen in connective tissue in many inflammatory disorders of skeletal muscle. Increased perimysial connective tissue reactivity, in particular, is a feature of some inflammatory myopathies associated with the presence of circulating anti-Jo1 or other anti-tRNA synthetase antibodies (Fig. 1.7f).

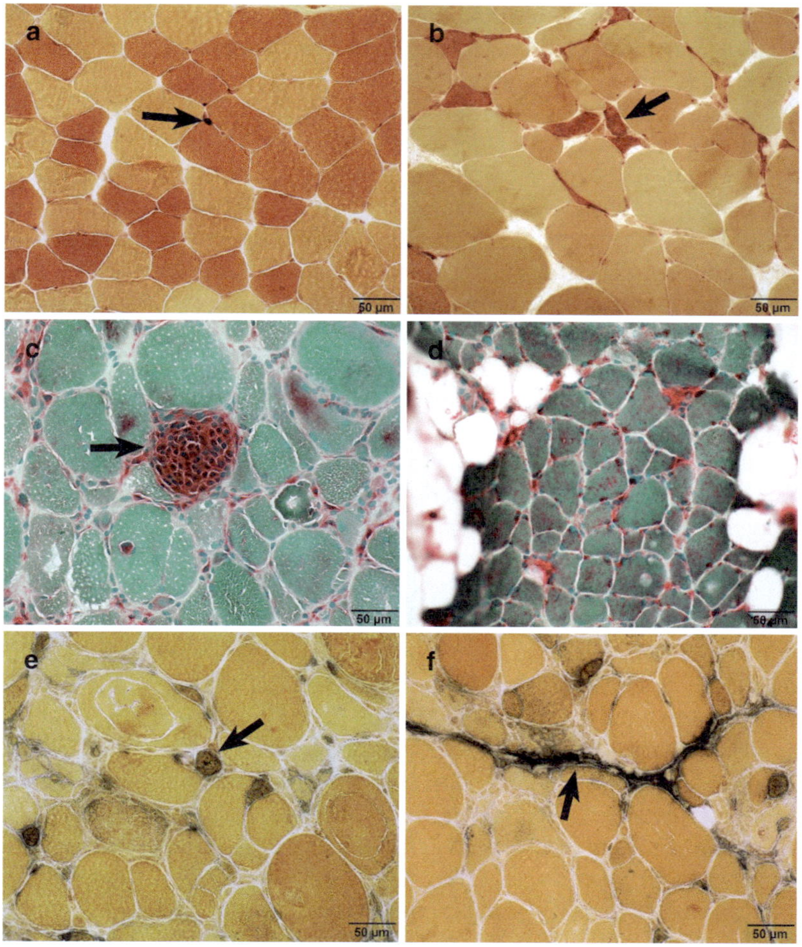

Fig. 1.7 Hydrolytic stains – esterase, acid phosphatase and alkaline phosphatase stains. (**a**) Normal skeletal muscle, esterase. The esterase stain highlight normal neuromuscular junctions (arrow). The brick-red reaction product in these structures is caused by the presence of the enzyme acetylcholinesterase, and serves as a reliable internal control for the esterase stain. (**b**) Denervation atrophy, esterase. The esterase stain is also an effective way to identify atrophic denervated myofibers (arrow), which stain with the same brick-red appearance as normal neuromuscular junctions. (**c**) Myophagocytosis, acid phosphatase. The acid phosphatase stain produces a bright red reaction product in areas of increased enzyme activity, and serves as a reliable marker for lysosomal activity. Activated macrophages contain numerous lysosomes and are highlighted in the acid phosphatase stain, as in the case of these macrophages engulfing the sarcoplasm of a necrotic muscle fiber (arrow). (**d**) Hydroxychloroquine myopathy, acid phosphatase. Abnormal lysosomal activity is a feature of some toxic myopathies. The excessive lysosomal activity in this muscle from a patient with hydroxychloroquine myopathy is responsible for the increased acid phosphatase reactivity in the sarcoplasm of many of these myofibers. (**e**) Myofiber regeneration, alkaline phosphatase. The alkaline phosphatase stain produces a dense black reaction product. This figure highlights areas of abnormal alkaline phosphatase reactivity associated with myofiber regeneration (arrow). (**f**) Inflammatory myopathy, alkaline phosphatase. Abnormal perimysial connective tissue reactivity (arrow) is a feature of inflammatory myopathies associated with the presence of anti-Jo1 and other anti-synthetase antibodies

The ***nicotinamide adenine dinucleotide-tetrazolium reductase (NADH-TR) stain*** is an extremely useful member of the "oxidative" family of stains. The NADH-TR enzyme is a flavoprotein involved in electron transfer in the normal respiratory chain. Both mitochondrial and cytosolic forms of NADH-TR are present in human skeletal muscle, the latter associated with sarcoplasmic reticulum. The NADH-TR staining reaction is based upon the enzymatic removal of hydrogen from exogenous NADH substrate, and the transfer of that hydrogen to nitro blue tetrazolium. The transfer of hydrogen to nitro blue tetrazolium, in turn, generates an insoluble dark blue reaction product, which marks the site of enzyme activity. Sections are coverslipped with an aqueous mounting medium [1, 11, 14]. Mitochondria have NADH-TR activity, and for this reason normal type 1 fibers stain more darkly than type 2 fibers. In optimally stained specimens, some differences in the staining intensity of type 2a versus type 2b fibers may be apparent, with type 2a fibers staining a bit more darkly than type 2b fibers, but this distinction is much more reliably made in the ATPase 4.6 stain, The NADH-TR stain is useful for demonstrating architectural abnormalities within muscle fibers, such as target/targetoid change, sarcoplasmic cores, moth-eaten fibers, sarcoplasmic "whorling", ring fibers and lobulated fibers (discussed later). Denervated myofibers are also variably highlighted in the NADH-TR stain. Abnormal mitochondrial aggregates are sometimes highlighted in the NADH-TR stain, although these are more reliably detected in the succinate dehydrogenase and/or cytochrome c oxidase stains, discussed below. The stain is also useful for the identification of tubular aggregates, structures that are derived from sarcoplasmic reticulum and are sometimes confused with ragged red change in Gomori trichrome-stained sections. An example of a normal NADH-TR stain is illustrated in Fig. 1.8a, and examples of abnormalities highlighted in the NADH-TR stain are illustrated later, under the heading "Interpretation of the Muscle Biopsy."

The ***succinate dehydrogenase (SDH) stain*** identifies a flavoprotein enzyme that is complex II in the mitochondrial respiratory chain. The enzyme is anchored to the inner mitochondrial membrane and is encoded exclusively by nuclear – as opposed to mitochondrial – DNA. SDH normally catalyzes the conversion of succinate to fumarate and the closely linked transfer of electrons to ubiquinone to form ubiquinol in the mitochondrial electron transport chain. In vitro, the SDH stain relies on the ability of SDH to release hydrogen from its sodium succinate substrate and reduce aqueous nitro blue tetrazolium to form a blue tetrazolium precipitate. The stained sections are coverslipped using an aqueous mounting medium [1, 11, 14, 15] The SDH stain is a specific stain for mitochondria, and a much more sensitive marker for mitochondrial aggregation than either the Gomori trichrome stain or the NADH-TR stain. Myofibers harboring abnormal mitochondrial aggregates appear as "ragged blue" fibers in the SDH stain. A normal SDH stain and an SDH stain in a patient with abnormal mitochondrial accumulation are illustrated in Fig. 1.8b, c.

The enzyme ***cytochrome c oxidase (COX)*** is complex IV in the mitochondrial respiratory chain. The enzyme is composed of multiple subunits, three of which are encoded by mitochondrial DNA in mammalian tissue. The COX complex is located in the inner mitochondrial membrane, where it transfers electrons from the cytochrome c protein to molecules of dioxygen to form water. The COX stain is based on the ability of the enzyme to transfer electrons from an artificial diaminobenzidine tetra hydrochloride substrate to produce an insoluble brown diaminobenzidine precipitate (Fig. 1.8d). Stained sections are coverslipped using an organic mounting medium [1, 11, 14, 15]. Like SDH, COX is a specific marker for mitochondria. Its usefulness in diagnostic work is based on the fact that many mitochondrial disorders are associated with COX deficiency, characterized by failure of affected myofibers to stain in the COX preparation (Fig. 1.8e). In most mitochondrial disorders associated with COX deficiency, SDH reactivity is preserved, and staining sections sequentially for COX and then SDH activities [15] makes detection of COX-deficient fibers a bit easier, with COX-deficient fibers standing out as blue fibers surrounded by brown-staining fibers with intact COX activity (Fig. 1.8f). COX-deficient fibers are common in a number of conditions including primary mitochondrial disorders, including inclusion body myositis and polymyositis with mitochondrial abnormalities [23]. COX deficient myofibers are also seen in some cases of dermatomyositis, wherein there is a selective loss COX activity in perifascicular myofibers [23, 24]. COX is a fairly unstable enzyme, and care must be taken to distinguish artifactual loss of COX activity associated with improper handling of muscle tissue from true COX deficiency; this staining pattern is illustrated later in Fig. 1.24c, under the discussion of Artifacts in Skeletal Muscle Biopsies.

Two standard enzyme histochemical procedures are available for the detection of enzymes associated with glycogen metabolism – muscle-specific phosphorylase (myophosphorylase) and phosphofructokinase. ***Myophosphorylase*** is an enzyme that catalyzes the conversion of glycosyl residues in glycogen to glucose-1-phosphate, which is then used in the generation of ATP. Detection of myophosphorylase is based on the ability of the enzyme to add glucose residues to a glycogen primer in the presence of a large amount of glucose-1-phosphate substrate (the reverse of the reaction sequence that occurs *in vivo*). The resultant glycogen is then stained with Lugol's iodine solution, resulting in a gray-brown reaction product. Sections are coverslipped using an aqueous mounting medium [11, 16]. Patients with myophosphorylase deficiency (type V glycogen storage disease, also known as McArdle's disease) classically present with histories of cramps, exercise intolerance and episodes of rhabdomyolysis following vigorous exercise. In muscle biopsies from such patients, no phosphorylase reaction product is detectable in intact muscle fibers, which appear yellow under the microscope. Myophosphorylase is a labile enzyme that is subject to artifactual degradation, and it is important to distinguish such artifactual losses of enzyme activity from true phosphorylase deficiency. Smooth muscle cells in intramuscular blood vessels express a different isoform of phosphorylase than skeletal muscle, and the identification of residual phosphorylase activity in blood vessel walls serves as an internal control that distinguishes artifactual loss of enzyme activity from selective myophosphorylase deficiency. Of note, the reaction product in the myophosphorylase stain will fade over time, and it is helpful to make a notation of a "positive" result on the slide label. The color of the reaction product can be restored by re-incubating the section in Lugol's solution.

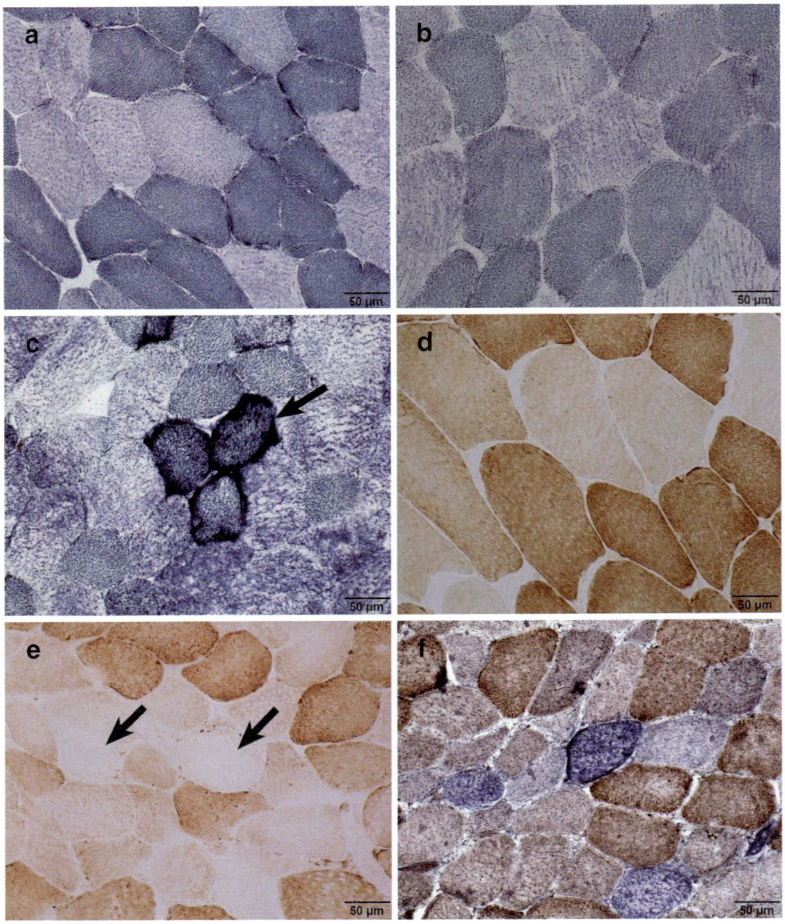

Fig. 1.8 Oxidative stains – NADH-TR, succinate dehydrogenase (SDH) and cytochrome c oxidase (COX). (**a**) Normal muscle, NADH-TR. The NADH-TR stain is highlights both mitochondria and sarcoplasmic reticulum. It is a useful stain for highlighting a wide range of structural sarcoplasmic abnormalities. In normal muscle, as illustrated here, type 1 fibers stain more intensely than type 2 fibers. (**b**) Normal muscle, SDH. The SDH stain has the same reaction product as the NADH-TR stain, and appears very similar to the NADH-TR stain in normal muscle. Unlike the NADH-TR stain, the SDH stain only highlights mitochondria, and is a more sensitive stain for highlighting abnormal mitochondrial aggregates. Owing to their greater numbers of mitochondria, type 1 fibers stain more intensely than type 2 fibers. (**c**) Mitochondrial myopathy, SDH. Abnormal mitochondrial accumulation is associated with intense blue sarcoplasmic reactivity in the SDH stain (arrow). (**d**) Normal muscle, cytochrome c oxidase (COX). The COX stain is another stain that highlights only mitochondria, in this case with a brown reaction product. In normal muscle, the pattern of COX reactivity parallels that of SDH reactivity, with type 1 fibers staining more intensely than type 2 fibers. (**e**) Mitochondrial myopathy, COX. Many mitochondrial myopathies are characterized by abnormalities in COX activity (complex IV in the mitochondrial respiratory chain). Affected muscle fibers in such cases fail to react when stained for COX reactivity (arrows). (**f**) Mitochondrial myopathy, sequential stain for COX and SDH. The sequential COX-SDH stain increases the sensitivity of detection of COX-deficient myofibers. In patients with mitochondrial myopathies associated with COX deficiency, the myofibers that fail to stain for COX activity do not precipitate a reaction product, and retain enzyme activity. If subsequently stained for SDH reactivity, the COX-deficient myofibers stand out as blue-staining fibers surrounded by brown, COX-reactive fibers

Phosphofructokinase (PFK) is a glycolytic pathway enzyme that converts fructose-6-phosphate to fructose-1,6-diphosphate. Patients with PFK deficiency (type VII glycogen storage disease, or Tarui's disease) have a clinical presentation similar to that of patients with myophosphorylase deficiency. The PFK stain is based on the conversion of exogenous fructose-6-phosphate to fructose-1,6-diphosphate by endogenous PFK. A metabolite of fructose-1,6-diphosphate – diphosphoglyceric acid – is formed *in vitro*, which then reacts with exogenous nicotinamide adenine dinucleotide to generate reduced nitro blue tetrazolium, the latter forming the usual blue precipitate. Sections are coverslipped using an organic mounting medium [1, 11, 17]. PFK is a labile enzyme that deteriorates rapidly in improperly handled biopsies. Patient sections stained for PFK should include a negative control (no added substrate) and a control section using fructose-1,6-diphosphate as a substrate, the latter always generating a blue reaction product, even if the patient is PFK-deficient. Patient sections stained for PFK activity should always be paired with a normal control section.

A final enzyme histochemical stain that is routinely performed in our laboratory is the ***myoadenylate deaminase (MAD) stain***. MAD is an enzyme that removes an ammonia molecule from adenosine monophosphate (AMP) to convert AMP to inosine monophosphate. Deficiency of the enzyme should be suspected when patients fail to generate a normal amount of ammonia during exercise testing. The clinical significance of MAD deficiency appears to vary from patient to patient. While some patients with MAD deficiency are asymptomatic, MAD deficiency has been associated in other patients with a clinical syndrome of exercise intolerance and exercise-induced muscle cramps and pain, and, in severe cases, rhabdomyolysis. A susceptibility to malignant hyperthermia syndrome has been suggested by some authors [25, 26]. The MAD stain is based on the generation of ammonia from an exogenous AMP substrate and subsequent reduction of nitro blue tetrazolium to form a blue reaction product. Staining for MAD is always paired with a negative control, in which aqueous citrate is added to the reaction in place of AMP substrate. Stained sections are coverslipped using an aqueous mounting medium [1, 18]. In patients with MAD deficiency, no blue reaction product is present in the sections stained with the AMP substrate. In addition to detecting MAD deficiency, the MAD stain reliably highlights tubular aggregates (see discussion of abnormal sarcoplasmic inclusions under "Interpretation of the Biopsy", below).

Non-enzymatic Staining of Fixed Skeletal Muscle (Paraffin Sections)

Although most of the useful diagnostic information in muscle biopsies at the light microscopic level is provided by the evaluation of stained cryostat sections, properly processed paraffin embedded tissue can also be of help in some conditions, particularly those characterized by the presence of inflammatory infiltrates and microorganisms. The morphology of inflammatory cells is generally better preserved in fixed, paraffin embedded tissue than in cryostat sections, and immunohistochemical markers (discussed below) often label inflammatory cells more clearly in paraffin-embedded tissue than in frozen tissue. Paraffin sections of skeletal muscle biopsies are routinely stained with ***H&E***, ***Masson trichrome*** and ***Congo red*** stains in our laboratory. The H&E and Congo red stains have the same applications in paraffin sections as they do in cryostat sections. The Masson trichrome stain is a sensitive stain for highlighting connective tissue in paraffin sections. An additional stain, the ***Morin stain***, has proven to be helpful in the detection of aluminum deposits in patients with macrophagic myofasciitis (see discussion of cellular infiltrates under "Interpretation of the Biopsy", below) [27].

Immunohistochemical Stains

Immunohistochemical staining is a technique that allows one to localize specific proteins in tissue sections. The procedure has broad applications in all areas of anatomic pathology, and now plays an indispensable role in the evaluation of a wide range of muscle disorders [1, 28, 29]. In brief, immunohistochemical staining involves incubation of a tissue section with a primary antibody directed against the protein of interest, followed by incubation of the tissue with a secondary antibody that recognizes the primary immunoglobulin molecule and, finally, labeling the secondary antibody with a molecule that can be visualized under the microscope. Both fluorescent and non-fluorescent labels are commercially available. Technical aspects of immunohistochemical staining are presented in detail in other references [1], and will not be reviewed here. Automated procedures are now available for immunohistochemical staining, greatly improving turnaround time for this procedure.

Demonstration of many of the proteins of interest in the evaluation of skeletal muscle generally requires the use of frozen sections, although some recent work has suggested that paraffin embedded tissue may also be used for this purpose [30]. These include virtually all of the sarcolemmal proteins of interest in the evaluation of suspected muscular dystrophies, as well as major histocompatibility complex class I (MHC1) antigen and terminal complement complex (C_{5b-9}), the latter two stains of special importance in the evaluation of suspected inflammatory muscle diseases. Staining for MHC class I has been particularly valuable in identifying cases of inflammatory myopathy associated with minimal changes in routine frozen and paraffin sections. Patterns of abnormal MHC1 reactivity associated with inflammatory myopathies are illustrated in Fig. 1.9a, b. The abnormal protein aggregates that characterize some muscle diseases (e.g., myofibrillar myopathies) are also most reliably demonstrated in cryostat sections. Many of the more common inflammatory cell markers, in contrast, are better demonstrated in paraffin embedded tissue. The immunohistochemical markers commonly employed in our laboratory in the evaluation of muscle biopsies, the preferred tissue for staining and the significance of each of these markers, are listed in Table 1.1.

As in the cases of the enzyme histochemical stains discussed previously, it is essential that appropriate control sections be available whenever immunohistochemical staining is performed, in order to minimize the possibility of either false negative or

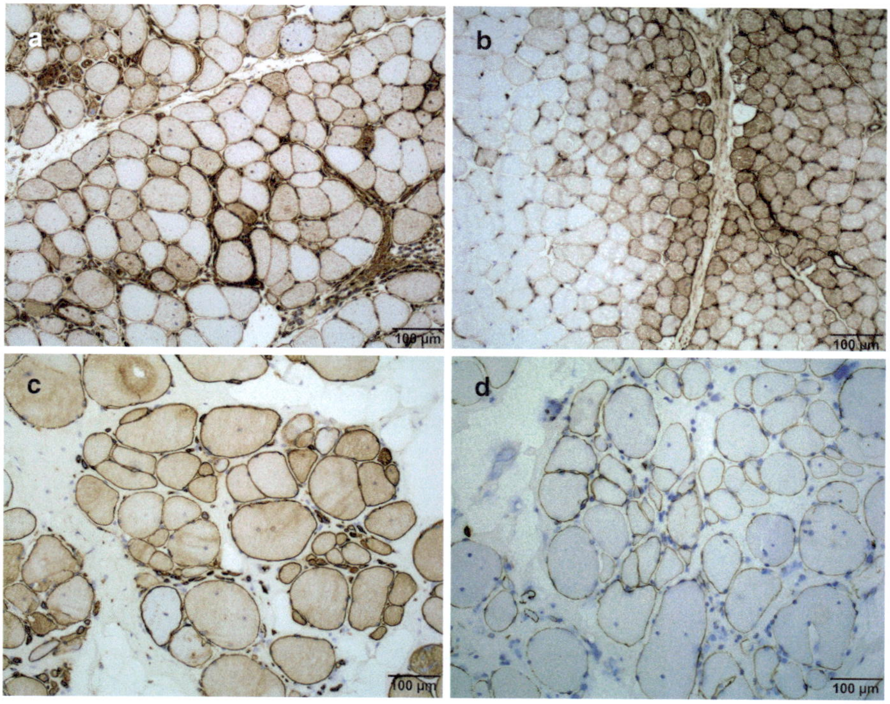

Fig. 1.9 Immunohistochemical staining of skeletal muscle. (**a**) Polymyositis, MHC class 1 (MHC1). MHC1 staining has been an invaluable tool in the assessment of suspected inflammatory myopathies. Sarcolemmal MCH1 reactivity can be seen in injured muscle fibers in a wide variety of conditions, but in classical polymyositis, one usually sees generalized reactivity involving both injured and morphologically normal fibers. Similar patterns of diffuse reactivity can be seen in inclusion body myositis and in some cases of dermatomyositis, related "overlap" inflammatory myopathic processes and in some dystrophies. (**b**) Dermatomyositis, MHC1. In many cases of dermatomyositis, one encounters selective staining of the sarcolemma in perifascicular myofibers, as shown here. In other patients with dermatomyositis, more diffuse sarcolemmal reactivity can be seen. (**c**) Becker muscular dystrophy, β-spectrin. When staining muscle biopsies for one of the dystrophy-associated membrane proteins, it is important to ensure that abnormalities in sarcolemmal staining are due to a specific protein abnormality rather than a nonspecific loss of membrane integrity due to cell injury or artifact. In this field, sarcolemmal β-spectrin reactivity is well preserved. (**d**) Becker muscular dystrophy, dystrophin carboxy terminus. In a contiguous section of the muscle biopsy shown in **c**, there is considerable loss of sarcolemmal dystrophin reactivity. The presence of intact β-spectrin staining in the same area ensures that the loss of dystrophin staining is caused by a true dystrophin abnormality rather than by nonspecific muscle fiber damage or an artifactual loss of immunoreactivity

false positive staining. These control sections should always include normal tissue stained for the protein of interest as well as negative controls. In addition, in the evaluation of sarcolemmal proteins in suspected muscular dystrophies, it is essential to ensure that the sarcolemma has not been artifactually disrupted by poor freezing technique or nonspecific myofiber injury. To accomplish this, sections stained for

Table 1.1 Antibodies, Preferred tissue, and Significance

Antibody	Preferred tissue	Significance
MHC class 1	Cryostat sections	Diffuse upregulation in polymyositis, inclusion body myositis, some cases of dermatomyositis; selective perifascicular upregulation in some cases of dermatomyositis
C_{5b-9}	Cryostat sections	Capillary reactivity seen in dermatomyositis, myopathy with pipestem capillaries, diabetes mellitus
β-spectrin	Cryostat sections	Essential control stain to ensure membrane integrity when evaluating muscle for sarcolemmal dystrophy-associated proteins
Dystrophin epitopes (rod domain, carboxy terminus, amino terminus)	Cryostat sections	Evaluation of suspected Duchenne / Becker dystrophy and other dystrophin-related disorders
Sarcoglycans (α, β, γ, δ)	Cryostat sections	Evaluation of suspected sarcoglycanopathies (LGMD* types 2C, 2D, 2E, 2F)
Caveolin-3	Cryostat sections	Evaluation of suspected LGMD* type 1C, rippling muscle disease, unexplained hyperCKemia
Dysferlin	Cryostat sections	Evaluation of suspected LGMD* type 2B, Miyoshi myopathy and related myopathies
α-dystroglycan	Cryostat sections	Evaluation of suspected congenital muscular dystrophies, LGMD* types 2I and 2M
Merosin (80 kDa and 300 kDa epitopes)	Cryostat sections	Evaluation of suspected merosin-deficient congenital muscular dystrophies
Collagen VI	Cryostat sections	Evaluation of suspected Ullrich or Bethlem myopathies
Collagen IV	Cryostat sections	Control stain for collagen VI staining
Emerin	Cryostat or paraffin sections	Evaluation of suspected Emery-Dreifuss muscular dystrophy
CD3	Paraffin sections	Pan T-lymphocyte marker
CD4	Paraffin sections	Helper T-lymphocyte marker
CD8	Paraffin sections	Cytotoxic/killer T-lymphocyte marker
CD20	Paraffin sections	B-lymphocyte marker
CD68	Paraffin sections	Macrophage marker
Desmin	Cryostat or paraffin sections	Evaluation of suspected myofibrillar myopathies
αB-crystallin	Cryostat or paraffin sections	Evaluation of suspected myofibrillar myopathies

[a]*LGMD* Limb Girdle Muscular Dystrophy

any dystrophy-associated sarcolemmal protein (e.g., dystrophin) should always be accompanied by patient sections stained in parallel for β-spectrin, a protein that is always present in the sarcolemma. The presence of intact β-spectrin reactivity in a given myofiber ensures that there has not been an artifactual or nonspecific disruption of the integrity of the sarcolemma. An example of normal β-spectrin staining and abnormal dystrophin staining in a patient with Becker muscular dystrophy is illustrated in Fig. 1.9c, d.

Electron Microscopy

Although less widely used in general pathology practice than in the past, electron microscopy continues to play a role in the evaluation of skeletal muscle biopsies. As noted in the section on the initial processing of skeletal muscle biopsies, electron microscopic evaluation of skeletal muscle is performed on fixed, resin-embedded tissue. In our laboratory, small sections of the same isometrically clamped, formalin-fixed muscle segment that is used for paraffin histology are post-fixed in glutaraldehyde and embedded in an Epon® medium. Delayed fixation or other improper handling of the biopsy can introduce significant artifacts into the tissue that hamper interpretation of fine structural changes. Prior to the preparation of thin sections for electron microscopy, 1.5 μm semithin sections of the tissue blocks are stained with toluidine blue and evaluated by light microscopy to select the optimum areas for ultrastructural study. Longitudinal sections of this tissue generally provide the most useful diagnostic information. Once an appropriate area has been identified in the semithin sections, thin (100 nm) sections are obtained from the block, placed on a copper grid, and stained with uranyl acetate-lead citrate [31]. The cross sectional area of the sections submitted for electron microscopy is quite small compared to the usual cryostat or paraffin sections, and sampling limitations should always be kept in mind when evaluating tissue ultrastructurally. Electron microscopy should never be used as a stand-alone diagnostic technique, but rather must be interpreted in the context of changes at the light microscopic level and the clinical history.

As in the case of the light microscopic evaluation of muscle biopsies, proper interpretation of changes at an ultrastructural level is based on a thorough knowledge of normal skeletal muscle morphology, particularly the appearance of the contractile apparatus (Fig. 1.10), sarcotubular structures, storage material, mitochondria, sarcolemma and nuclei. The observer should also be familiar with the appearance of surrounding connective tissue and the morphology of interstitial blood vessels.

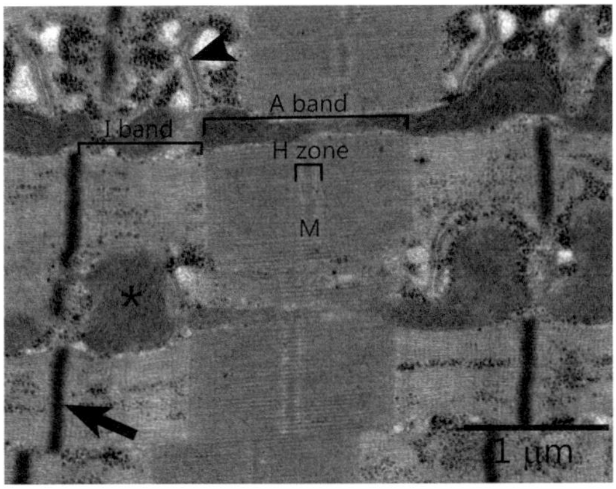

Fig. 1.10 Electron micrograph of normal sarcomeric structures. The sarcomere is the basic contractile unit of skeletal muscle, and familiarity with the appearance of normal sarcomeres is the foundation for interpreting the various structural abnormalities that one can see in diseased muscle. The normal sarcomere is bordered on each end by densely staining Z-bands (arrows), biochemically complex structures that contain a-actinin and a multitude of additional proteins, including those that anchor actin, titin and nebulin filaments. Immediately adjacent to the Z-band, one encounters a lightly-staining region known as the "isotropic" (I) band, composed of actin filaments and various accessory proteins (including nebulin and titin). The sarcomere's I-bands flank a darker staining area in the central region of the sarcomere known as the "anisotropic" (A) band, composed of myosin (thick) filaments, a number of accessory proteins and, at its junction with the I-band, variable numbers of overlapping actin filaments. In the center of each A-band, a lighter staining area called the H-zone is present, composed portions of the myosin filaments that are not overlapping with actin filaments. A central line (M) bisects the H-zone, composed of the creatine kinase and various proteins that anchor myosin filaments and cross-link proteins in the A-band on the other side of the M line. Mitochondria (*) as well as T-tubules (arrowhead) and adjacent cisternae of sarcoplasmic reticulum are also visible in this field

Interpretation of the Biopsy

Proper interpretation of skeletal muscle biopsies begins, ideally, with familiarity with the patient's clinical history, including age, presenting symptoms, duration of disease, family history, imaging studies and any laboratory studies (e.g., CK levels). Clinical information may be lacking at the time biopsies are submitted to the laboratory, and in such cases, the pathologist should make every effort to contact the referring physician to obtain that information. Changes that should be noted in the biopsy include: (1) patterns of myofiber atrophy or hypertrophy; (2) the presence of myofiber degeneration, necrosis or regeneration; (3) changes in the location and appearance of myofiber nuclei and; (4) structural sarcoplasmic abnormalities, including sarcoplasmic whorling, myofiber myofibrillar disarray, inclusions and vacuolar change; (5) connective tissue changes; (6) abnormal cellular infiltrates and (7) alterations related to poor specimen preservation. These are discussed in more detail in the paragraphs below.

Myofiber Atrophy and Hypertrophy

The size and shape of individual myofibers should be noted and documented in the biopsy report. It is important to remember that myofiber size is influenced by the age of the patient, and myofiber diameters, particularly in pediatric patients, should be measured and compared to published normal ranges. ***Myofiber atrophy*** is a common alteration in muscle biopsies, occurring in disuse, denervation and many myopathic disorders. If atrophy is present, the ***shapes of the atrophic myofibers*** should be noted. Angular atrophic myofibers are typical in cases of denervation atrophy and most cases of type 2 myofiber atrophy in mature skeletal muscle (Fig. 1.11a), while more rounded atrophic fibers are typical of denervation in infants with spinal muscular atrophy type 1 (Fig. 1.11b) and in many myopathic processes. Profound myofiber atrophy, manifested by the presence of compact myonuclear clusters, is common in long-standing denervation, and can also be seen in some myopathic processes, notably myotonic dystrophy. The ***distribution of the atrophic myofibers*** should also be documented. The presence of groups of contiguous atrophic myofibers (group atrophy) is a feature of denervation atrophy (Fig. 1.11c), while the presence of selective atrophy of myofibers at the periphery of muscle fascicles (perifascicular atrophy) is a feature of dermatomyositis and several other related inflammatory myopathic disorders (Fig. 1.11d). The histochemical subtype(s) of the atrophic fibers should also be noted; as one might expect, the ATPase stains play a critical role in identifying the subtype(s) of the atrophic fibers. ***Selective atrophy of type 2 myofibers*** is a common change in skeletal muscle biopsies, typically associated with disuse atrophy and/or hypercortisolism (Fig. 1.12a). The atrophy in such cases preferentially involves type IIb myofibers; the reason for this selective involvement of fast twitch glycolytic fibers remains unclear. Selective atrophy of type 1 fibers is much less common than type 2 atrophy, but can be seen in patients with myotonic dystrophy type 1. Selective "smallness" of type 1 fibers is also a feature of congenital fiber type disproportion and many other congenital myopathies. The term "hypotrophy" is sometimes used to describe the small size of the myofibers in such cases, based on the notion that the affected fibers have not undergone atrophy, but rather never reached normal diameters (Fig. 1.12b). Mixed type 1 and type 2 atrophy is a feature of neurogenic atrophy (Fig. 1.12c), but is also present in biopsies of many primary myopathic processes. Widespread myofiber atrophy is also a feature of myopathy with thick filament loss; the atrophic fibers in such cases can be mistaken for denervated fibers, but are distinguished from denervated myofibers by a widespread loss of sarcoplasmic ATPase reactivity. ***Myofiber hypertrophy*** is a feature of many muscular dystrophies and other chronic myopathic diseases, and can also be seen in biopsies from individuals engaged in weight-bearing exercise and in some cases of chronic denervation. Paradoxically hypertrophic type 1 myofibers are common in the infantile pattern of denervation seen in spinal muscular atrophy type I (Fig. 1.12d).

Myofiber Degeneration, Necrosis and Regeneration

Muscle fiber degeneration, necrosis and regeneration are common in a wide range of primary myopathic disorders, including inflammatory myopathies and other immune-mediated myopathic processes, most types of muscular dystrophy, metabolic myopathies associated with acute myofiber injury, and many myopathies caused by exogenous myotoxic insults. The sarcoplasm of ***degenerating myofibers*** can appear hypercontracted, dense and homogeneously staining in H&E and Gomori trichrome-stained cryostat sections or can appear paler than the sarcoplasm of adjacent normal fibers (Fig. 1.13a). The delicate intermyofibrillar network seen in normal fibers is obscured in degenerating fibers. As degeneration proceeds to frank necrosis, the sarcoplasm

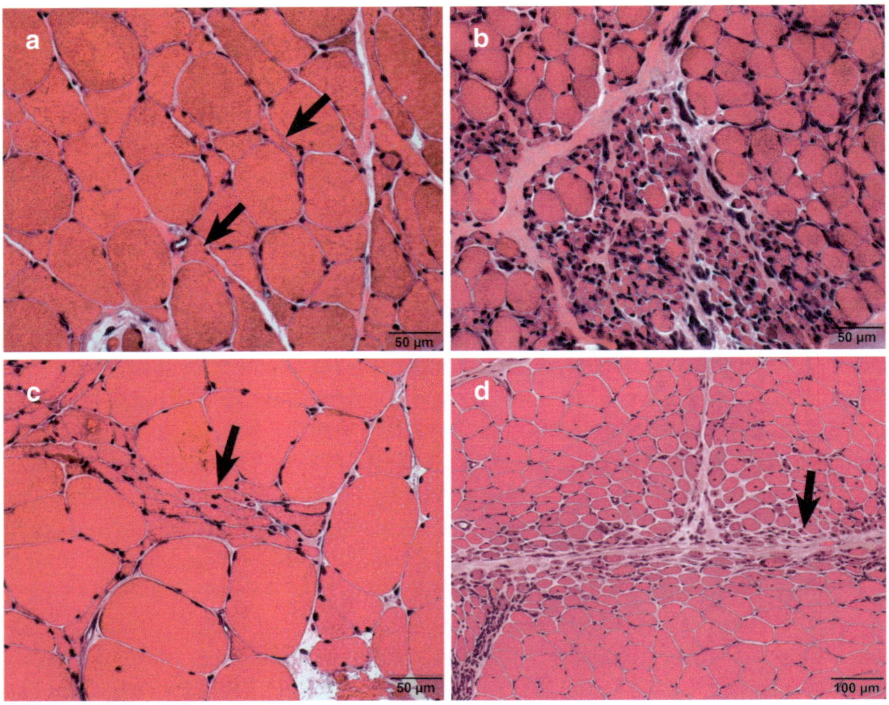

Fig. 1.11 Common patterns of myofiber atrophy. (**a**) Denervation atrophy, H&E. Neurogenic atrophy in mature skeletal muscle is characterized by the presence of atrophic myofibers with an angular profile in cross sections (arrow). This pattern can be difficult to distinguish from type 2 myofiber atrophy in H&E-stained sections. (**b**) Denervation atrophy in infancy, H&E. Denervation atrophy in young infants is characterized by the presence of groups of rounded, rather than angular, atrophic myofibers. This infantile pattern of denervation atrophy is seen most frequently in patients with infantile spinal muscular atrophy (SMA type 1). (**c**) Group atrophy in denervation atrophy, H&E. In many cases of denervation atrophy in mature muscle, angular atrophic myofibers occur in clusters, a pattern known as group atrophy (arrow). The presence of group atrophy helps one to distinguish denervation atrophy from type 2 myofiber atrophy even in H&E-stained sections. (**d**) Perifascicular atrophy in dermatomyositis, H&E. Selective atrophy of myofibers at the periphery of a muscle fascicle, termed perifascicular atrophy (arrow), is often seen in biopsies from patients with dermatomyositis and related inflammatory myopathic disorders (e.g. lupus myositis) (Panel **d** courtesy of Chunyu Cai, MD, PhD)

becomes fragmented, and is eventually invaded by macrophages, a process termed ***myophagocytosis*** (Fig. 1.13b). It is important to recognize that macrophagic invasion of such fibers is a nonspecific host reaction to the myofiber necrosis, and should not be interpreted as evidence of an inflammatory myopathic disorder (discussed below). The cytoplasm of ***regenerating myofibers***, in contrast, is basophilic, owing to the presence of sarcoplasmic ribonucleoproteins engaged in protein synthesis. The nuclei of regenerating myofiber tend to be enlarged, with finely dispersed chromatin and discernible nucleoli (Fig. 1.13c). It is not uncommon for regenerative change to occur in muscle fibers that contain residual necrotic sarcoplasm, the former typically manifesting as a rim of basophilic sarcoplasm at the edge of a central area of necrosis (Fig. 1.13d).

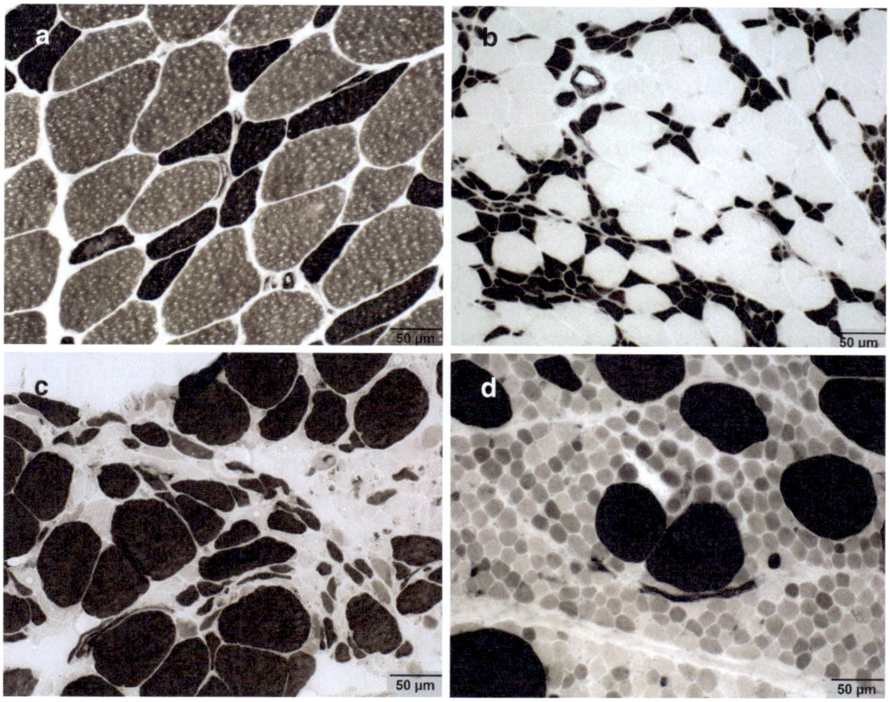

Fig. 1.12 Fiber type-specific patterns of myofiber atrophy and hypertrophy. (**a**) ATPase 9.4, type 2 myofiber atrophy. Selective atrophy of type 2 myofibers is a very common pattern of myofiber atrophy. Common clinical features in most of the long list of conditions associated with type 2 atrophy are disuse and elevated corticosteroid levels. (**b**) Type 1 myofiber atrophy/hypotrophy, ATPase 4.3. Selective "smallness" of type 1 myofibers is less common than selective type 2 myofiber atrophy. It is most commonly encountered in congenital fiber size disproportion and other congenital myopathic disorders where it is usually referred to as "hypotrophy" rather than atrophy, based on the assumption that the fibers have never reached a normal diameter during their development. Small type 1 fibers are also often present in biopsies from patients with myotonic dystrophy, type 1. (**c**) Denervation atrophy, ATPase 4.3. Mixed type 1 and type 2 myofiber atrophy is a characteristic feature of neurogenic atrophy. It is also common in many myopathic disorders, but in the latter conditions, the affected fibers are usually rounded rather than angular. (**d**) Infantile spinal muscular atrophy, ATPase 4.3. Myofiber hypertrophy involving both type 1 and type 2 fibers is commonly seen in chronic myopathic processes as well as in many cases of chronic neurogenic atrophy. Selective type 1 myofiber hypertrophy, illustrated here, is usually present in biopsies from infants with SMA type 1

Changes in the Location and Appearance of Myofiber Nuclei

As noted previously and illustrated earlier in Fig. 1.3, myofiber nuclei normally lie just beneath the sarcolemma. ***Increased numbers of internalized nuclei*** – defined by the presence of internalized nuclei in >3% of myofibers in transverse of areas away from myotendinous insertion sites – are common in many chronic myopathic and neuropathic disorders, where they usually coexist with myofiber hypertrophy, myofiber splitting and other chronic sarcoplasmic alterations discussed in the next section. Internalized nuclei are also common in regenerating muscle fibers. Internalized – often centrally-situated - nuclei are a defining feature of the ***centronuclear myopathies***, a genetically and clinically heterogeneous group of congenital myopathies with presentations that range from severe neonatal weakness with respiratory failure and early death - e.g. X-linked myotubular myopathy (Fig. 1.14a) - to adult-onset, much more slowly progressive weakness. A number of genetic abnormalities, variably associated with X-linked, autosomal dominant or autosomal recessive inheritance patterns, have been described [32]. Mutations in the gene encoding the ryanodine receptor, best known for its association with central core disease and susceptibility to malignant hyperthermia syndrome, have also been associated with abnormal numbers of central / internalized nuclei [33]. Internal nuclei are also a common feature of ***myotonic dystrophy***, particularly myotonic dystrophy type 1 (DM1) (Fig. 1.14b). Biopsies from patients with congenital-onset DM1 may be extremely difficult to distinguish from those with congenital onset variants of centronuclear myopathy [34].

Changes in the appearance of myofiber nuclei should also be noted in the biopsy report. As mentioned previously, ***enlarged nuclei*** with finely dispersed chromatin and conspicuous nucleoli are a feature of myofiber regeneration. Although difficult to appreciate at the light microscopic level, a number of different ***intranuclear inclusions*** can be seen under the electron microscope in a number of different neuromuscular disorders, including inclusion body myositis [35], oculopharyngeal muscular dystrophy [36], inflammatory myopathies associated with the presence of anti-synthetase antibodies [37] and some cases of nemaline myopathy [38] (see discussion of "nemaline bodies" under Abnormal Sarcoplasmic Inclusions, below).

Sarcoplasmic Abnormalities

A wide variety of other sarcoplasmic structural alterations can be seen in muscle biopsies. These include (1) various forms of ***myofibrillar disarray***, (2) abnormal ***sarcoplasmic inclusions*** and (3) ***vacuolar change***.

<u>Patterns of myofibrillar disarray</u> include myofiber splitting, sarcoplasmic "whorling", target/targetoid change, central cores, multiminicores, ring fibers, lobulated (trabecular) change, moth-eaten change and whorled fibers. Target/targetoid change and sarcoplasmic cores are similar from a morphological standpoint but have very different clinical implications. ***Myofiber splitting*** is particularly common in hypertrophic fibers (Fig. 1.15a), and is a feature of chronic myopathic and some

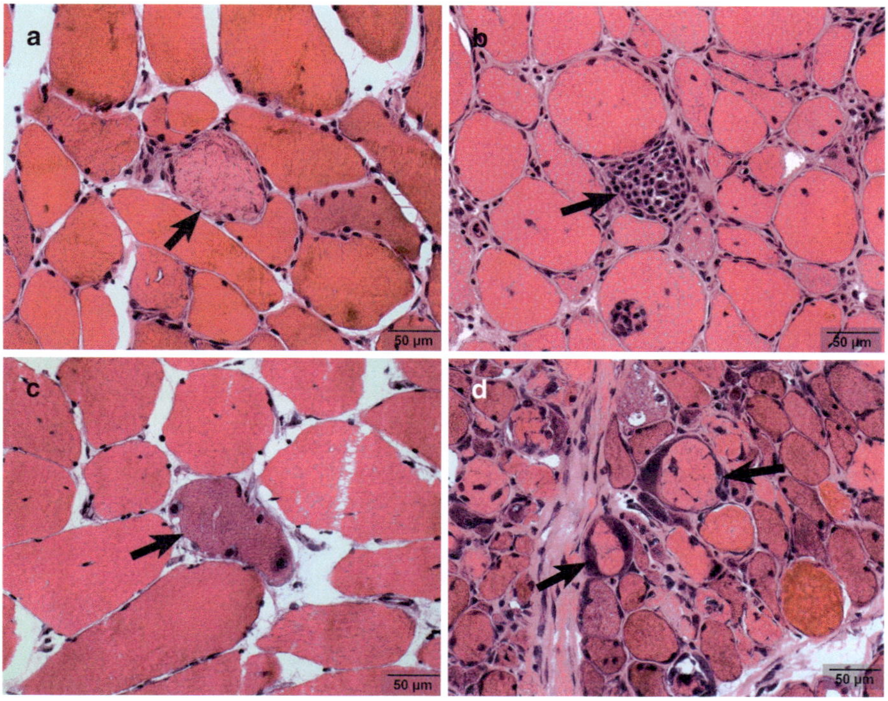

Fig. 1.13 Myofiber degeneration, necrosis and regeneration. (**a**) Degenerating myofiber, H&E. As myofibers degenerate, their sarcoplasm often becomes pale (arrow) and the normal intermyofibrillar network is obscured. In other instances, the sarcoplasm of degenerating myofibers can stain more darkly than that of normal myofibers due to the presence of denatured proteins. (**b**) Myophagocytosis, H&E. Once a myofiber becomes necrotic, its sarcoplasm becomes fragmented and undergoes phagocytosis by macrophages (arrow). (**c**) Regenerating myofiber, H&E. The sarcoplasm of regenerating myofibers is basophilic (arrow), owing to the presence of ribonucleoproteins engaged in protein synthesis. The nuclei of regenerating myofibers are enlarged, and often contain conspicuous nucleoli. (**d**) H&E, mixed myofiber necrosis and regeneration. Myofiber necrosis and regeneration often occur as segmental changes, and it is not uncommon to see evidence of regenerative sarcoplasmic basophilia (arrow) adjacent to areas of sarcoplasmic necrosis in the same myofiber

neuropathic conditions. Split fibers are also a normal feature of myotendinous insertion sites, and in this location should not be interpreted as evidence of a myopathic disorder. Myofiber splitting is often accompanied by other chronic architectural abnormalities, including increased numbers of internalized nuclei, internalized capillary loops, and irregular areas of sarcomeric disarray, the last imparting a *"whorled"* appearance to the sarcoplasm of affected fibers in transverse sections (Fig. 1.15b). This pattern of sarcomeric disarray is common in dystrophic processes, but can also be seen in long-standing chronic neurogenic disorders. The NADH-TR stain, as noted earlier, is a useful stain for demonstrating a number of important sarcoplasmic abnormalities. ***Target/targetoid change*** is characterized by the presence of a fairly well-demarcated zone of pallor and decreased oxidative enzyme activity caused by disorganization of sarcomeres and an absence of mitochondria,

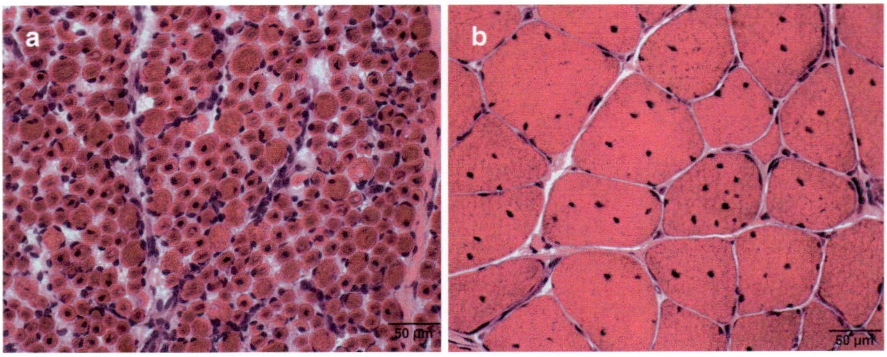

Fig. 1.14 Abnormalities in the location of myofiber nuclei. (**a**) H&E, X-linked myotubular myopathy. In normal skeletal muscle in both infants and older individuals, the vast majority of the myofiber nuclei lie just beneath the sarcolemma. Internalized nuclei are common near myotendinous insertion sites in normal muscle, and are also common in chronic myopathic and neuropathic processes. X-linked myotubular myopathy, illustrated here, is one of a group of hereditary congenital myopathies characterized by abnormally increased numbers of centrally-situated nuclei. (**b**) Myotonic dystrophy type 1, H&E. Myotonic dystrophy is another form of hereditary myopathy associated with increased numbers of internalized nuclei. In biopsies from older patients with this condition, a significant number of myofibers contain multiple, randomly distributed internalized nuclei. In cases of myotonic dystrophy presenting in infancy, the histological changes may be difficult to distinguish from myotubular myopathy and other congenital centronuclear myopathies

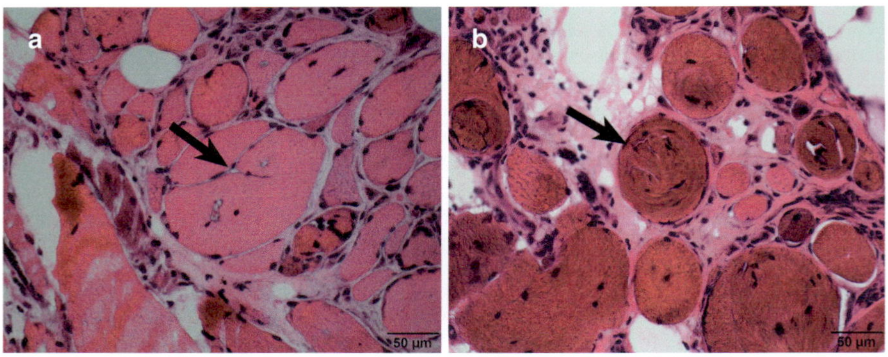

Fig. 1.15 Patterns of myofibrillar disarray: myofiber splitting and sarcoplasmic "whorling". (**a**) Myofiber splitting, H&E. Myofiber splitting is a common, nonspecific change in chronic myopathic disorders, and can also be seen as a secondary change in chronic neurogenic atrophy. The "splitting" (arrow) typically occurs in hypertrophic fibers, and is associated with the presence of internalized nuclei and, in some cases, internalized capillary loops. (**b**) Sarcoplasmic whorling, H&E. "Whorling" of sarcoplasmic elements (arrow) is another common change seen in a wide range of chronic myopathic conditions. Like myofiber splitting, with which it usually coexists, this pattern of sarcomeric disarray is most common in hypertrophic myofibers and is associated with internalized nuclei

usually near the center of the myofiber in transverse sections. Target fibers are distinguished from targetoid fibers by the presence of a thin zone of increased oxidative enzyme activity at the edge of the region of decreased oxidative enzyme activity, while "targetoid" fibers lack this hyperintense border. Both of these structures are best visualized in NADH-TR-stained cryostat sections (Fig. 1.16a) and in sections stained for mitochondrial enzyme activity. Target formation is usually restricted to type I myofibers and is most commonly seen in chronic denervation, although it can also be produced by tendon transection. At an ultrastructural level, targets extend for a considerable distance along the long axis of the affected fiber and are characterized by an absence of mitochondria and variable degrees of sarcomeric disarray and Z-band streaming. Sarcoplasmic cores are another important pattern of myofibrillar disarray, and can take the form of central cores or so-called multiminicores (also known as minicores). As the name suggests, ***central cores*** are classically located in the central area of the sarcoplasm of transversely sectioned fibers, but can also occupy a more eccentric position. Like target fibers, cores are characterized by a well-demarcated zone of decreased oxidative enzyme activity (Fig. 1.16b). They are the defining morphological feature of central core disease, a congenital myopathy associated in a significant number of patients with a ryanodine receptor (RYR1) mutation and susceptibility to malignant hyperthermia syndrome [39]. Like target fibers, their distribution is limited to type I fibers. Ultrastructurally, two forms of central cores have been described. The so-called unstructured cores are characterized by sarcomeric disarray and Z-band streaming similar to that seen in target fibers. "Structured" cores, on the other hand, are characterized by the presence of readily discernable sarcomeres that are usually shorter than the sarcomeres in the adjacent non-core areas and contain wider, more irregular Z-bands. ***Multiminicores*** are also characterized by zones of decreased oxidative enzyme activity but, unlike targets and central cores, tend to be multiple and smaller (Fig. 1.16c), with an orientation perpendicular to the long axis of the affected myofiber. Multiminicores are a feature of a family of congenital myopathies known as multiminicore (or multicore) myopathies. A significant percentage of cases of congenital myopathies with a multiminicore morphology have been associated with a mutation in the gene encoding selenoprotein N1, although other variants also occur. Although not initially felt to be associated with a risk of malignant hyperthermia, some patients with multiminicore change have been shown to carry a mutation in the RYR1 gene and, with it, susceptibility to malignant hyperthermia syndrome [40]. Although uncommon, multiminicore-like structures can also occasionally be encountered in patients with chronic denervation. ***Moth-eaten change*** is a common, nonspecific change that is also characterized by the presence of irregular areas of decreased oxidative enzyme activity (Fig. 1.16f). Moth-eaten change can be difficult to distinguish from multiminicores in some cases. ***Lobulated*** (or ***trabecular***) fibers are myofibers that have an abnormally coarsely-staining intermyofibrillar network that is also best demonstrated in the NADH-TR stain (Fig. 1.17a). This pattern is caused by abnormal aggregation of mitochondria, thought to be associated with a defect in the normal "anchoring" of mitochondria near Z-bands. The lobulated change typically preferentially affects type 1 myofibers, which are often atrophic. While not specific for any one myopathic disorder, they are particularly common in patients with the autosomal recessive form of limb girdle muscular dystrophy associated with

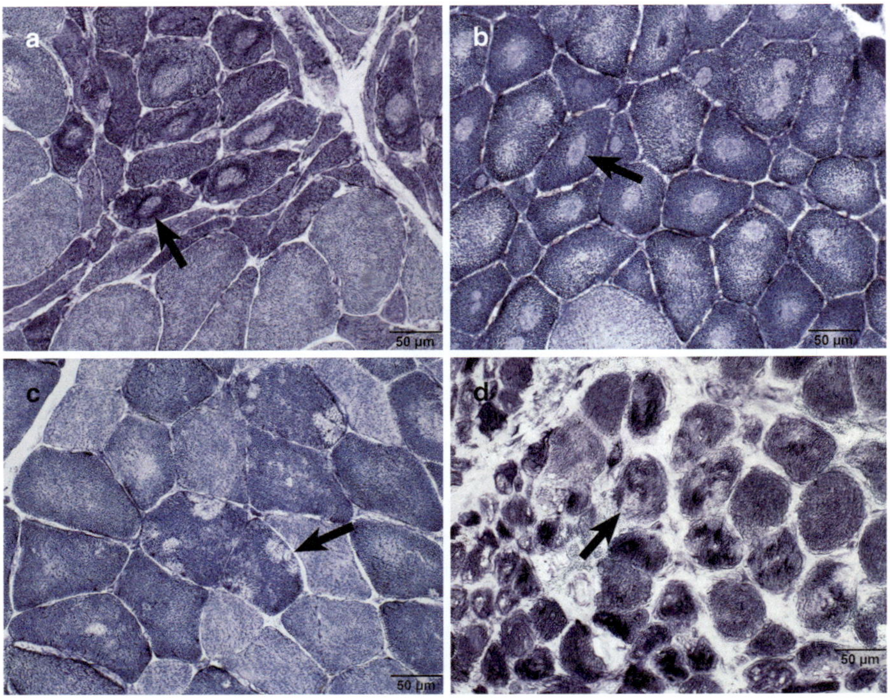

Fig. 1.16 Patterns of myofibrillar disarray, continued: target/targetoid fibers, central cores, multiminicores and moth-eaten change. (**a**) Target fibers in chronic denervation, NADH-TR. The NADH-TR stain is an excellent stain for highlighting abnormalities in myofibrillar elements. Target fibers are common in chronic peripheral neuropathies, and are characterized by a fairly well-demarcated zone of decreased oxidative enzyme activity surrounded by a rim of increased enzyme activity (arrow). "Targetoid" fibers are similar to target fibers, but lack the peripheral zone of increased enzyme activity. (**b**) Central core disease, NADH-TR. Central cores, the hallmark of central core disease, are also best seen in oxidative stains, where they appear as a well-defined area of decreased enzyme activity (arrow). Despite their name, in some myofibers, the cores can lie in a more peripheral position. Patients with central cores are at increased risk for ryanodine receptor abnormalities and susceptibility to malignant hyperthermia syndrome. (**c**) Multiminicore disease, NADH-TR. Multiminicores, as the name suggests, appear as multiple, irregular areas of decreased oxidative enzyme activity (arrow). Multiminicore disease, although not originally felt to be associated with an increased risk of malignant hyperthermia syndrome, can also be associated with ryanodine receptor abnormalities. (**d**) Moth-eaten change, NADH-TR. Moth-eaten change refers to the presence of irregular, usually ill-defined areas of decreased oxidative enzyme activity (arrow) This is a nonspecific degenerative alteration encountered in a wide range of myopathic processes. Moth-eaten change can be difficult to distinguish from multiminicores, but is usually less widely distributed than the multiminicores seen in cases of multiminicore myopathy

calpain-3 deficiency (LGMD 2A) [41, 42]. They have also been reported in other dystrophic processes, including facioscapulohumeral dystrophy, and have been described as the predominant change in a subset of elderly patients with limb girdle weakness in the absence of a defined protein abnormality [43]. ***Ring fibers*** are another example of myofibrillar disarray, characterized by the presence of a peripheral rim of improperly oriented myofibrils encircling a central region of well-preserved sarcoplasm, best demonstrated in oxidative (Fig. 1.17b) and PAS stains. Ring fibers are often smaller and stain more intensely in H&E and Gomori trichrome stains than their normal counterparts. Although commonly associated with myotonic dystrophy, they can be seen in a wide range of myopathic processes, and sometimes as isolated incidental changes.

Abnormal sarcoplasmic inclusions can occur in muscle fibers, and their presence can provide important clues to the nature of the neuromuscular disorder. Many of these are recognizable in Gomori trichrome-stained cryostat sections, supplemented by other stains. ***Ragged red change*** in the Gomori trichrome stain is a hallmark of abnormal mitochondrial accumulation. As mentioned previously, the mitochondrial aggregates have a granular, faintly basophilic appearance in H&E sections. The membrane-rich mitochondria are highlighted red in the Gomori trichrome stain, producing the characteristic ragged red appearance (Fig. 1.18a). Mitochondrial stains, particularly the SDH stain, highlight mitochondrial aggregates with even greater sensitivity than the trichrome stain, and should always be

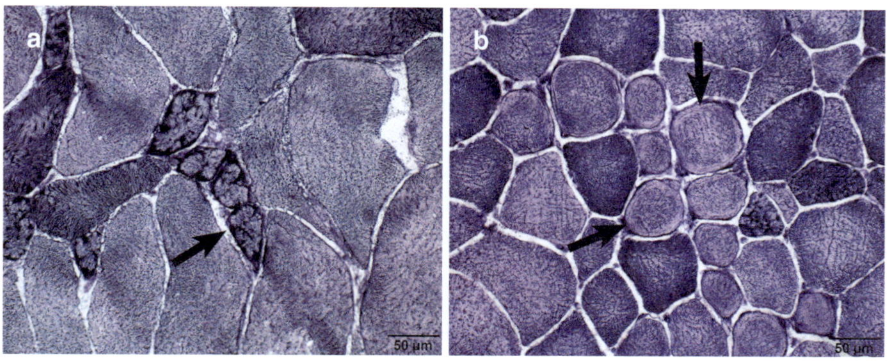

Fig. 1.17 Patterns of myofibrillar disarray, continued: lobulated fibers and ring fibers. (**a**) Lobulated fibers, NADH-TR. Lobulated fibers (arrow), sometimes designated as "trabecular" fibers, are characterized by coarsening of the intermyofibrillar network, best appreciated in oxidative stains. Lobulated fibers can be seen in a number of different myopathic disorders, and are often conspicuous in patients with facioscapulohumeral muscular dystrophy and in autosomal recessive limb girdle muscular dystrophy caused by calpain-3 deficiency (LGMD 2A). They have also been described as the predominant change in a subset of elderly patients with limb girdle weakness in the absence of a defined protein abnormality. The affected fibers are usually type 1 myofibers, and are smaller than neighboring normal myofibers. (**b**) Ring fibers, NADH-TR. Ring fibers, sometimes designated as spiral annulets or "Ringbinden", are characterized by a peripheral zone of circumferentially-oriented myofibrils (arrow) surrounding a central area of normally oriented myofibrils. They are most commonly seen in patients with myotonic dystrophy, but can be encountered as nonspecific changes in a wide range of chronic myopathic processes

used to confirm the mitochondrial nature of the inclusions. Ragged red change is also a feature of some inflammatory myopathies (inclusion body myositis [35, 44], polymyositis with COX-deficient myofibers [45], and is common in paraspinous muscles [46] and in muscle biopsies from older adults [47]. ***Tubular aggregates*** are membrane rich inclusions derived from redundant collections of sarcoplasmic reticulum that are also highlighted in the trichrome stain (Fig. 1.18b). These inclusions are sometimes mistaken for ragged red change, but tend to be better-demarcated than the mitochondrial aggregates in ragged red fibers. Like mitochondrial aggregates, they are highlighted in NADH-TR stained sections, but lack SDH and COX activity and, in contrast to mitochondrial aggregates, are typically restricted to type 2 myofibers (except in some of the rare familial tubular aggregate myopathies, in which they occur in type 1 fibers). Tubular aggregates are usually sporadic, incidental findings, but have also been associated with a number myopathic conditions, including some forms of periodic paralysis and myotonia [48]. Hereditary forms of tubular aggregate myopathy have also been documented, with symptoms that include progressive weakness, exercise-induced myalgias and cramps, and weakness with myasthenic features. In addition to highlighting membrane-rich sarcoplasmic accumulations, the Gomori trichrome stain is also useful for highlighting a variety of protein-rich inclusions. ***Nemaline bodies*** are a feature of the nemaline myopathies, a clinically and genetically heterogeneous group of congenital myopathies that are characterized by the presence of small rod-like structures (nemaline "rods") in the sarcoplasm of affected myofibers [49]. These structures contain a high concentration of the Z-disc protein α-actinin, stain dark-red to blue in the Gomori trichrome stain, and often aggregate at the periphery of the affected myofiber (Fig. 1.19a). Nemaline bodies can be difficult to identify at the light microscopic level in some biopsies, for which reason we routinely perform electron microscopy on any biopsy in which a nemaline myopathy (or other congenital myopathy) is suspected. Nemaline bodies can also be seen as incidental structures, particularly in the vicinity of myotendinous insertion sites and in extraocular muscles. ***Cytoplasmic bodies*** are fairly distinctive inclusions that are especially common in patients with inclusion body myopathies and myofibrillar myopathies (discussed below) [50]. They have been described in earlier publications as a distinguishing feature of a heterogeneous group of conditions termed "cytoplasmic body myopathies", some examples of which are now classified as variants of myofibrillar myopathy or inclusion body myopathy. They can also be encountered in patients with myopathy related to ipecac abuse [51] and as incidental findings in otherwise normal muscle. Cytoplasmic bodies are eosinophilic in H&E stained sections, and stain red to dark green in the Gomori trichrome stain (Fig. 1.19b); a pale halo is usually discernable at their periphery. They have a very distinctive ultrastructural appearance, with a darkly staining, dense filamentous core surrounded by a halo of thin radiating filaments. ***Spheroid bodies*** are another type of proteinaceous inclusion that can be seen in many of the same conditions that are associated with cytoplasmic bodies. They tend to be larger and more irregular than classical cytoplasmic bodies, but can be probably be thought of as a variant of the latter. Spheroid bodies are particularly conspicuous in spheroid body myopathy, a variant of myofibrillar myopathy associated with

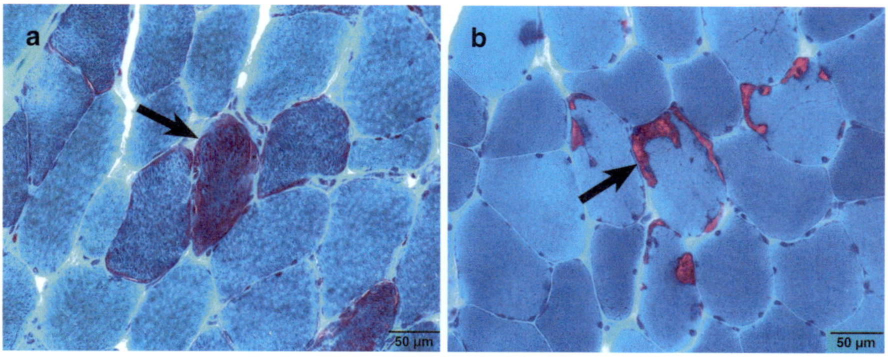

Fig. 1.18 Abnormal sarcoplasmic inclusions: ragged red change and tubular aggregates. (**a**) Ragged red change, Gomori trichrome. The Gomori trichrome stain is an invaluable tool for demonstrating a variety of abnormal sarcoplasmic inclusions. One of the best known examples is ragged red change (arrow), caused by the presence of abnormal mitochondrial aggregates. Such changes are the hallmark of many mitochondrial myopathies, but are also common in inclusion body myositis, polymyositis with mitochondrial abnormalities, in muscle biopsies from elderly patients, and in orbital and paraspinous muscles. Myofibers with ragged red change are also reliably highlighted in sections stained for succinate dehydrogenase activity. (**b**) Tubular aggregates, Gomori trichrome. Tubular aggregates (arrow) are structures composed of redundant collections of sarcoplasmic reticulum. Like mitochondrial membranes, the sarcoplasmic reticulum has an affinity for the red dye used in the Gomori trichrome stain. Tubular aggregates are sometimes confused with ragged red change, but tend to be better demarcated and, unlike ragged red change, usually restricted to type 2 fibers. They are NADH-TR reactive but lack mitochondrial enzyme activity

mutations in the gene encoding myotilin [52]. ***Reducing bodies*** are well-circumscribed, darkly-staining eosinophilic inclusions in H&E-stained sections that, like cytoplasmic bodies, stain dark red in the Gomori trichrome stain. They are distinguished from the latter by their dark reaction product in the menadione nitroblue tetrazolium stain [53]. Reducing bodies are a prominent feature in reducing body myopathies, hereditary myopathies caused by mutations in the *FHL1* gene [54]. Some myopathic disorders, exemplified by the myofibrillar myopathies, are characterized by the presence of ***larger, irregular proteinaceous aggregates***. The staining properties of these aggregates is variable, but most appear as irregular eosinophilic hyaline deposits in H&E sections (Fig. 1.19c). The inclusions can range from dark green to red in color in trichrome-stained cryostat sections, and in some cases stain faintly in Congo red stains. In the case of myofibrillar myopathies, the inclusions are often immunoreactive for desmin (Fig. 1.19d), as well as a number of other proteins [55, 56]. Abnormal proteinaceous aggregates are also a feature of sporadic inclusion body myositis [57] and hereditary inclusion body myopathies [58].

Sarcoplasmic vacuoles of various types are a feature of a number of different muscle diseases and, in some cases, are the defining feature of a specific myopathic disorder. One must be careful to distinguish true sarcoplasmic vacuoles from clear spaces caused by ice crystal artifact. Some vacuoles are distinguished by conspicuous ***lysosomal activity***, best demonstrated in cryostat sections stained for acid phosphatase activity. These include acid maltase deficiency (type II glycogen storage disease) (Fig. 1.20a, b) and two hereditary X-linked conditions (Danon myopathy, associated with deficiency of the LAMP-2 protein [59], and X-linked myopathy with excessive autophagy [60, 61]. Vacuolar change and increased lysosomal activity are also a feature of some amphiphilic cationic myopathies, most notably those associated with exposure to chloroquine or hydroxychloroquine. ***Rimmed sarcoplasmic vacuoles*** are a feature of hereditary and sporadic inclusion body myopathies, myofibrillar myopathies, oculopharyngeal muscular dystrophy and some forms of hereditary limb girdle muscular dystrophy and distal myopathy. Classical rimmed vacuoles contain membranous material that is highlighted in the Gomori

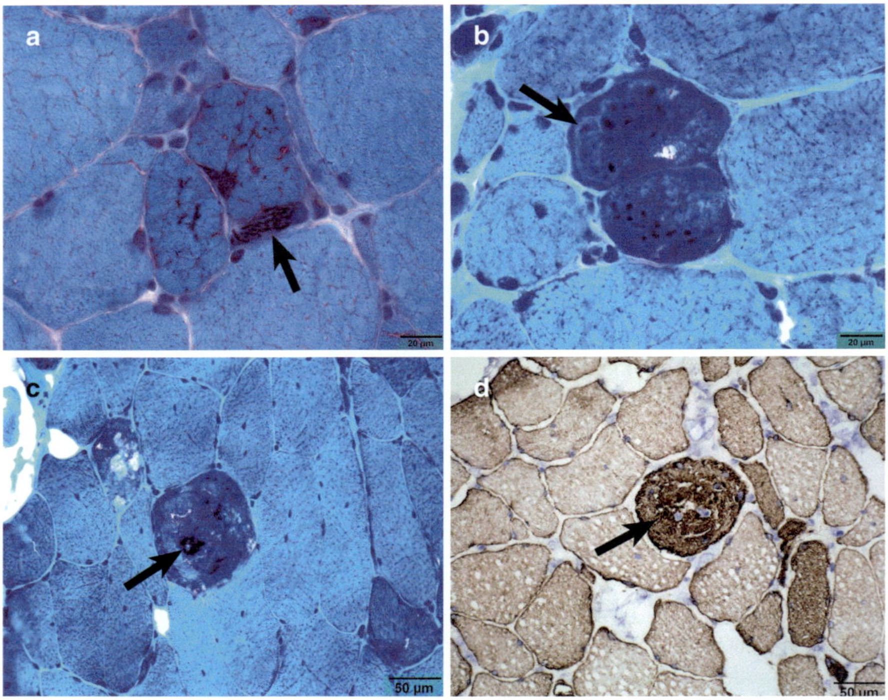

Fig. 1.19 Abnormal sarcoplasmic inclusions, continued: nemaline rods, cytoplasmic bodies and other proteinaceous aggregates. (**a**) Nemaline myopathy, Gomori trichrome. Nemaline rods are structures that are derived from abnormal sarcomeric Z-band material. They are the defining morphological feature of a clinically and genetically heterogeneous group of congenital myopathies known as nemaline myopathies. They can also be seen as incidental structures in a number of other myopathic processes and in normal skeletal muscle at myotendinous insertion sites. Nemaline rods typically cluster in subsarcolemmal areas (arrow). (**b**) Cytoplasmic bodies, Gomori trichrome. Cytoplasmic bodies are small proteinaceous inclusions that can be seen in a number of different myopathies, but are especially conspicuous in myofibrillar myopathies and inclusion body myopathies. The classic cytoplasmic body has a core that stains blue in the Gomori trichrome stain, surrounded by a clear halo (arrow). (**c**) Protein aggregate in myofibrillar myopathy, Gomori trichrome. Large, irregular proteinaceous inclusions, like cytoplasmic bodies, are common in myofibrillar myopathies and inclusion body myopathies. Their appearance ranges from red to blue-green in the Gomori trichrome stain (arrow). (**d**) Protein aggregate in myofibrillar myopathy, desmin stain. Immunohistochemical staining is a useful technique for identifying specific protein entities in the proteinaceous deposits seen in the trichrome stain. Desmin reactivity (arrow) is particularly common, although a variety of other proteins are often also present

trichrome stain, and gives the vacuoles their classical "rimmed" appearance (Fig. 1.20c). They are of lysosomal origin, and often have some acid phosphatase reactivity, although this is typically less intense than that seen in vacuoles in acid maltase deficiency. Amyloid is demonstrable in some examples, but this is variable. At an ultrastructural level, the rimmed vacuoles of inclusion body myositis contain bundles of characteristic "tubulofilamentous" structures measuring from 16–24 nm in diameter (Fig. 1.20d), usually accompanied by nonspecific lysosomal debris; accurate measurement of these tubulofilamentous structures is essential to avoid

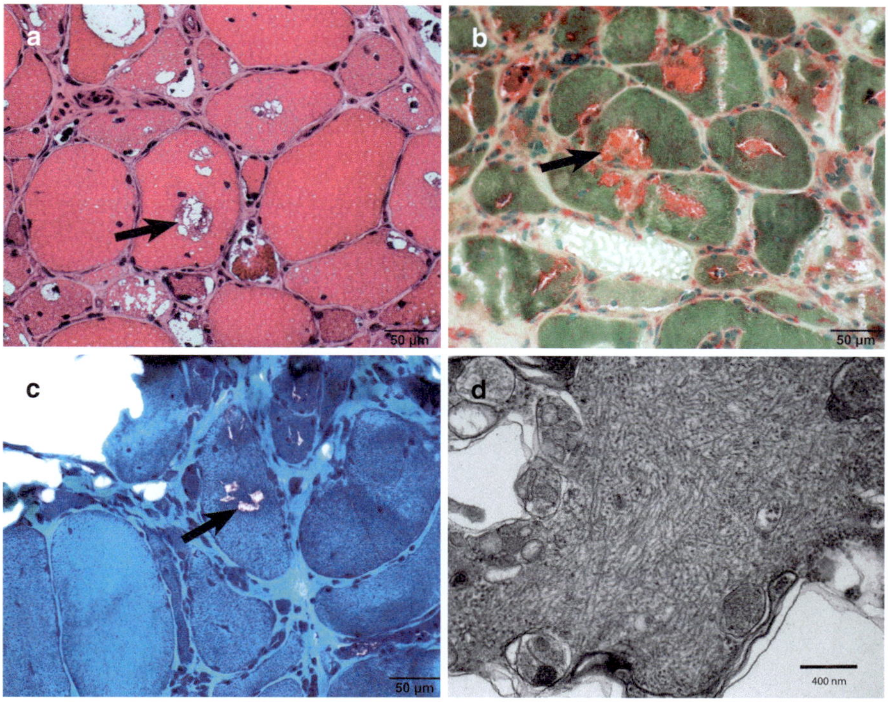

Fig. 1.20 Sarcoplasmic vacuoles: Acid maltase deficiency and inclusion body myositis. (**a**) Acid maltase deficiency, H&E. Acid maltase deficiency, also known as glycogen storage disease type 2, is characterized by the presence of vacuolar change (arrow). In adult cases, the vacuolar change is less dramatic than those seen in infantile cases (Pompe disease), and can vary considerably from muscle to muscle. The vacuoles contain stainable glycogen. (**b**) Acid maltase deficiency, acid phosphatase. In acid maltase deficiency, much of the abnormal glycogen accumulates within lysosomes, and is therefore associated with areas of abnormal acid phosphatase reactivity (arrow). Similar patterns of vacuolar change associated with abnormal lysosomal activity can also be seen in Danon myopathy and X-linked myopathy with excess autophagy. (**c**) Inclusion body myositis, Gomori trichrome. Rimmed vacuoles (arrow) are a characteristic feature of sporadic inclusion body myositis, hereditary inclusion body myopathies, myofibrillar myopathies, oculopharyngeal muscular dystrophy and some distal myopathies. The vacuoles typically contain abundant membranous debris, as well as an interesting array of proteins. The membranous debris has an affinity for the red dye in the Gomori trichrome stain. (**d**) Inclusion body myositis, EM. Under the electron microscope, the rimmed vacuoles in muscles from patients with inclusion body myositis often contain inclusions composed of filaments with diameters ranging from 16 to 24 mm. It is important to distinguish these larger filaments from collections of smaller actin and myosin filaments that can be seen in any injured myofiber

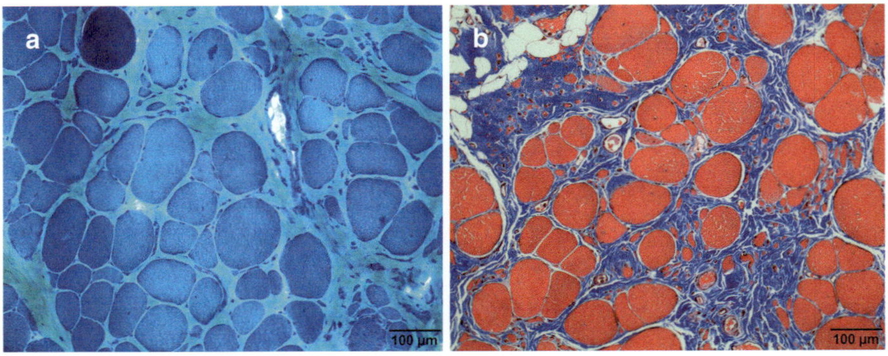

Fig. 1.21 Interstitial fibrosis. (**a**) Duchenne muscular dystrophy, Gomori trichrome. Increased endomysial connective tissue is a feature of many chronic myopathic disorders, including most muscular dystrophies. The abundant endomysial collagen in this biopsy stains light green in a cryostat section stained with the Gomori trichrome stain. (**b**) Duchenne muscular dystrophy, Masson trichrome. The endomysial collagen in a paraffin section from the same patient is highlighted dark blue in the Masson trichrome stain, contrasting sharply with the red color that the stain gives to the sarcoplasm of adjacent myofibers

confusion with the disrupted myosin and/or actin filaments that are often seen in injured myofibers. ***Non-lysosomal vacuoles*** are a feature of some of the non-lysosomal glycogen storage diseases, as well as some forms of periodic paralysis. Properly performed PAS stains reliably highlight the glycogen in vacuoles associated with glycogen storage diseases, while those associated with periodic paralysis are devoid of glycogen.

Changes in Connective Tissue

Endomysial fibrosis is commonly seen in chronic neuromuscular disorders (Fig. 1.21). Changes of this type are particularly common in chronic myopathic conditions, but can also be seen in severe, long-standing denervation. As muscle injury progresses, the areas previously occupied by skeletal muscle fibers are sometimes replaced by adipose tissue. In some biopsies, these connective tissue changes are so extensive that it is impossible to determine the nature of the underlying neuromuscular disease, and the biopsy must be designated simply as “end-stage muscle”.

Cellular Infiltrates

Inflammatory infiltrates are a common change in muscle biopsies, particularly in patients with myopathic disorders. The most common inflammatory cells are lymphocytes and macrophages (histiocytes), although other cell types – plasma cells, neutrophils and eosinophils – are sometimes encountered. ***Infiltrating lymphocytes*** are particularly important to recognize in muscle biopsies. Lymphocytic infiltrates can be encountered in any of the muscle compartments – endomysium, perimysium and even in epimysial connective tissue – and their distribution can provide important clues to the nature of the muscle disease. Endomysial lymphoid infiltrates are a feature of polymyositis (Fig. 1.22a), classically associated with lymphocytic invasion of non-necrotic myofibers by CD8-reactive T-lymphocytes. Identical patterns of endomysial inflammation are also seen in inclusion body myositis and in polymyositis with mitochondrial abnormalities. Perimysial lymphocytic infiltration (Fig. 1.22b), in contrast, is often seen in dermatomyositis and related inflammatory myopathic disorders, such as systemic lupus erythematosus-associated myositis, as well as in cases of primary inflammation of fascial connective tissue (fasciitis). While the presence of lymphocytic infiltration can be an important clue to the presence of an inflammatory myopathy responsive to immunomodulatory therapy, it is important to note that they can also be seen in myopathic processes that do not respond to immunosuppression, including inclusion body myositis, some muscular dystrophies (notably facioscapulohumeral dystrophy, dysferlin deficiency, merosin-deficient congenital muscular dystrophy and occasional dystrophinopathy cases). Conversely, lymphocytic infiltrates are not always present in biopsies from patients with immune-mediated myopathic disorders (e.g. immune-mediated necrotizing myopathies), and may be absent even in biopsies from patients with conventional inflammatory myopathies (e.g., polymyositis) due to "sampling error". ***Macrophages*** are almost invariably present in conditions associated with muscle fiber necrosis, where they engulf necrotic fibers, as illustrated earlier in Fig. 1.13b, and sometimes infiltrate the connective tissue adjacent to damaged myofibers. In such conditions, macrophages are a nonspecific host reaction to muscle fiber injury, and, as noted earlier, should not be misinterpreted as evidence of a primary inflammatory myopathic process. Less commonly, macrophages can be a component of a primary inflammatory process, exemplified by cases of macrophagic myofasciitis (Fig. 1.22c) an inflammatory muscle disease caused by the intramuscular injection of vaccines containing aluminum adjuvant [27], and in cases of granulomatous myositis.

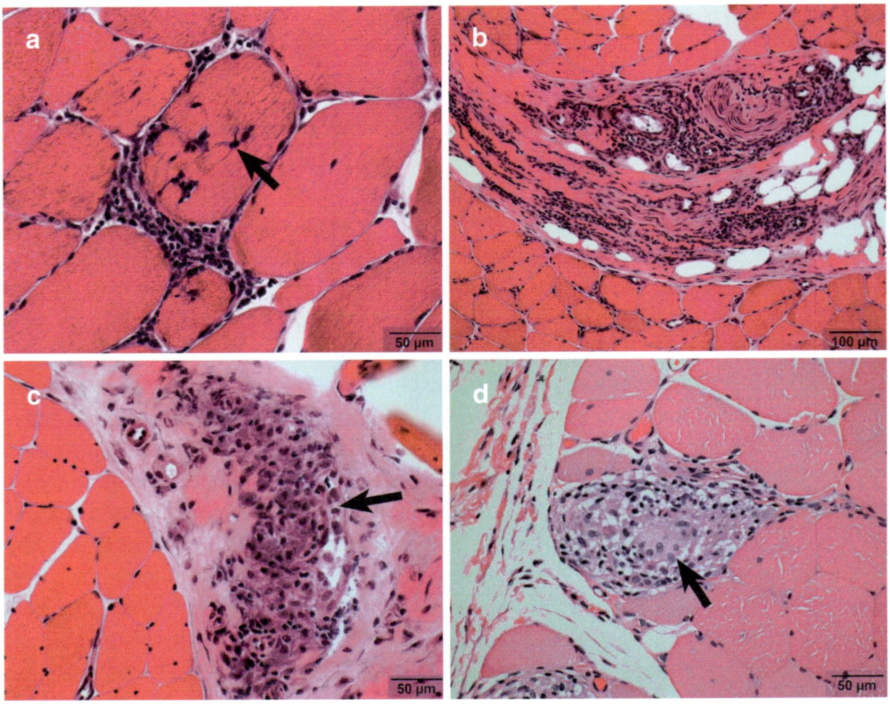

Fig. 1.22 Inflammatory infiltrates. (**a**) Endomysial inflammation with lymphocytic myofiber invasion in polymyositis, H&E. Lymphocytic infiltration of the endomysium is a feature of polymyositis and inclusion body myositis, and can also be seen in some forms of muscular dystrophy. Invasion of adjacent myofibers by lymphocytes (arrow) is seen in polymyositis and inclusion body myositis, but not in muscular dystrophies. (**b**)**,** Perimysial inflammation, H&E. Lymphocytic infiltration of the perimysial is common in dermatomyositis and related inflammatory myopathies, and is also a feature of some cases of fasciitis. (**c**) Macrophagic myofasciitis, H&E. Macrophages (arrow) are most often encountered in skeletal muscle as a host response to muscle fiber injury, but in some inflammatory conditions, including macrophagic myofasciitis, are the primary inflammatory cell. The cytoplasm of the macrophages in macrophagic myofasciitis has a characteristic granular, basophilic appearance. (**d**) Granulomatous inflammation, H&E. Granulomas are compact aggregates of activated macrophages, often associated with multinucleate giant cells (arrow). Granulomatous inflammation in skeletal muscle is a feature of sarcoidosis and a number of other non-infectious entities, but its presence should always prompt a search for microorganisms, particularly acid fast bacilli or fungi

Macrophagic infiltration associated with ***granulomatous inflammation*** can be seen in the muscles of patients with sarcoidosis (Fig. 1.22d), and, less commonly, in patients with thymoma, Crohn's disease, and isolated granulomatous myositis [62, 63]. Granulomatous inflammation can also be encountered in patients with inflammatory myopathy associated with the presence of anti-mitochondrial antibodies [64] and in some vasculitic disorders (discussed below). Finally, the possibility of an infectious process should always be excluded in patients with evidence of granulomatous inflammation. Enzyme histochemical staining for acid phosphatase reactivity and immunohistochemical staining for CD68 reliably highlight the macrophagic infiltrates in cases of granulomatous myositis and other conditions. ***Plasma cells*** are less commonly encountered in muscle biopsies than either macrophages or lymphocytes. They may be conspicuous in cases of myositis associated with Sjogren's syndrome. ***Eosinophils*** can be seen in small numbers in inflammatory myopathies of various types, but are not usually conspicuous. Well-developed eosinophilic infiltrates have been reported in as an idiopathic focal lesion ("focal eosinophilic myositis"), as a manifestation of parasitic infection and in rare examples of muscle involvement in systemic hypereosinophilic syndrome [65] and in allergic granulomatosis [66]. They have also been reported in limb girdle muscular dystrophies associated with calpain-3 mutations [67] and γ-sarcoglycan mutations [68]. ***Neutrophilic infiltrates*** are also fairly uncommon in muscle biopsies. Their presence should prompt careful search for a bacterial or fungal infection. Sterile neutrophilic myositis has been reported in Sweet's syndrome [69] associated with hematologic malignancies and myelodysplastic disorders.

Vascular Changes

A variety of important diagnostic changes can be seen in the blood vessels in skeletal muscle biopsies. ***Amyloid deposits***, discussed earlier, are often associated with vessel walls in patients with amyloid myopathies. ***Thickening of vascular basal laminae*** is common in aging, hypertension and diabetes mellitus, and is also a conspicuous change in patients with an uncommon immune-mediated disorder designated necrotizing myopathy with pipestem capillaries [70]. Thickened basal laminae have a homogeneous, lightly eosinophilic appearance in H&E stains, appear pale green in Gomori trichrome-stained cryostat sections, and are highlighted in PAS stains. Thickened basal laminae are easily identified at an ultrastructural level (Fig. 1.23a), where it is often split and reduplicated. ***Dermatomyositis*** is associated with areas of reduced capillary density, deposition of terminal complement complex (C_{5b-9}) in perifascicular capillaries and, at an ultrastructural level, the presence of characteristic ***tubuloreticular inclusions*** in the cytoplasm of endothelial cells (Fig. 1.23b). For completeness, it should be noted that, while capillary C5b-9 deposition is a feature of a dermatomyositis and some additional immune-mediated myopathic processes, it is also commonly seen in endomysial capillaries in patients with diabetes mellitus in the absence of immune-mediated muscle injury [71]. ***Vasculitis*** can be seen in skeletal muscle in patients with a number systemic disorders, including polyarteritis nodosa, allergic granulomatosis (Churg-Strauss disease), rheumatoid arthritis, systemic lupus erythematosus and related connective tissue disorders. A spectrum of morphological patterns can be seen in cases of vasculitis, ranging from simple lymphocytic infiltration of vessel walls to fibrinoid necrosis and leukocytoclastic change (Fig. 1.23c). Vasculitis associated with

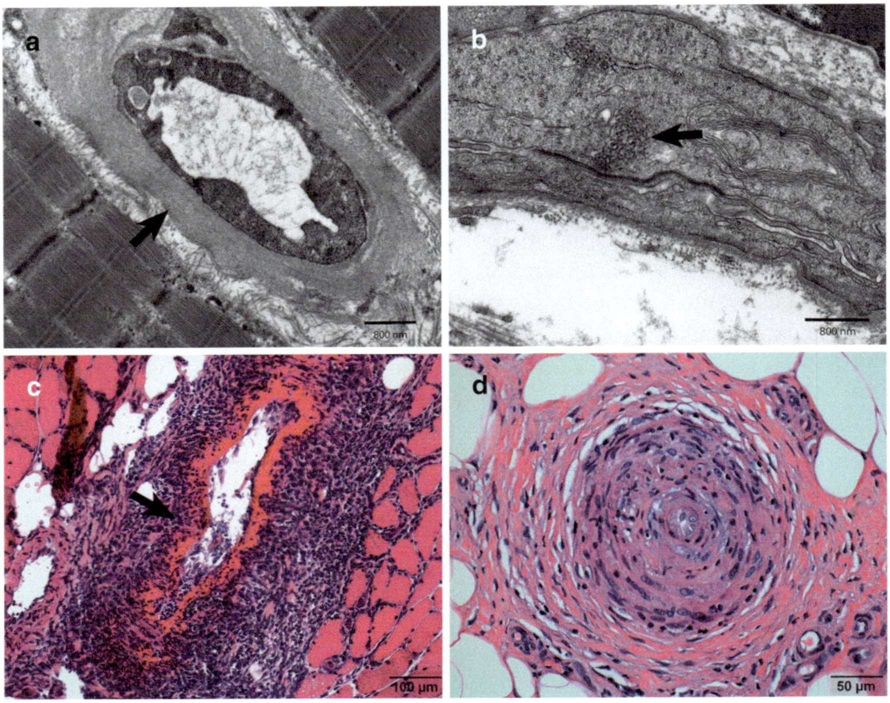

Fig. 1.23 Vascular changes. (**a**) Microvascular sclerosis, EM. Thickening of vascular basal laminae (arrow) can occur as a consequence of aging, but can also be an indicator of diabetes mellitus or hypertension. Basal lamina thickening has also been described in a variant of inflammatory myopathy known as necrotizing myopathy with pipestem capillaries. PAS stains are a useful technique for demonstrating basal lamina thickening at the light microscopic level. (**b**) Endothelial tubuloreticular inclusions in dermatomyositis, H&E. Tubuloreticular inclusions (arrow) in the cytoplasm of endothelial cells are a classical feature of dermatomyositis and related disorders such as lupus-associated myositis. (**c**) Necrotizing vasculitis, H&E. Necrotizing vasculitis is characterized by the presence of vessel wall inflammation associated with fibrinoid necrosis (arrow), the latter a brightly eosinophilic staining pattern caused by altered plasma proteins that have leaked into the wall of the injured vessel. (**d**) Remote vasculitic injury, H&E. When a vessel has been injured by vasculitis, cellular elements in the vessel wall proliferate in an attempt to repair the damage. The end result is often a markedly thickened, fibrotic vessel wall with an abnormally small lumen

granulomatous inflammation can be seen in patients with Wegener's granulomatosis and allergic granulomatosis. It is important to remember that vasculitis is a multifocal, rather than a diffuse, process, and that diagnostic changes may not be present in a single biopsy from a patient with a systemic vasculitic process. In such cases, serial sections of the specimen may disclose areas of vasculitis not represented in the initial sections. Search for evidence of remote vascular damage (e.g. asymmetrical fibrosis of the vessel wall, disruption of the elastic lamella or remote occlusion of the vessel lumen) may also provide clues to the presence of vasculitis (Fig. 1.23d). In the final analysis, a "negative" biopsy should never be taken as proof that that the possibility of vasculitis has been excluded.

Artifacts in Skeletal Muscle Biopsies

As noted in the comments on the proper acquisition of muscle biopsies, improper handling of muscle tissue at the time of biopsy, during transport to the laboratory or during processing in the laboratory can produce a range of artifacts ranging from alterations that are annoying but otherwise inconsequential to changes that preclude meaningful interpretation of the biopsy. An unfortunate and avoidable artifact commonly introduced at the time of biopsy is ***cautery artifact***. The cauterized muscle fibers have a condensed, dark appearance in H&E and trichrome stains (Fig. 1.24a) and are, predictably, devoid of normal enzyme activity. ***Formalin artifact***, cause by accidental exposure of fresh tissue destined for frozen section histology is another abnormality encountered in muscle tissue, particularly those submitted from institutions with less experience in performing neuromuscular biopsies. The affected myofibers in such cases stain diffusely red in the Gomori trichrome stain rather than green (Fig. 1.24b). There is typically a significant loss of enzyme activity in such cases, even after very brief, inadvertent exposure to formalin. An ***artifactual loss of enzyme activity*** can be seen in muscle tissue that has been transported in excess saline, or in which processing in the laboratory has been delayed. Some stains, including those for glycolytic pathway enzymes, are particularly sensitive to delayed processing, and "negative" reactions in such cases should be interpreted with caution. Prolonged immersion of fresh muscle into excess saline also tends to leach glycogen from the sarcoplasm. Mitochondrial enzymes, particularly cytochrome c oxidase, are also susceptible to artifactual degradation, which typically appears as a loss of enzyme activity at the edges of the tissue (Fig. 1.24c). ***Ice crystal artifact*** is a common change in specimens that have been transported in excess saline. Ice crystal artifact is characterized by the presence of optically clear sarcoplasmic vacuoles of variable size and distribution (Fig. 1.24d), and can be confused with vacuoles associated with some vacuolar myopathies. Thawing and properly refreezing the tissue can sometimes reduce the amount of ice crystal artifact, although myofibers tend to shrink during this process. ***Drying artifact*** can occur if the fresh muscle segment is exposed to air for an excessive amount of time prior to freezing (Fig. 1.24e). Muscle fibers that have dried out tend to be rounded and retracted from the adjacent endomysium, and often have a pale, "smudgy" appearance in H&E stains. They usually stain poorly in enzyme histochemical preparations. Artifactual pallor is also commonly seen if fresh muscle has been immersed in

Fig. 1.24 Artifacts in skeletal muscle biopsies. (**a**) Cautery artifact, H&E. The use of an electrocautery instrument during excision of muscle tissue effectively "cooks" the myofibers, giving them a shrunken, dark, contracted appearance (arrow). This change precludes meaningful interpretation of the morphology of the affected tissue. (**b**) Formalin artifact, Gomori trichrome. Accidental immersion of fresh muscle into formalin causes the myofibers to stain red (arrow). These myofibers are effectively "fixed", and cannot be evaluated for the presence of enzyme activity or subtle changes in the intermyofibrillar network. (**c**) Artifactual loss of mitochondrial enzyme activity, sequential COX-SDH stain. Cytochrome c oxidase activity is often lost in muscles that have been subjected to drying or inadequate freezing during transport to the laboratory from remote locations. The artifactual loss of enzyme activity is most apparent at the edges of the tissue fragments (arrow). This pattern needs to be distinguished from the selective perifascicular loss of COX reactivity that can be seen in dermatomyositis. (**d**) Freezing artifact, H&E. Skeletal muscle that has been improperly frozen, or inadvertently thawed during transfer to the cryostat, contains irregular, optically clear vacuoles caused by the presence of ice crystals (arrows). These artifactual changes can be confused with true vacuolar change, and make evaluation of other morphological changes extremely difficult. (**e**) Drying artifact, H&E. Tissue that has been dried, as often happens when muscle is transported from a distant site, thawed and refrozen yields sections in which the muscle fibers are artifactually separated and stain poorly, particularly in enzyme histochemical preparations. If cryostat sections are allowed to air dry at room temperature for too long a time, they have a "smudgy", pale appearance in most stains. Abnormal sarcoplasmic pallor is also a feature of fresh muscle that has been immersed in excess saline prior to freezing. (**f**) Contraction artifact, EM. Immersion of fresh muscle tissue into aldehyde-based fixatives causes the muscle fiber to vigorously contract. This results in aggregation of normal contractile elements into amorphous, densely staining areas (arrow) that can obscure diagnostically significant changes in sarcomeric morphology, such as multiminicores. Contraction artifact can be minimized by clamping muscle segments *in situ* before excising them and placing them into fixative excess saline during transport to the laboratory. ***Contraction artifact*** can occur when muscle segments are placed into fixative for subsequent paraffin or resin embedding. In some instances, this results in only occasional dense, hypercontracted segments in longitudinally oriented myofibers, but in more extreme cases, can completely obscure sarcomeric morphology and hamper the evaluation of the muscle biopsy for multi-minicores or other pathological patterns of sarcomeric disorganization (Fig. 1.24f). Contraction artifact can be minimized by clamping the muscle segment *in situ* prior to excising it and placing it into fixative.

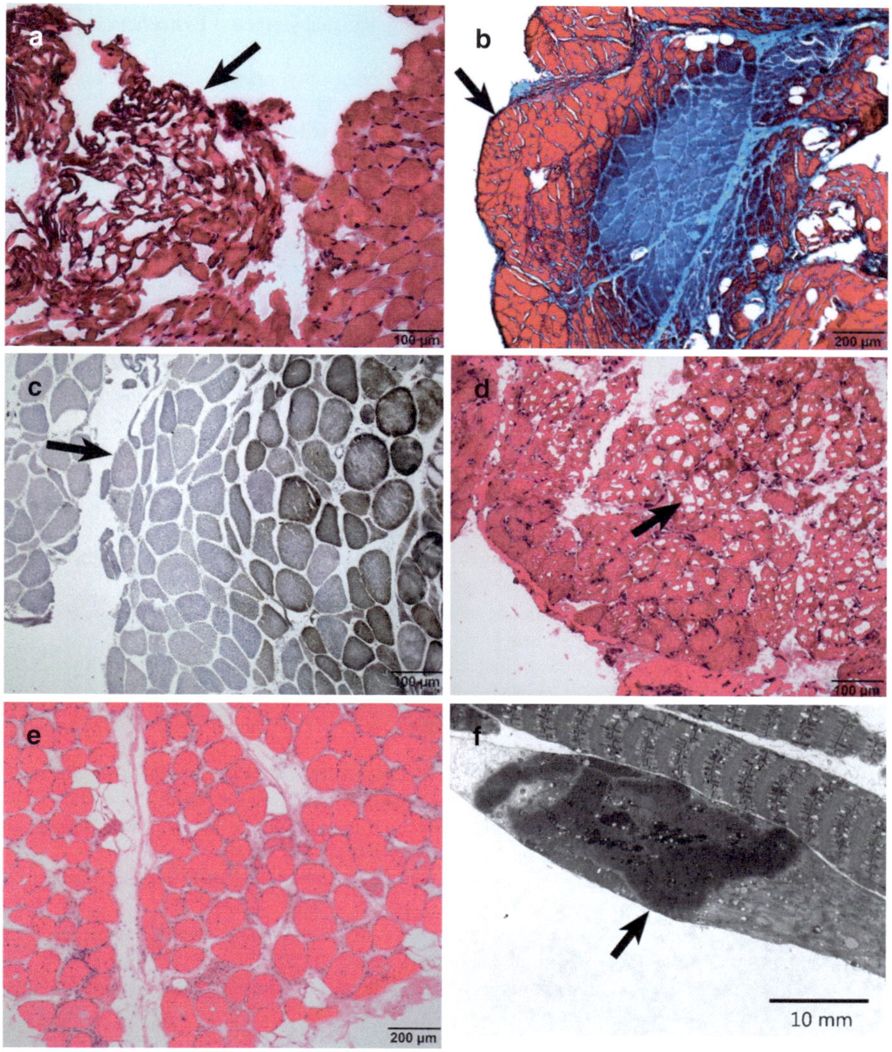

Acknowledgement The author gratefully acknowledges the many helpful suggestions from Drs. Lan Zhou and Chunyu Cai during the preparation of this chapter, and for special assistance provided by Dr. Zhou in the preparation of the section on muscle biopsy technique.

References

1. Dubowitz VS, Sewry CA, Oldfors A. Muscle biopsy a practical approach. Philadelphia. Sanders Elsevier: 4th ed; 2013.
2. Nance JR, Mammen AL. Diagnostic evaluation of rhabdomyolysis. Muscle Nerve. 2015;51(6):793–810.
3. Schiaffino S, Reggiani C. Fiber types in mammalian skeletal muscles. Physiol Rev. 2011;91(4):1447–531.
4. Staron RS, Hagerman FC, Hikida RS, Murray TF, Hostler DP, Crill MT, et al. Fiber type composition of the vastus lateralis muscle of young men and women. J Histochem Cytochem. 2000;48(5):623–9.
5. Engel WK. Focal myopathic changes produced by electromyographic and hypodermic needles. "Needle myopathy". Arch Neurol. 1967;16(5):509–11.
6. Edwards RH. Percutaneous needle-biopsy of skeletal muscle in diagnosis and research. Lancet. 1971;2(7724):593–5.
7. Edwards RH, Lewis PD, Maunder C, Pearse AG. Percutaneous needle biopsy in the diagnosis of muscle diseases. Lancet. 1973;2(7837):1070–1.
8. Edwards RH, Round JM, Jones DA. Needle biopsy of skeletal muscle: a review of 10 years experience. Muscle Nerve. 1983;6(9):676–83.
9. Engel WK, Cunningham GC. Rapid examination of muscle tissue. An improved trichrome method for fresh-frozen biopsy specimens. Neurology. 1963;13(11):919–23.
10. Round JM, Matthews Y, Jones DA. A quick, simple and reliable histochemical method for ATPase in human muscle preparations. Histochem J. 1980;12:707–10.
11. Sarnat HB. Muscle pathology and histochemistry. Chicago: American Society of Clinical Pathologists Press; 1983.
12. Barka T, Anderson PJ. Histochemistry theory and practice and bibliography. New York: Hoeber; 1963.
13. Engel KW, Cunningham GC. Alkaline phosphatase-positive abnormal muscle fibers of humans. J Histochem Cytochem. 1970;18:55–7.
14. De Paepe B, De Bleecker JL, Van Coster R. Histochemical methods for the diagnosis of mitochondrial diseases. Curr Protoc Hum Genet. 2009;19(2):1–19.
15. Ross JM. Visualization of mitochondrial respiratory function using cytochrome c oxidase/ succinate dehydrogenase double-labeling histochemistry. J Vis Exp. 2011;e3266:1–6.
16. Takeuchi T, Kuriaki H. Histochemical detection of phosphorylase in animal tissues. J Histochem Cytochem. 1955;3:153–60.
17. Bonilla E, Schotland DL. Histochemical diagnosis of muscle phosphofructokinase deficiency. Arch Neurol. 1970;8222:8–12.
18. Fishbein WN, Griffin JL, Armbrustmacher VW. Stain for skeletal muscle adenylate deaminase. An effective tetrazolium stain for frozen biopsy specimens. Arch Pathol Lab Med. 1980;104:463–6.
19. Brook MH, Engel WK. The histographic analysis of human muscle biopsies with respect to fiber types. 1. Adult male and female. Neurology. 1969;19(3):221–33.
20. Spuler S, Carl M, Zabojszcza J, Straub V, et al. Dysferlin-deficient muscular dystrophy features amyloidosis. Ann Neurol. 2008;63(3):323–8.
21. Milone M, Liewluck T, Winder TL, Pianosi PT. Amyloidosis and exercise intolerance in ANO5 muscular dystrophy. Neuromuscul Disord. 2012;22(1):13–5.
22. Clement CG, Truong LD. An evaluation of Congo red fluorescence for the diagnosis of amyloidosis. Hum Pathol. 2014;45:1766–72.
23. Chariot P, Ruet E, Authier FJ, Labes D, Poron F, Gherardi R. Cytochrome c oxidase deficiencies in the muscle of patients with inflammatory myopathies. Acta Neuropathol. 1996;91:530–6.
24. Alhatou M, Sladky JT, Bagasra O, Glass JD. Mitochondrial abnormalities in dermatomyositis: characteristic pattern of neuropathology. J Mol Histol. 2004;35:615–9.

25. Fishbein WN, Muldoon SM, Deuster PA, Armbrustmacher VW. Myoadenylate deaminase deficiency and malignant hyperthermia susceptibility: is there a realtionship? Biochem Med. 1985;34:344–54.
26. Fricker R, Bittner R, Böhm D, Shorney S, Gilly H, Kress HG. Malignant hyperthermia (MH) susceptibility and myoadenylate deaminase (MAD) deficiency. Eur J Anesth. 1997;14:82.
27. Chkheidze R, Burns DK, White CL 3rd, Castro D, Fuller J, Cai C. Morin stain detects aluminum-containing macrophages in macrophagic myofasciitis and vaccination granuloma with high sensitivity and specificity. J Neuropathol Exp Neurol. 2017;76:323–31.
28. Vogel H, Zamecnik J. Diagnostic immunohistology of muscle diseases. J Neuropathol Exp Neurol. 2005;64:181–93.
29. Tews DS, Goebel HH. Diagnostic immunohistochemistry in neuromuscular disorders. Histopathology. 2005;46:1–23.
30. Suriyonplengsaeng C, Dejthevaporn C, Khongkhatithum C, Sanpapant S, Tubthong N, Pindradap N, Srinark N, Waisayarat J. Immunohistochemistry of sarcolemmal membrane-associated proteins in formalin-fixed and paraffin-embedded skeletal muscle tissue: a promising tool for the diagnostic evaluation of comon muscular dystrophies. Diagn Pathol. 2017;12:19.
31. Bozzola JJ, Russell LD. Electron microscopy: principles and techniques for biologists. 2nd ed. Boston: Jones and Bartlett; 1992.
32. Romero NB. Centronuclear myopathies: a widening concept. Neuromuscul Disord. 2010;20:223–8.
33. Wilmshurst JM, Lillis S, Zhou H, Pillay K, Henderson H, Kress W, et al. RYR1 mutations are a common cause of congenital myopathies with central nuclei. Ann Neurol. 2010;68:717–26.
34. Sewry CA, Quinlivan RCM, Squier W, Morris GE, Holt I. A rapid immunohistochemical test to distinguish congenital myotonic dystrophy from X-linked myotubular myopathy. Neuromuscul Disord. 2012;22:225–30.
35. Lotz BP, Engel AG, Nishino H, Stevens JC, Litchy WJ. Inclusion body myositis. Observations in 40 patients. Brain. 1989;112:727–47.
36. Coquet M, Vital C, Julien J. Presence of inclusion body myositis-like filaments in oculopharyngeal muscular dystrophy. Ultrastructural study of 10 cases. Neuropathol Appl Neurobiol. 1990;16:393–400.
37. Stenzel W, Preuβe C, Allenbach Y, Pehl D, Junckerstorff R, Heppner FL, et al. Nuclear actin aggregatino is a hallmakr of anti-synthetase syndrome-induced dysimmune myopathy. Neurology. 2015;84:1346–54.
38. Koy A, Ilkovski B, Laing N, North K, Weis J, Mayatepek E, et al. Nemaline myopathy with exclusively intranuclear rods and a nobel mutation in ACTA1 (Q139H). Neuropediatrics. 2007;38:282–6.
39. Wu S, Ibarra MC, Malicdan MC, Murayama K, Ichihara Y, Nonaka I, et al. Central core disease is due to RYR1 mutations in more than 90% of patients. Brain. 2006;129:1470–80.
40. Ferreiro A, Monnier N, Romero NB, Leroy J-P, Bönneman C, Haenggeli C-A, Straub V, et al. A recessive form of central core disease, transiently presenting as multi-minicore disease, is associated with a homozygous mutation in the ryanodine receptor type 1 gene. Ann Neurol. 2002;51:750–9.
41. Figarella-Branger D, El-Dassouki M, Saenz A, Cobo AM, Malzac P, Tong S, et al. Myopathy with lobulated fibers: evidence for heterogeneous etiology and clincial presentation. Neuromuscul Dis. 2002;12:4–12.
42. Tsuburaya R, Suzuki T, Saiki K, Nonaka I, Sugito H, Hayashi YK, et al. Lobulated fibers in a patient with a 46-year history of limb-girdle muscle weakness. Neuropathology. 2011;31:455–7.
43. Weller B, Carpenter S, Lochmuller H, Karpati G. Myopathy with trabecular muscle fibers. Neuromuscul Dis. 1999;9:208–14.
44. Hilton-Jones D, Miller A, Parton M, Holton J, Sewry C, Hanna MG. Inclusion body myositis. Neuromuscul Dis. 2010;20:142–7.
45. Blume G, Pestronk A, Frank B, Johns DR. Polymyositis with cytochrome oxidase negative muscle fibres. Early quadriceps weakness and poor response to immunosuppressive therapy. Brain. 1997;120:39–45.
46. Wharton SB, Chan KK, Pickard JD, Anderson JR. Pearavertebral muscles in disease of the cervical spine. J Neurol Neurosurg Psychiatry. 1996;61:461–5.
47. Fayet G, Rouche A, Hogrel J-Y, Tomé FMS, Fardeau M. Age-related morphological changes in the deltoid muscle from 50 to 79 years of age. Acta Neuropathol. 2001;101:358–66.
48. Rosenberg NL, Neville HE, Ringel SP. Tubular aggregates. Their association with neuromuscular disease, including the syndrome of myalgias/cramps. Arch Neurol. 1985;42:973–6.

49. Romero NB, Sandaradura SA, Clarke NF. Recent advances in nemaline myopathy. Curr Opin Neurol. 2013;26:519–26.
50. Schröder JM, Sommer C, Schmidt B. Desmin and actin associated with cytoplasmic bodies in skeletal muscle fibers: immunohistochemical and fine structural studies, with a note on unusual 18- to 20-nm filaments. Acta Neuropathol. 1990;80:406–14.
51. Mateer JE, Farrell BJ, Chou SSM, Gutmann L. Reversible ipecac myopathy. Arch Neurol. 1985;42:188–90.
52. Foroud T, Pankratz N, Batchman AP, Pauciulo MW, Vidal R, Miravalle N, et al. A mutation in myotilin causes spheroid body myopathy. Neurology. 2005;65:1936–40.
53. Brooke MH, Neville HE. Reducing body myopathy. Neurology. 1972;22:829–40.
54. Schessl J, Taratuto AL, Sewry C, Battini R, Chin SS, Maiti B, et al. Clinical, histological and genetic characterization of reducing body myopathy caused by mutations in FHL1. Brain. 2009;132:452–64.
55. Nakano S, Engel AG, Wacklawik AJ, Emslie-Smith AM, Busis NA. Myofibrillar myopathy with abnormal foci of desmin positivity. I. Light and electron microscopy analysis of 10 cases. J Neuropathol Exp Neurol. 1996;55:549–62.
56. Olive M, Kley RA, Goldfarb MG. Myofibrillar myopathies: new developments. Curr Opin Neurol. 2013;26:527–35.
57. Askansas V, Engel WK, Nogalska A. Inclusion body myositis: a degenerative muscle disease associated with intra-muscle fiber multi-protein aggregates, proteasome inhibition, endoplasmic reticulum stress and decreased lysosomal degradation. Brain Pathol. 2009;19:493–506.
58. Broccolini A, Mirabella M. Hereditary inclusion body myopathies. Biochim Biophys Acta. 1852;2015:644–50.
59. Sugie K, Yamamoto A, Murayama K, Oh SJ, Takahashi M, Mora M, et al. Clinicopathological features of genetically confirmed Danon disease. Neurology. 2002;58:1773–8.
60. Kalimo H, Savontaus ML, Lang H, Paljarvi L, Sonninen V, Dean PB, et al. X-linked myopathy with excessive autophagy: a new hereditary muscle disease. Ann Neurol. 1988;23:258–65.
61. Ramachandran N, Munteanu I, Wang P, Ruggieri A, Rilstone JJ, Israelian N, et al. VMA21 deficiency prevents vacuolar ATPase assembly and causes autophagic vacuolar myopathy. Acta Neuropathol. 2013;25:439–57.
62. Le Roux K, Streichenberger N, Vial C, Petiot P, Feasson L, Bouhour F, et al. Granulomatous myositis: a clincial study of thirteen cases. Muscle Nerve. 2007;35:171–7.
63. Prieto-Gonzalez S, Grau JM. Diagnosis and classification of granulomatous myositis. Autoimmun Rev. 2014;13:372–4.
64. Maed MH, Tsuji S, Shimizu J. Inflammatory myopathies associated with anti-mitochondrial antibodies. Brain. 2012;135:1767–77.
65. Selva-O'Callaghan A, Trallero-Araguás E, Grau JM. Eosinophilic myositis: an updated review. Autoimmune Rev. 2014;13:375–8.
66. Vital A, Vital C, Viallard J-F, Ragnaud J-M, Canron MH, Lagueny A. Neuro-muscular biopsy in Churg-Strauss syndrome: 24 cases. J Neuropathol Exp Neurol. 2006;65:187–92.
67. Amato A. Adults with eosinophilic myositis and calpain-3 mutations. Neurology. 2008;70:730–1.
68. Baumeister SK, Todorovic S, Milać-Rašić V, Dekomien G, Lochmüller H, Walter MC. Eosinophilic myositis as presenting symptom in gamma-sarcoglycanopathy. Neuromuscul Disord. 2009;19:167–71.
69. Attias D, Laor R, Zuckermann E, Naschitz JE, Luria M, Misselevitch I, Boss JH. Acute neutrophilic myositis ins Sweet's syndrome: late phase transformation into fibrosing myositis and panniculitis. Hum Pathol. 1995;26:687–90.
70. Schröder NWJ, Goebel H-H, Brandis A, Ladhoff A-M, Heppner FL, Stenzel W. Pipestem capillaries in necrotizing myopathy revisited. Neuromuscul Disord. 2013;23:66–74.
71. Yell PC, Burns DK, Dittmar EG, White CL 3rd, Cai C. Diffuse microvascular C5b-9 deposition is a common feature in muscle and nerve biopsies from diabetic patients. Acta Neuropathol Commun. 2018;6(1):11.

Chapter 2
Peripheral Nerve Biopsy Evaluation

Chunyu Cai

Introduction

Surgical removal of a segment of nerve leads to a permanent loss of function in that nerve and in rare cases painful injury neuromas. Therefore, a nerve biopsy is usually performed only if clinical, laboratory, and electrophysiological studies have been done, yet failed to clarify the nature or the cause of the disease. A nerve should not be biopsied if it appears normal on electrophysiological study. The major indications for nerve biopsy are clinically suspected vasculitis and amyloidosis. These disease processes are patchy; thus negative findings in a nerve biopsy does not completely exclude the above conditions. Other indications for nerve biopsy include infections (e.g. leprosy), sarcoidosis, tumor, chronic inflammatory demyelinating polyneuropathy (CIDP) that does not fully meet the electrophysiologic criteria, and hereditary neuropathies that cannot be confirmed by genetic tests [1]. In general, nerve biopsies have a higher yield in acute, multifocal, asymmetrical and severe demyelinating conditions than in chronic, symmetric and axonal types. A concomitant muscle biopsy from the same incision is advised as it may substantially increase the diagnostic yield for systemic disease processes such as vasculitis [2], amyloidosis and sarcoidosis, and causes very little additional discomfort to the patient. The muscle biopsy may also provide useful diagnostic information by confirming denervation changes in the muscle and excluding a primary myopathic process. In this chapter, we summarize biopsy procedure, specimen processing, common morphologic findings, and their diagnostic implications in peripheral nerve biopsies.

C. Cai (✉)
Department of Pathology, University of Texas Southwestern Medical Center, Dallas, TX, USA
e-mail: chunyu.cai@UTSouthwestern.edu

L. Zhou et al. (eds.), *A Case-Based Guide to Neuromuscular Pathology*,
https://doi.org/10.1007/978-3-030-25682-1_2

Nerve Biopsy Acquisition

The choice of the site and the nerve for biopsy should be made based on the clinical and electrophysiological findings. One should choose a nerve which is affected by the disease to increase the biopsy yield and to reduce the risk of neuroma formation. Distal sensory nerves such as sural nerve, superficial peroneal nerve, and superficial radial nerve are preferred as these nerves are frequently affected by inflammatory and amyloid neuropathies, and the biopsy of these nerves do not cause motor deficit. Sural nerve is the most commonly biopsied nerve. It can be biopsied alone at the lateral aspect of the distal leg with a 5-cm longitudinal incision made between the fibula and the Achille's tendon ending distally just proximal to the lateral malleolus.

Sural nerve is frequently biopsied along with gastrocnemius muscle via a single 5-cm longitudinal incision made over the midline of posterior distal leg. The biopsy is done under local anesthesia with a monitored anesthesia care. A length of 4–5 cm of nerve is biopsied. Shorter nerve biopsy specimen may hamper diagnosis yet will leave an identical sensory deficit. The risk of post-biopsy bleeding and infection is minimal. The patient may have transient irritating discomfort at the biopsy site. The sensory loss at the dorsolateral aspect of the foot usually improves with time. The neuroma formation is very rare. A combined superficial peroneal nerve and peroneus brevis muscle biopsy via a single incision may be done if the superficial peroneal nerve is more affected by the disease than the sural nerve. Superficial radial nerve biopsy is rarely done; it can be helpful when a multiple mononeuropathy only affects upper limbs. When a nerve disease (lesion) predominantly involves a proximal nerve such as sciatic nerve, median nerve at the upper arm, lumbosacral plexus, or brachial plexus, magnetic resonance neurography (MRN)-targeted fascicular nerve biopsies may be performed in a tertiary medical center by a surgeon with special expertise after communication with treating neurologist and radiologist [3].

Specimen Processing Procedure

The biopsied nerve is divided into 3 parts, a fresh specimen, a formalin fixed specimen for paraffin embedding, and a glutaldehyde fixed specimen for resin embedding, toluidine blue stain, and electron microscopy (EM). The glutaldehyde fixed specimen is superior in demonstrating myelin morphology but also most susceptible to stretching, compression and delayed fixation artifacts. The specimen must be handled with extreme care. We recommend first clamping the middle 2 cm segment of nerve in situ. Then 1 cm of nerve proximal to the clamp is excised, wrapped in a 4 × 4 gauze sponge moistened with 4 ml normal saline, and placed in a sealed container as a fresh specimen. A 1-cm nerve fragment distal to the clamp is tied at both ends with sutures, excised and tied onto wooden tongue depressor so that the nerve is straight but not overstretched, and placed in a sealed container of 10% phosphate-buffered neutral formalin for paraffin embedding. The middle clamped segment (Fig. 2.1) is placed in a sealed container with chilled 3% glutaraldehyde for resin embedding and EM. The specimens are placed on ice for subsequent transfer from operating room to pathology laboratory, usually within 2 hours.

Once in pathology laboratory, the fresh specimen is snap frozen in isopentane cooled in liquid nitrogen. Frozen sections can be cut and stained with hematoxylin and eosin (H&E) immediately for rapid screening of vasculitis or inflammation. The formalin specimen is divided into 3–4 cross and longitudinal pieces for paraffin embedding. The glutaldehyde specimen is carefully cut out from the clamp, divided into 3 cross and 1 longitudinal pieces and further fixed in glutaldehyde overnight before epoxy resin embedding and semithin sections.

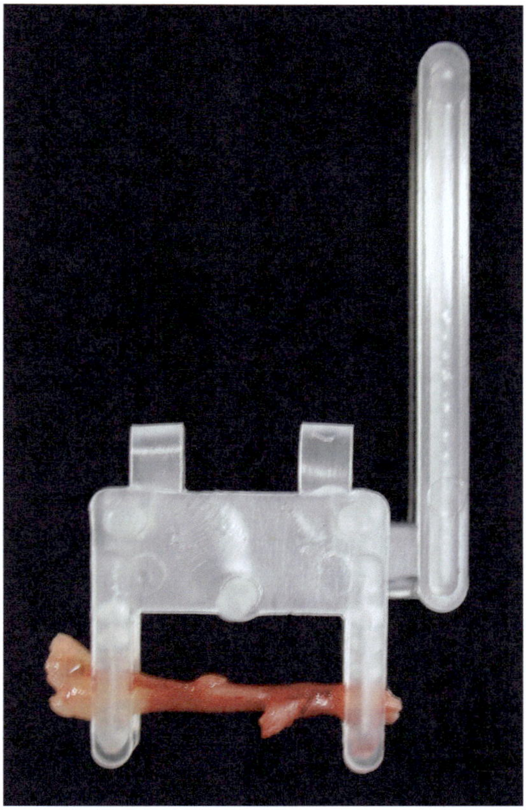

Fig. 2.1 Properly clamped peripheral nerve is fixed in glutaldehyde for resin embedding and EM processing

Routine Stains and Utilities

In our laboratory, frozen, formalin fixed and paraffin embedded (FFPE), and glutaldehyde fixed and resin embedded nerve biopsies specimens are routinely evaluated with a panel of stains as listed below.

- Frozen nerve specimen
  - H&E
  - Modified Gomori trichrome
  - Crystal violet
  - Congo red
- FFPE nerve specimen
  - H&E
  - Masson trichrome
  - Periodic acid Schiff (PAS)
  - Congo red
- Glutaldehyde fixed, resin embedded specimen
  - Toluidine blue stained thick sections for light microscopy
  - Toluidine blue stained thin sections for electron microscopy

Serial section of multiple levels on H&E stained cryostat and FFPE sections is recommended for the detection of vasculitis or inflammation. Congo red stain is performed on both cryostat and FFPE sections to increase the rate of detection for amyloidosis.

Hematoxylin and Eosin (H&E)

H&E stain provides the initial and most important morphological assessment of nerve histology, and is routinely performed on both the frozen and FFPE specimens. H&E stain is excellent in identifying vasculitis, inflammation and neoplasm, but generally offers limited value in assessing myelin or axon pathology.

One of the most important task of nerve biopsy evaluation is to identify evidence of vasculitis. The 2012 Chapel Hill Consensus Conference provides an updated classification of vasculitis [4]. Pertaining to peripheral nerve, vasculitis can be broadly dichotomized into infectious (e.g. leprosy, fungus) and noninfectious etiologies. Noninfectious vasculitis are further classified into systemic and nonsystemic vasculitic neuropathies (NSVN) [5, 6]. Morphology varies depending on the size of the vessels involved. Fibroid necrosis is more commonly seen in large ((>100 micron) to medium sized (40–100 microns) epineurial arteries [7] in polyarteritis nodosum, Churg-Strauss syndrome, Wegener's granulomatosis, ANCA associated vasculitis, or collagen vascular diseases (e.g. lupus, rheumatoid arthritis, etc.). Leukocytoclasia or perivascular lymphocytic cuffing are more commonly seen in smaller vessel (<40 microns) vasculitis such as collagen vascular disease, microscopic polyangiitis [7] and NSVN [8, 9]. NSVN can only be diagnosed on a nerve biopsy and encompasses a heterogeneous and expending group of diseases such as painless diabetic radiculoplexus neuropathies, postsurgical inflammatory neuropathy, and Wartenberg migratory sensory neuropathy [5]. Subclassification of NSVN relies on clinical information and cannot be differentiated by histology alone. Takayasu arteritis, Kawasaki diseases and antiglomerular basement membrane disease do not involve peripheral nerves [5].

Acute vasculitis ***Fibrinoid necrosis with associated inflammation*** of blood vessel wall is the most definitive histological evidence of acute necrotizing vasculitis. It appears as amorphous, refractile material within arterial wall that deeply stain with eosin (Fig. 2.2a). On EM, these fibrinoid material is composed of electron dense fibrin strands with cross banding of 20.8 nm periodicity [10] (Fig. 2.2b). The origin of the fibrinoid material is believed to be polymerised fibrinogen which has permeated through the injured endothelial cell layer [11]. It should be noted that fibrinoid necrosis without inflammation can be seen in nonvasculitic conditions such as malignant hypertension [10, 12, 13] and complement mediated hypersensitivity reaction [14]. ***Transmural inflammation accompanied by karyorrhexis debris (leukocytoclasia)*** (Fig. 2.3a) carries a similar diagnostic implication as fibrinoid necrosis as definitive evidence of active vasculitis. The presence of inflammatory cells in the vessel wall or ***perivascular cuffing*** (Fig. 2.3b) of lymphocytes, while a frequent finding in vasculitis involving smaller arteries and veins, is less specific and can be seen in a variety of non-vasculitic inflammatory neuropathies including chronic inflammatory demyelinating polyneuropathy (CIDP) [15], paraneoplastic syndrome [16], as well as many other systemic inflammatory conditions. When in doubt, additional deeper levels are recommended. Presence of luminal thrombosis, endothelial damage, perivascular hemosiderin, disruption of internal elastic lamina (by elastin special stain) or separation/disruption of smooth muscle cells in media (by smooth muscle actin immunostain) support the diagnosis of vasculitis [6].

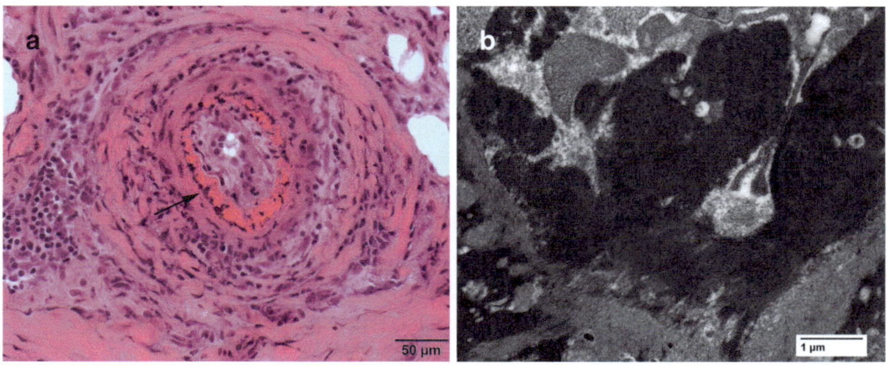

Fig. 2.2 Fibrinoid necrosis of medium sized epineurial artery. (**a**) H&E. (**b**) EM. (Images from a 78-year-old patient with rheumatoid arthritis, who presented with mononeuritis multiplex)

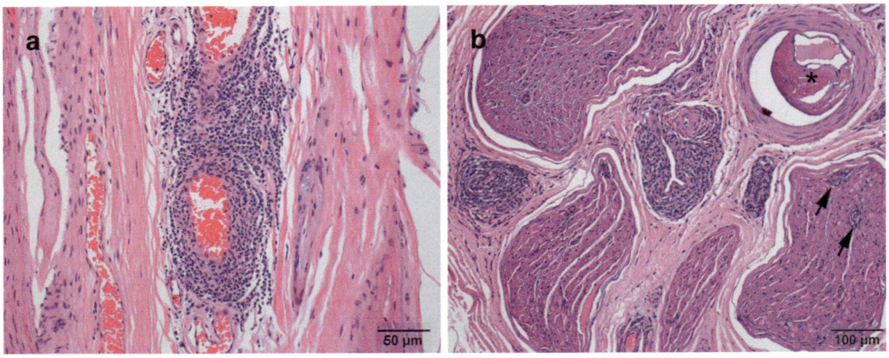

Fig. 2.3 Vessel wall inflammation. (**a**) Transmural inflammation with karyorrhexis debris is diagnostic for vasculitis. (**b**) Transmural and perivascular lymphocytic cuffing in a patient with a clinical diagnosis of diabetic amyotrophy. Panel B also shows endoneurial perivascular inflammation (arrows) and an atherosclerotic plaque within the lumen of an epineurial artery (∗)

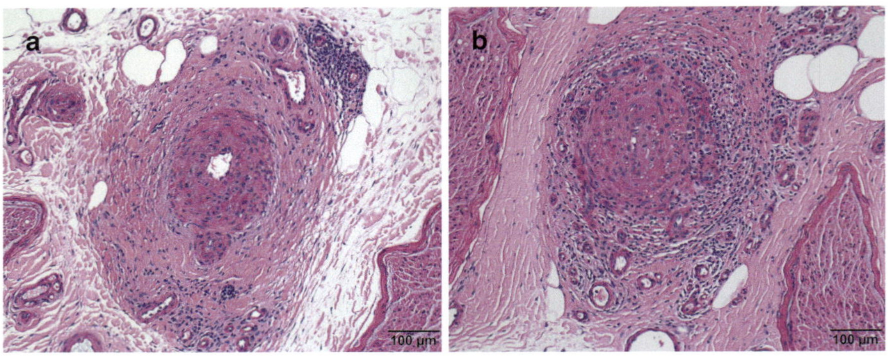

Fig. 2.4 Chronic vascular remodeling changes supportive of prior vasculitis. (**a**) PAS stain shows a medium sized epineurial artery with marked intimal and adventitia fibrosis. Two smaller vessels in the upper right corner show perivascular lymphocytic cuffing. (**b**) PAS stain of an epineurial artery with completely occluded lumen and neovascularization within and outside the lumen. (Sural nerve biopsy from a 63-year-old female with rheumatoid arthritis and progressive polyneuropathy)

Chronic vascular damage with repair Features of chronic vascular damage/repair include intimal hyperplasia, fibrosis of media, adventitia fibrosis (Fig. 2.4a), and chronic thrombosis with recanalization (Fig. 2.4b). With the presence of mononuclear inflammatory cells in the wall, these chronic vascular remodeling changes can serve as definitive evidence for vasculitis [6]. Since vasculitis is a multifocal process, additional sections or adjacent block near vessels with chronic remodeling change may demonstrate adjacent active vasculitic changes. ***Increased epineurial vessel density:*** In sural nerve, epineurial vessel number stay relatively constant throughout ages in normal person (mean 58, range 34–76), but is significantly increased in patients with vasculitic neuropathies (mean 108, range 47–179),

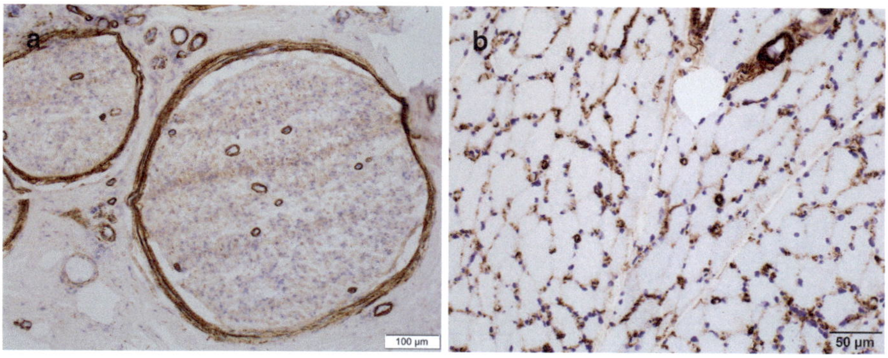

Fig. 2.5 Diffuse terminal complement complex (C5b-9) deposition in nerve (**a**) and muscle (**b**) small vessels and capillaries in a 49-year-old patient with poorly controlled diabetes

microvasculitic neuropathies (mean 110.8, range 85–131), and diabetes (Mean 106, range 85–131) [17]. The endoneurial vessel number remains remarkably constant [18]. Thus, a prominently increased number of epineurial vessels may serve as a suggestive feature for vasculitis or microvasculopathy, particularly when they are clustered or growing within the wall of vessels or perineurium (Fig. 2.4b). Increased epineurial vessels can also be seen in a significant number of nerve biopsies with mixed axonal and demyelinating features [17] and paraneoplastic syndrome [16]. Overall this is a relatively nonspecific finding that by itself conveys limited diagnostic implication. ***Arteriolosclerosis:*** Prominent thickening of the wall of endoneurial vessels is commonly associated with hypertension or diabetes. Diffuse deposition of terminal complement complex (C5b-9) in both nerve endothelial vessels and muscle capillaries is a rather characteristic feature of diabetic microangiopathy and not an indication of immune-mediated vascular injury [19] (Fig. 2.5).

Endoneurial perivascular inflammation Selective endoneurial perivascular mononuclear inflammation without significant epineurial inflammation is an uncommon finding in peripheral nerve biopsies and is a supportive feature of CIDP or Guillain-Barre syndrome (GBS) in the appropriate clinical context [16, 20]. It has also been reported in paraneopalstic syndrome [21], immune checkpoint inhibitor associated neuropathy [22], and leprosy [23]. ***Individually scattered endoneurial inflammation*** is difficult to discern on H&E. Immunostain highlighted T cells can be found in CIDP, chronic idiopathic axonal polyneuropathy, vasculitic neuropathy, as well as normal controls, thus of limited diagnostic value [24].

Perineurium pathology Inflammation that preferentially involves perineurium is associated with leprosy, which is rare in the United States but can be seen in countries with relative high incidence of leprosy, such as India, Brazil, and Indonesia [25]. Anecdotal case reports on idiopathic perineuritis [26, 27], cryoglobulinemia [28], and epidemic toxic oil syndrome [29] with preferential perineurium inflammation have been reported. Sarcoid peripheral neuropathy often shows inflammation

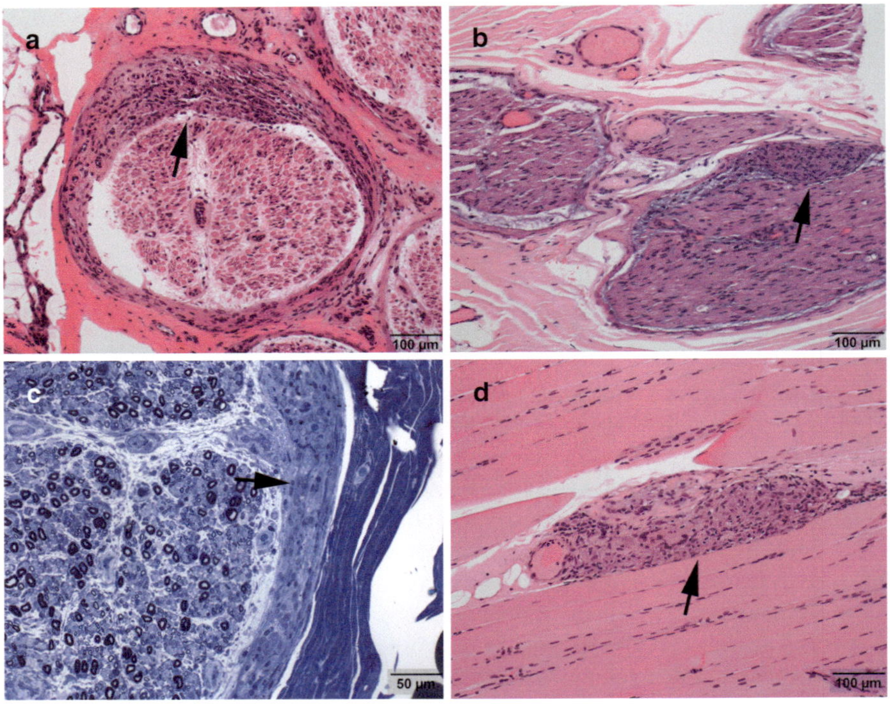

Fig. 2.6 Sarcoid perineuritis. (**a**) H&E stained cryostat section of the sural nerve shows inflammation and irregular thickening of perineurium (arrow). (**b**) Granuloma (arrow) is apparent on the paraffin fixed longitudinal nerve section. (**c**) Toluidine blue stained plastic section shows that the granulomatous inflammation (arrow) is centered on the perineurium and blood vessels. (**d**) Granulomas are also identified in the concomitant muscle biopsy. (Images from a 21-year-old patient with sarcoidosis and peripheral neuropathy)

and thickening of the perineurium [30] (Fig. 2.6). Vasculitis or other ischemic injury to the nerve fascicules can cause thickening of the perineurium, and sometimes the formation of ***injury neuroma***, characterized by the presence of microfascicles within or beyond the perineurium [31] (Fig. 2.7), even the appearance of perineuritis [32]. Injury neuromas due to trauma or prior surgery are typically larger, composed of numerous haphazardly arranged microfascicles replacing an entire fascicle or nerve. In patients with diabetic peripheral neuropathy, thickening of perineurial basal lamina and atrophy of perineurial cells (Fig. 2.8) were considered by some as a more characteristic feature of diabetic neuropathy than arteriolosclerosis [33]. ***Perineurial calcifications*** may be seen as an age related change but is more frequent and can be marked at younger age in patients with diabetic neuropathy [34] (Fig. 2.8).

Neoplasms Schwannoma, perineurioma, and neurofibroma are common peripheral nerve neoplasms that are usually excised as mass lesions and treated as general surgical pathology specimens rather than nerve biopsy. In rare occasions, lymphoma may secondarily involve a peripheral nerve and present as atypical lymphoid

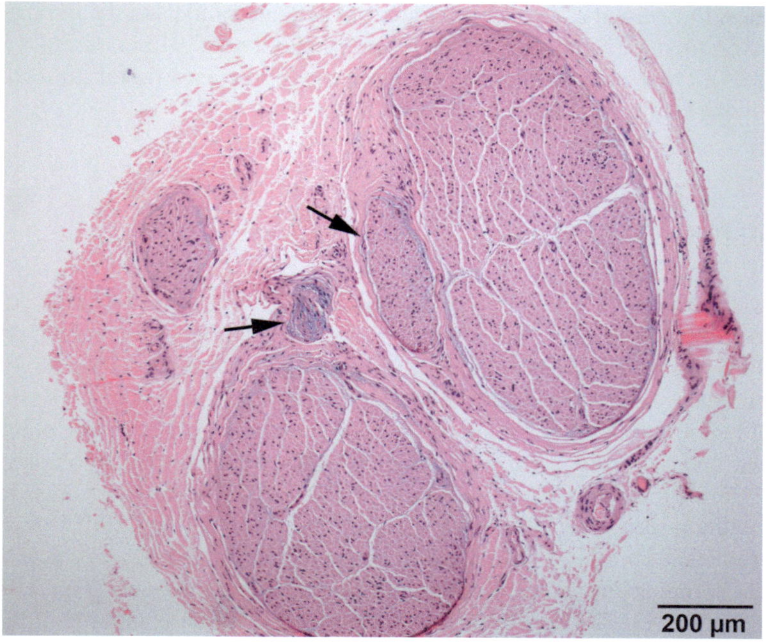

Fig. 2.7 Injury neuromas (arrows) in sural nerve biopsies are more commonly associated with prior ischemic damage rather than traumatic injury. (Image from a 57-year-old patient who presented with foot drop)

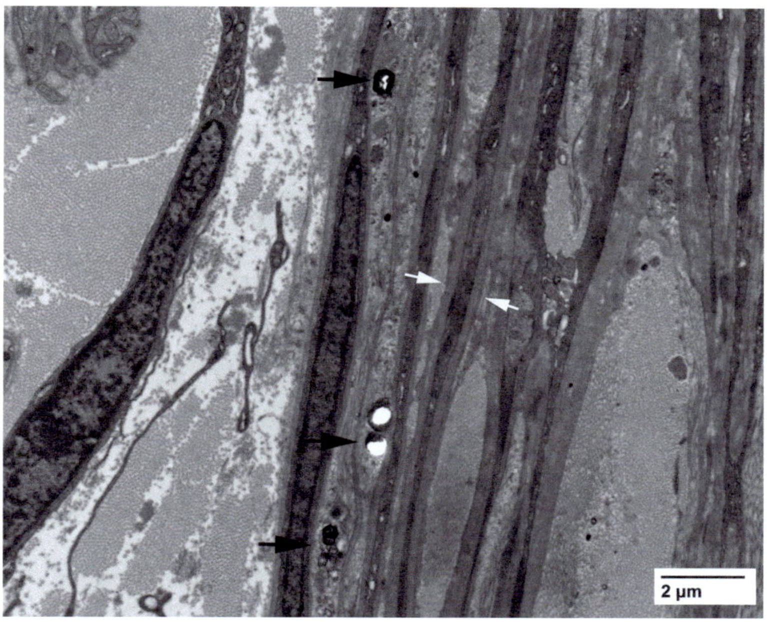

Fig. 2.8 Perineurial calcifications (black arrows) and markedly thickened basal lamina (white arrows) in a 31-year-old patient with type I diabetes

infiltrates. Intravascular B cell lymphoma can be quite subtle and the findings may be limited to small aggregates of atypical lymphoid cells within vascular lumen (Fig. 38.1). Once noticed, the diagnosis can usually be established through additional immunohistochemistry and clinical history.

Congo Red Stain

Amyloid deposits can be subtle and difficult to differentiate from hyaline on H&E stained sections (Fig. 2.9a). We routinely perform Congo red stain on both cryostat and FFPE sections of all nerve biopsies to evaluate for amyloidosis. Amyloid tends to accumulate within or around epi- or endoneurial blood vessels or in the subperineurial regions. On Congo red stained section, amyloid deposits appear orange red under regular light (Fig. 2.9b) and yellow-green birefringence under polarized light (Fig. 2.9c). A thioflavin S or T special stain is more sensitive than Congo red but requires fluorescence scope to view the amyloid deposits (Fig. 2.9d). Amyloid is also prominent on crystal violet special stain (Fig. 2.9e) and strongly accumulate terminal complement complex detectable by C5b-9 immunostain (Fig. 2.9f). On plastic section (Fig. 2.9g) and EM, the amyloid deposits are composed of haphazardly arranged fibrils. The diameter of the fibrils vary widely and range from 8–24 nanometers depending on the types of amyloid (Fig. 2.9h, i). The most common form of primary acquired amyloid neuropathy is due to immune light chain (AL) deposition that can be highlighted by Kappa or Lambda immunohistochemistry. These patients usually are over 50 years of age and have lymphoproliferative disorders, plasma cell dyscrasias or monoclonal gammopathies. Secondary amyloidosis due to infection or chronic inflammation (AA) usually does not cause polyneuropathy [35]. Patients with hereditary amyloidosis usually present early in their 30–40s but can be later. Vast majority is caused by transthyretin point mutations. The amyloid deposits are negative for immunoglobin light chains but positive on transthyretin (prealbumin) immunostain (Fig. 2.9j). Other rare forms of hereditary amyloidosis involve mutations in gesolin, apolipoprotein A1, fibrinogen A alpha chain, or lysozyme. Amyloid classification can be determined by liquid chromatography-mass spectrometry [36] followed by genetic testing.

Toluidine Blue Stained Plastic Sections

Toluidine blue stained 1.5 μm plastic section from resin embedded nerve blocks provides an accurate assessment of the number of myelinated axons and provides higher contrast and finer detail in myelin and axon morphology than frozen or FFPE specimens. Thick sections, in combination with EM when necessary, is the most important tool in determining whether the dominant pathology of a nerve is axonal degeneration, demyelination or mixed. ***Features of axonal degeneration***

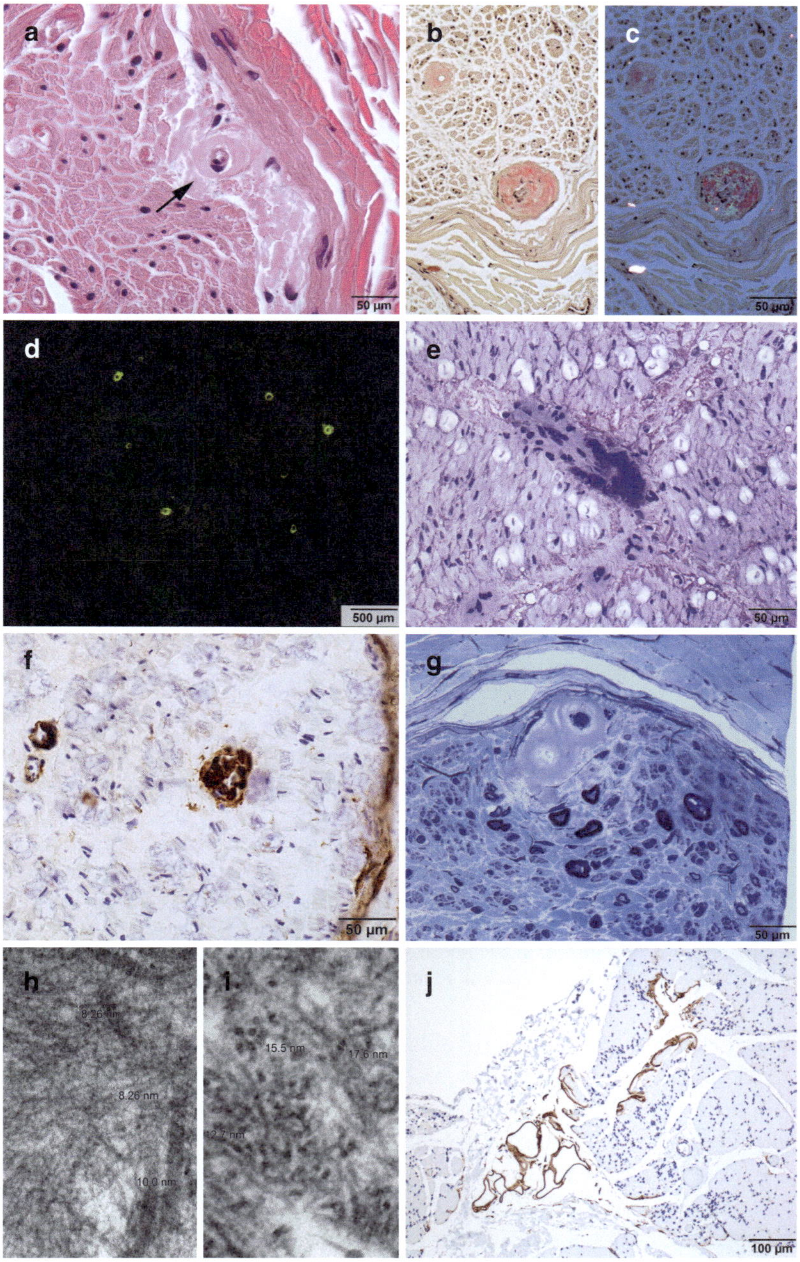

Fig. 2.9 Amyloid neuropathies. (**a**) H&E. (**b**) Congo red stain, nonpolarized light. (**c**) Congo red stain, polarized light. (**d**) Thioflavin S stain viewed under green fluorescence light. (**e**) Crystal violet stain. (**f**) C5b-9 immunostain. (**g**) Toluidine blue stained thick section. (**h**) Amyloid fibril on EM from a patient with transthyretin amyloidosis. (**i**) Amyloid fibril on EM from a patient with non-AL, non-transthyretin amyloidosis. (**j**) Transthyretin stain on the concomitant muscle biopsy from the patient with transthyretin amyloidosis

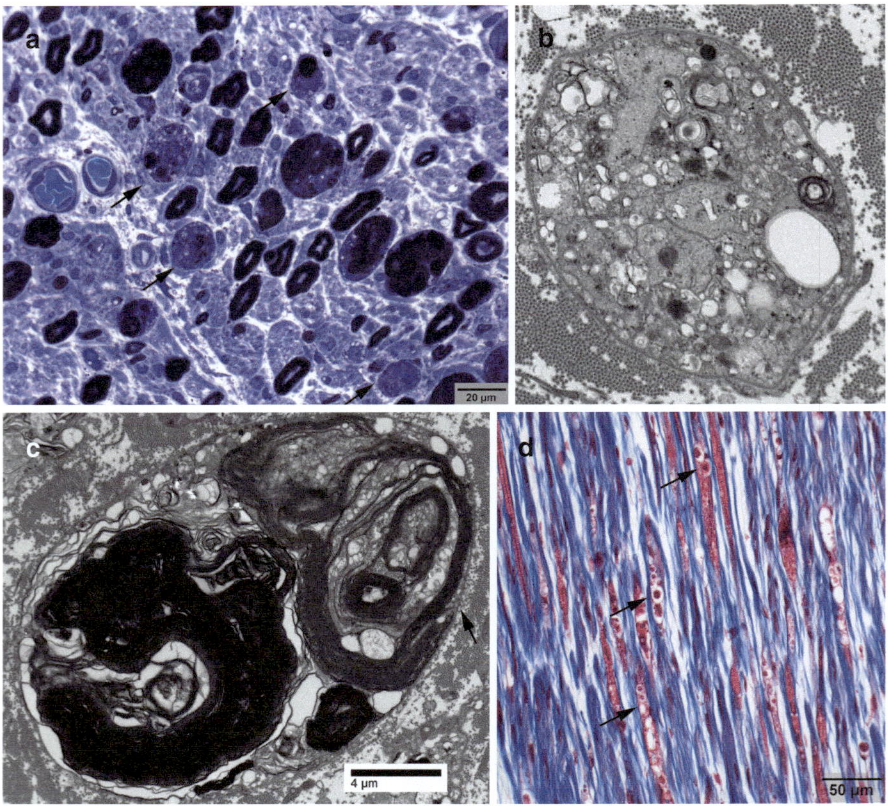

Fig. 2.10 Myeline ovoids are feature of active axonal degeneration of myelinated axons. (**a**) On toluidine blue stained thick section, myelin ovoids are round structures containing myelin debris (arrows). (**b, c**) On electron microscopy, myelin ovoids are composed of myelin debris at various stages of digestion still confined within the Schwann cell basal lamina (arrow) (**d**) Strings of myelin ovoids can be visualized on trichrome stained longitudinal section (arrows). (Images are from a 32-year-old patient with acute motor and sensory axonal neuropathy)

and regeneration are myelin ovoids (Fig. 2.10) and regenerating clusters (Fig. 2.11), respectively, which are readily identifiable on toluidine blue stained thick sections. They will be discussed in more detail in the EM section. ***Features of demyelination*** include naked axons, thinly myelinated axons, and segmental demyelination. Naked axons may be difficult to appreciate on light microscopy and often requires electron microscopy. Thinly myelinated axons (Fig. 2.12a, b) can be seen in regenerating clusters or regenerating axons, thus not a reliable feature of demyelination. Segmental demyelination is best appreciated on teased fiber analysis but can also be seen on longitudinally embedded toluidine stained thick sections. It should be noted though segmental demyelination is not specific for primary demyelination and can be seen in many primarily axonal processes such as diabetic neuropathy, porphyria, uremic neuropathy [37], even vasculopathies [38], these are referred to as "secondary segmental demyelination". The hallmark of ***chronic demyelination*** is the presence of true onion bulbs (Fig. 2.12c,

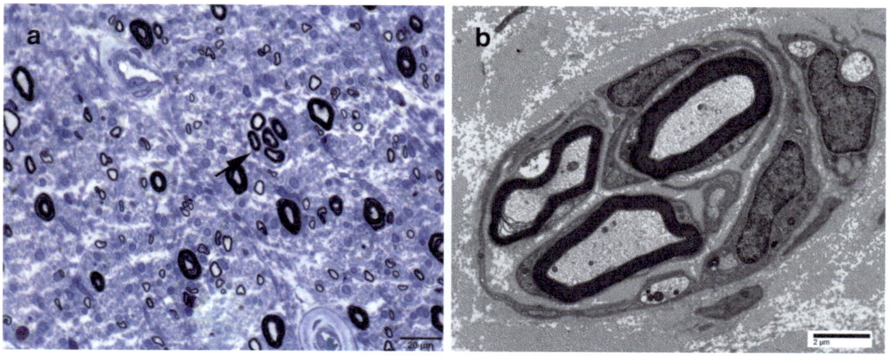

Fig. 2.11 Regenerating cluster forms in the regenerating phase following axonal degeneration, thus considered an evidence of axonopathy. (**a**) Toluidine blue. (**b**) Electron microscopy

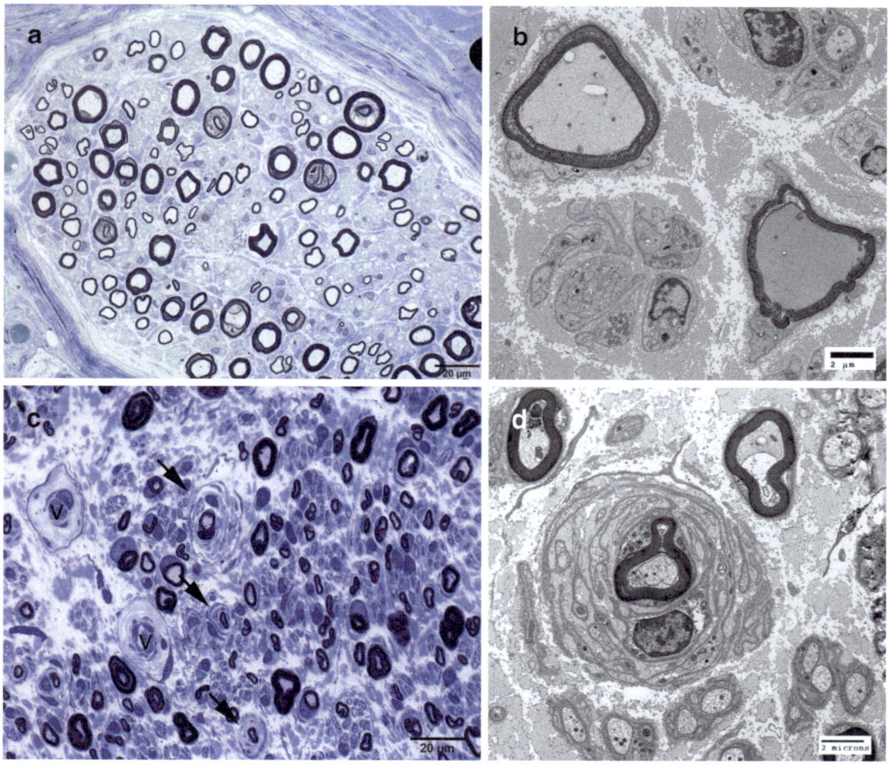

Fig. 2.12 Features of demyelination. (**a**, **b**) are images from a patient with CIDP. (**a**) Toluidine blue stained thick section show numerous thinly myelinated axons in a background without myelin ovoids or regenerating clusters. (**b**) EM shows that the axons are intact and not associated with regenerating clusters. (**c**, **d**) are images from a separate patient with CIDP. (**c**) Toluidine blue stained thick section shows multiple well-formed onion bulbs (arrows). "v" indicate vessels.(**d**) EM shows that the onion bulbs are composed of a central thinly myelinated axon surrounded by multiple layers of supernumerary Schwann cell processes. No other myelinated or unmyelinated axons are present within the onion bulb to suggest a regenerating cluster

d), which results from repeated cycles of demyelination and re-myelination that leads to the buildup of multiple concentric layers of Schwann cell processes and their basal lamina. In practice, determination of primary axonal degeneration versus demyelination often relies on the dominant pathology of the nerve, e.g. occasional thinly myelinated fibers in a background of frequent myelin ovoids and regenerating clusters are likely axonal, while abundant thinly myelinated axons or onion bulbs with minimal associated axonal degeneration supports primary demyelination. When comparable amount of axonal and myelin alterations are present, a descriptive "mixed axonal and demyelinating features" is rendered. This is a nonspecific but relatively common finding in patients with diabetic peripheral neuropathy.

Differential fascicular loss of myelinated axons (Fig. 2.13) is commonly considered an indirect evidence of vasculitic neuropathy. However, it can be seen in CIDP (also referred to as "multifocal loss" of myelinated fibers [16]) and chronic nerve compression [39]. ***Subperineurial edema*** is an abnormal finding in sural nerve readily detectable on H&E but best viewed on toluidine blue stained plastic sections (Fig. 2.13). It is generally considered an indicator for inflammatory neuropathies such as vasculitis, CIDP and GBS. The degree of edema is more prominent in inflammatory neuropathies with recent onset [40]

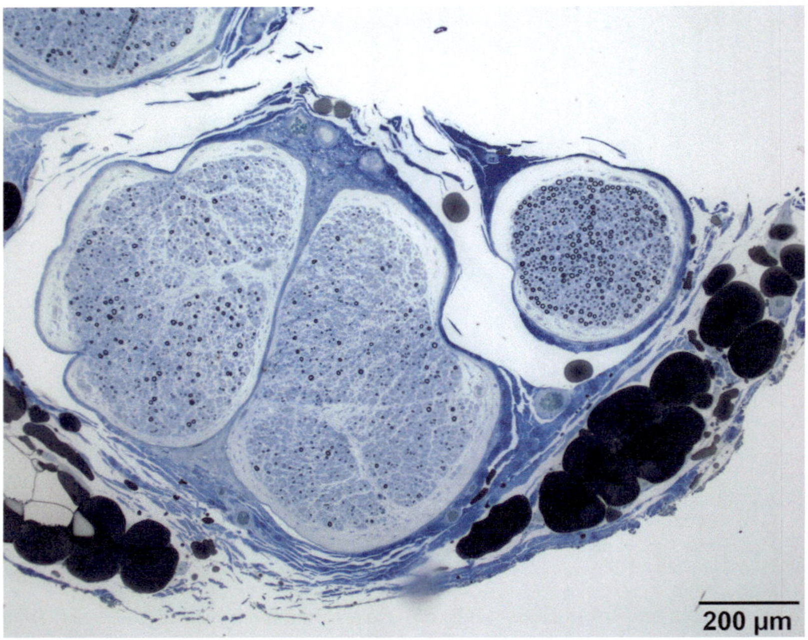

Fig. 2.13 Differential fascicular loss of axons. Toluidine blue section shows severe depletion of axons in the left two fascicles but well preserved axons in the fascicle on the top right. All fascicle show prominent subperineurial edema. (Sural nerve biopsy from a 17-year-old patient with axonal neuropathy)

but has no correlation with the severity of axon loss. However, subperineurial edema is nonspecific and has been well documented in many non-inflammatory conditions such amyloidosis [41], lead poisoning [42], thiamine deficiency [43], immune checkpoint inhibitor chemo reagents [22], chronic nerve compression [39], as a non-exhaustive list.

Electron Microscopy (EM)

While thick section viewed at the light microscopy resolution can provide a general assessment of large myelinated axon density, myelin thickness, and the presence of ovoids, regenerating clusters, and well-formed onion bulbs, many important diagnostic features can only be assessed by EM, such as macrophage mediated demyelination, presence of naked axons or early degenerating axons, true onion bulb versus pseudo-onion bulb, and integrity and density of unmyelinated axons. We perform electron microscopy on most of nerve biopsies when an etiologic diagnosis (e.g. vasculitis, amyloidsis) is not apparent on routine histological sections. In each case multiple 1.5 μm thick sections from a total of four resin embedded nerve blocks are first reviewed by light microscopy. The most representative block is selected, from which 100 nanometer thin sections are cut, mounted on a copper grid, stained, and viewed by electron microscopy.

Features of axonal degeneration and regeneration When an axon is injured, most often by trauma or ischemia, the axon and its myelin sheath distal to the injury site undergo a sequence of events referred to as ***Wallerian degeneration***. The neuron is still viable which will then attempt to regenerate the axon from the proximal stump, forming regenerating cluster. The very first sign of axonal degeneration is ***increased organelles*** (mainly mitochondria) due to cessation of axonal transport, occurring within 12–24 hours of axon injury (Fig. 2.14a). This is followed by degeneration of the axoplasm with loss of structure, rarification, and eventually disappearance of the axon (Fig. 2.14b, c). The myelin sheath subsequently collapses and degenerates, forming ***myelin ovoids*** (Fig. 2.14d). The initial phase of myelin degeneration occurs in the Schwann cell cytoplasm, the remnants are then removed by macrophages (Fig. 2.14e). The macrophages can be distinguished from Schwann cells by their filopodia (arrows) and the lack of a basement membrane. The Schwann cell unit devoid of myelinated axon collapses (Fig. 2.14f). Regeneration occurs at the viable tip of the proximal stump, where a growth cone is formed and extends multiple axon sprouts. Meanwhile, Schwann cells proliferate within the original basement membrane tube and guide axon growth, forming ***Bands of Büngner*** (Fig. 2.14g). The ***regenerating cluster*** follows when individual axon sprout becomes associated with a Schwann cell which produces its own basement membrane and myelin. The original basement membrane tube is usually degenerated by this time (Fig. 2.14h). The axon sprouts that do not reach a target will disappear, while usually one dominant regenerating axon will remain. The myelin sheath of the regenerating axon is thin-

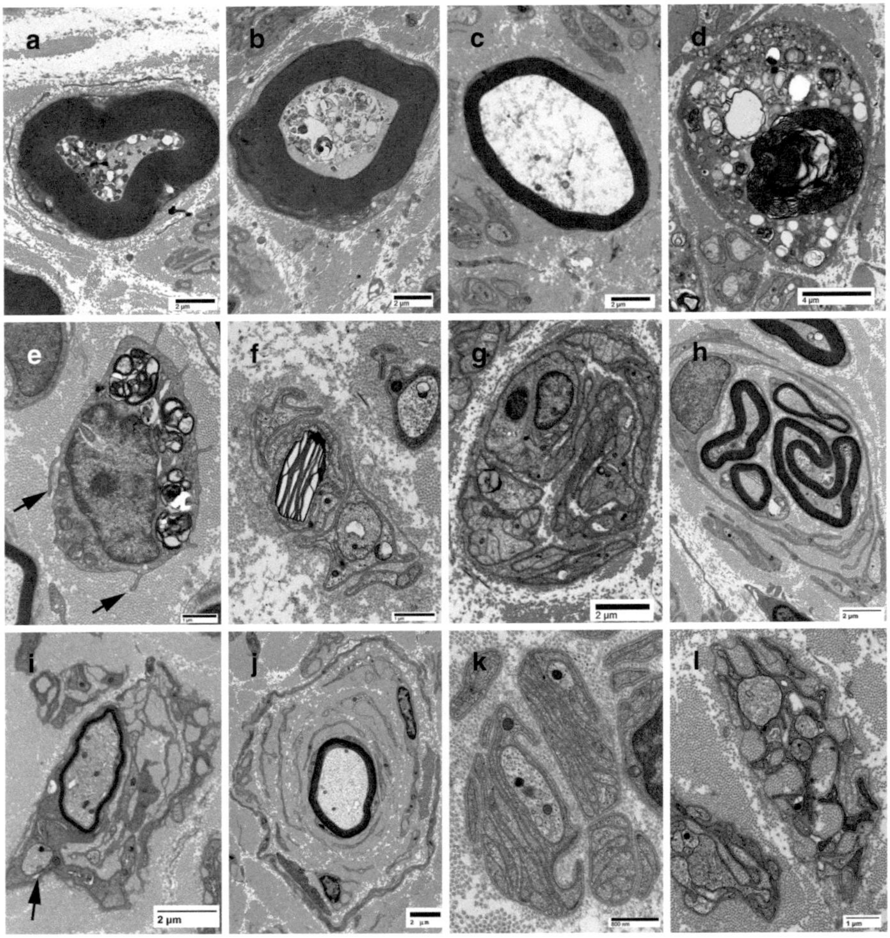

Fig. 2.14 Features of axonal degeneration/regeneration on EM. (**a**) Early degenerating axon with increased organelle. (**b, c**) Mid to late degenerating axons with degeneration and dissolution of axoplasm. (**d**) Myelin ovoid. (**e**) Macrophage containing myelin debris. Arrows indicate filopodia. (**f**) Collapsed Schwann cell unit devoid of axon. The presence of Reich granule at the center indicates this was a myelinating Schwann cell with an axon. (**g**) Bands of Bungner. (**h**) Regenerating cluster (**i**) Pseudo-onion bulb contain unmyelinated axons (arrow) within the Schwann cell processes and is a feature of axonopathy. (**j**) True onion bulb does not contain unmyelinated axons and is a feature of chronic demyelination. (**k**) Stacked Schwann cell processes and (**l**) Clustered collagen pockets indicate loss of unmyelinated axons

ner than normal axons of similar caliber and gives the appearance of a ***Pseudo-onion bulb,*** a central thinly myelinated axon surrounded by proliferating, sometimes concentric Schwann cell processes (Fig. 2.14i). Pseudo-onion bulbs are thus considered a feature of axonopathy rather than demyelination. The presence of unmyelinated axons within the Schwann cell processes differentiate pseudo-onion bulbs (Fig. 2.14i arrow) from a true onion bulb (Fig. 2.14j). ***Stacked Schwann cell pro-***

cesses is a feature of degeneration of unmyelinated axons (Fig. 2.14k). The flatness of Schwann processes and the lack of a common basal lamina tube differ from bands of Büngner. Occasional ***collagen pockets*** can be seen in normal sural nerve but clustered collagen pockets indicate unmyelinated axonal loss (Fig. 2.14l).

Features of demyelination ***Macrophage mediated demyelination***, characterized by macrophage entering Schwann cell basement membrane and directly contacting or stripping the myelin sheath off an intact axon (Fig. 2.15a), is considered a definitive diagnostic feature of active immune mediated demyelination (e.g. GBS or CIDP). Macrophage mediate demyelination is rarely seen in peripheral nerve biopsies, however, as axons do not stay demyelinated for long in CIDP, and peripheral nerve biopsy is rarely done in the acute phase of GBS. The diagnosis of CIDP on a nerve biopsy often relies more on the presence of prominent endoneurial lymphohistiocytic inflammation, and evidence of demyelination of intact associated axons. Individual axon devoid of myelin sheath (also referred to as "***naked axons***") comparable in size to adjacent myelinated axons is a feature of demyelination (Fig. 2.15b). Care should be taken not to confuse naked axons with nodes of Ranvier, which are the gap areas between two adjacent myelinating Schwann cells where the axon is not covered by myelin sheath. Node of Ranvier is a normal structure, not evidence of demyelination, and can be differentiated from a naked axon by the presence of nodal processes (Fig. 2.15c). ***Onion bulb*** is a feature of chronic demyelination and has been discussed in the section above. ***Vesicular degeneration of myelin*** in a well preserved nerve biopsy specimen is considered evidence of demyelination. However, in most situations encountered in nerve biopsy, it is more likely a result of delayed fixation artifact (Fig. 2.15d). Widely spaced myelin and uncompacted myelin are rare myelin abnormalities but have important diagnostic implications when detected. ***Widely spaced myelin (WSM)*** refers to increased space between myelin laminae (Fig. 2.15e). Majority of WSM cases are associated with Waldenstrom's macroglobulinemia with circulating IgM paraprotein against myelin associated glycoprotein (anti-MAG) activity [44]. A minority of cases have been reported in association with IgM monoclonal gammopathy of undetermined significance and anti-MAG activity. ***Uncompacted myelin*** refers to separation of the major dense lines of myelin (Fig. 2.15f) and is most frequently reported in association with POEMS syndrome [45]. It has also been reported in dysglobulinemic neuropathies [46], Waldenström's macroglobulinemia [44], monoclonal gammopathies [47], and a range of hereditary neuropathies with mutations in myelin associated proteins [48, 49].

Other Miscellaneous EM findings and artifacts ***Polyglucosan bodies*** are round, laminated intra-axonal inclusions that are morphologically identical to corpora amylacea and Lafora bodies (Fig. 2.16a). They are strongly PAS positive and diastase resistant (Fig. 2.16b, c). On EM, polyglucosan bodies are composed mostly of filamentous polysaccharide (Fig. 2.16d–f). While frequent polyglucosan bodies in multiple nerve fascicles are diagnostic for adult polyglucosan disease in the case featured by the Fig. 2.16, the finding of isolated polyglucosan

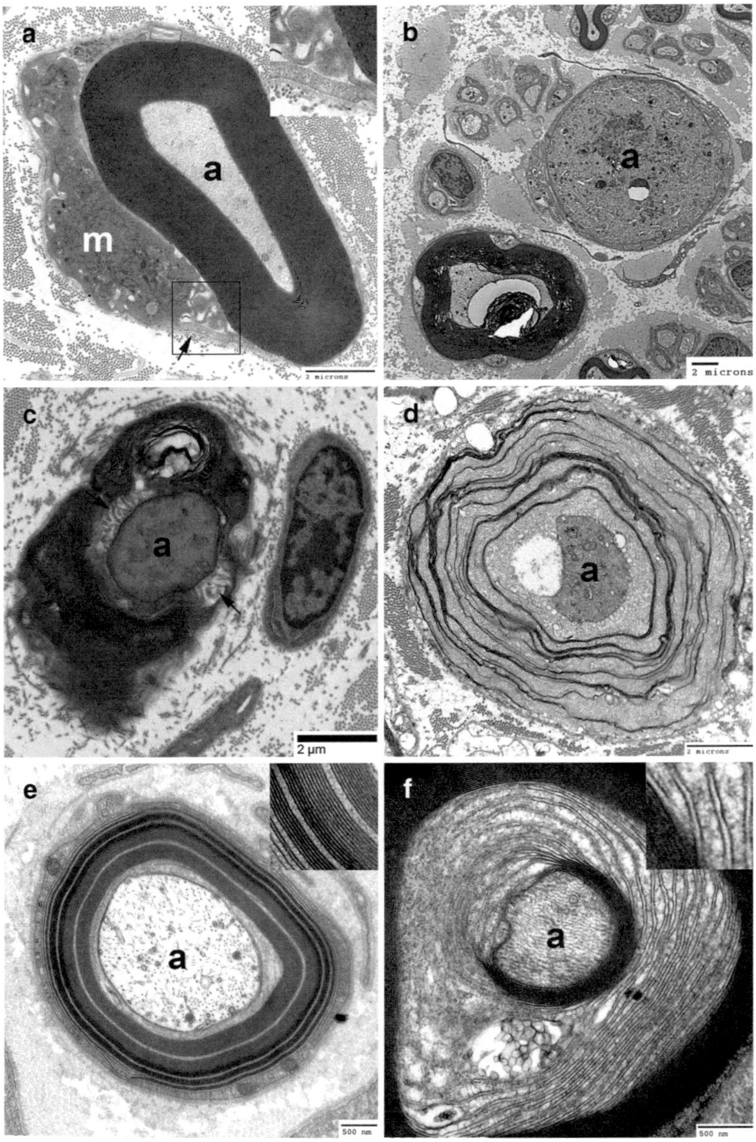

Fig. 2.15 Features of demyelination on EM. (**a**) Macrophage mediated demyelination. A macrophage (m) is within the basement membrane (arrow) of a Schwann cell containing a myelinated axon (a). The macrophage filopodia are in direct contact of the myelin sheath (inset) (Image from a 74-year-old man with fulminant GBS). (**b**) Naked axon (a) in a patient with CIDP. (**c**) Not all large unmyelinated axon profile represents demyelination. Axon segment at the node of Ranvier is unmyelinated. The presence of nodal processes (arrows) distinguishes node of Ranvier from naked axons. (**d**) Vesicular myelin degeneration due to delayed fixation artifact in an infant autopsy nerve. (**e**) Widely spaced myelin is associated with Waldenstrom Macroglobulinemia with anti-MAG IgM and characterized by increased space between myelin laminae (inset). (**f**) Uncompacted myelin is associated with POEMS syndrome and characterized by separation of the major dense line (inset). (Image panels **a**, **d**, **e**, and **f** are provided by Dr. Robert E. Schmidt, Department of Pathology and Immunology, Washington University School of Medicine at St. Louis, MO)

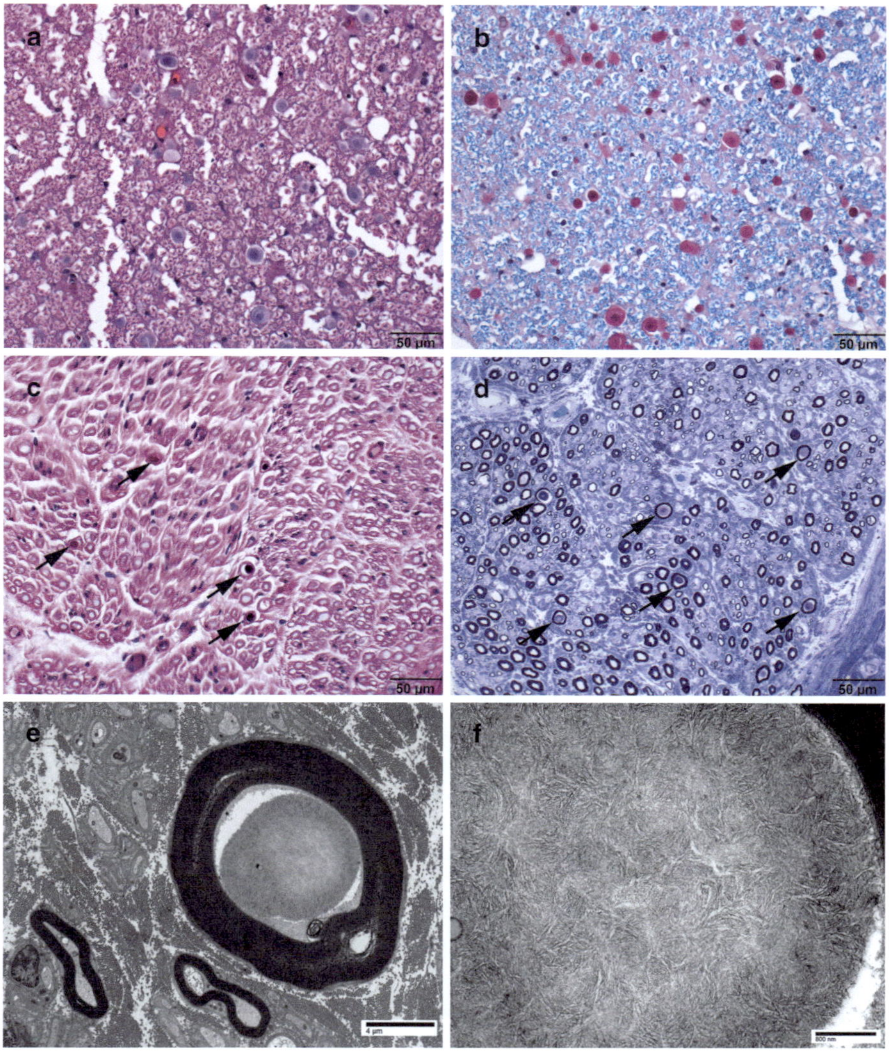

Fig. 2.16 Images of polyglucosan bodies from an autopsy patient who died from adult polyglucosan disease at age 49 years. H&E (**a**) and Luxol-fast blue/PAS stains (**b**) show numerous polyglucosan bodies throughout the central nervous system (Images A&B are from the dorsal column of spinal cord). PAS stain (**c**) and toluidine blue stained thick sections of the peroneal nerve (**d**) show multiple intra-axonal polyglucosan bodies. On electron microscopy (**e**, **f**), the polyglucosan bodies are mainly composed of filamentous polysaccharide

body is less specific and can also be seen as a common age related nonspecific change in normal person [50]. ***Renaut bodies*** are whorled structures located in the subperineurial regions (Fig. 2.17a, b). On EM they are composed of collagen, intermediate filaments, and fibroblast processes (Fig. 2.17c). Renaut body can be seen in normal person as an age related change [51]. Frequent Renaut bodies are associated with chronic nerve impingement [52] and may provide

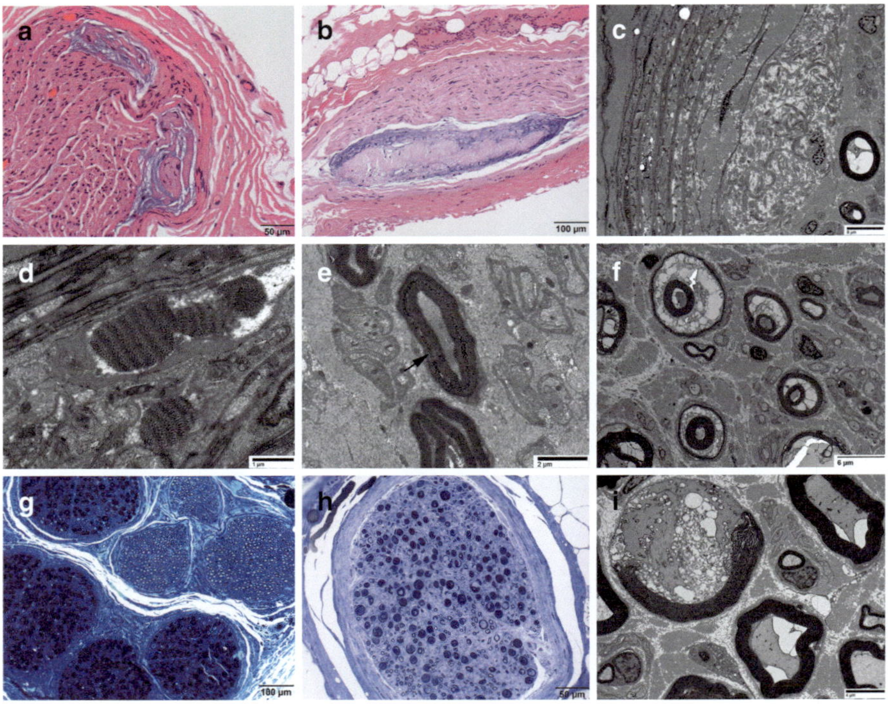

Fig. 2.17 Miscellaneous findings and artifacts. (**a–c**) Renaut bodies on H&E stained cross section (**a**), longitudinal section (**b**) and EM (**c**). (**d**) Luse body (fibrous long spacing collagen) on EM. (**e**) Schmidt-Lanterman incisure (arrow). (**f**) In poorly preserved specimen, the Schmidt-Lanterman spaces are often markedly enlarged. (**g–i**): compression artifacts due to rough handling. (**g**) Toluidine blue stained thick section shows compression artifacts of the four fascicles on the left. (**h**) Large myelinated axons are most susceptible to compression artifacts. Smaller myelinated axons are better preserved. (**i**) Artifactually damaged myelin may retract from the axon and create half myelin

diagnostic value in peripheral nerves resected due to chronic neurogenic pain. ***Luse bodies*** are fusiform structures composed of fibrous long-spacing collagen that resemble raccoon tail on EM (Fig. 2.17d). Luse bodies are originally described by Luse in Schwannomas [53]. In sural nerve biopsies, they are typically found in the perineurium or endoneurium and represent a nonspecific finding that carries no diagnostic implications. They can be seen in normal nerves [54, 55] and a range of neoplastic and non-neoplastic conditions. ***Schmidt-Lanterman incisures*** are cleft like space of noncompaction that is normally present within the myelin sheath (Fig. 2.17e). In poorly preserved or fixed nerve specimens, the Schmidt-Lanterman incisures are often enlarged and may contain disrupted or vesicular myelin (Fig. 2.17f). ***Reich Pi granules.*** Small Pi granules are a normal component of Schwann cells associated with myelinated axons. In Schwann cell units devoid of axons, the presence of large Pi granules indicates loss of myelinated axons (Fig. 2.14f). ***Crush artifacts:*** The myelin sheath is composed of semi-liquid lipid-protein bilayers with no mechanic strength, and thus highly subject to prefixation manipulation damages. A common compression artifact is "blue blobs", which may selectively affect some fascicles of a nerve (Fig. 2.17g) or a subset of fibers within a fascicle (Fig. 2.17h). Large myelinated axons are most susceptible to compression damage. On EM, the broken myelin sheath may retract and create a half ring around the axon (Fig. 2.17i), which should not be mistaken with myelinopathy.

Teased Fiber Analysis

Teased fiber analysis is the preferred method in differentiating primary from secondary segmental demyelination, and is more sensitive in detecting tomacula. However, fiber teasing is quite laborious and a sufficient number of cases is required for performers to maintain technical skill and proficiency. Many centers consider nerve fiber teasing to be insufficiently informative to justify its cost in routine evaluation of sural nerve biopsies [1]. In one study, teased fiber analysis added critical information to other classical techniques in only 4/102 cases [56]. At our institution, we have essentially stopped requesting teased fiber analysis for routine nerve biopsy evaluation.

Special Stains and Utilities

A variety of special stains can be utilized to highlight certain structures in peripheral nerve biopsy. ***Gomori's trichrome*** stain is performed on cryostat section of peripheral nerve and stains myelin red and collagen blue, thus may provide a quick assessment of the density and distribution of myelinated axons (Fig. 2.18). ***Masson's trichrome*** similarly stains myelin red on formalin fixed nerve segment and can well demonstrate myelin ovoids on longitudinal sections (Fig. 2.10d). ***Periodic acid Schiff (PAS)*** stains basement membrane in blood vessels and perineurium (Fig. 2.4), and also intensely stain polyglucosan bodies (Fig. 2.16c). ***Elastin (Verhoeff-van Gieson, or VVG)*** stain highlights internal elastic lamina of arteries in case where chronic vascular damage is suspected. ***Crystal violet*** stain can help highlight amyloid and metachromatic deposits in metachromatic leukodystrophy. ***Modified Grocott's methenamine silver (GMS)*** and ***acid fast bacillus (AFB)*** stains are occasionally performed when granulomatous inflammation is present to exclude fungal or mycobacteria organisms. ***Fite*** stain helps demonstrate mycobacterium leprae and other weakly acid fast bacteria.

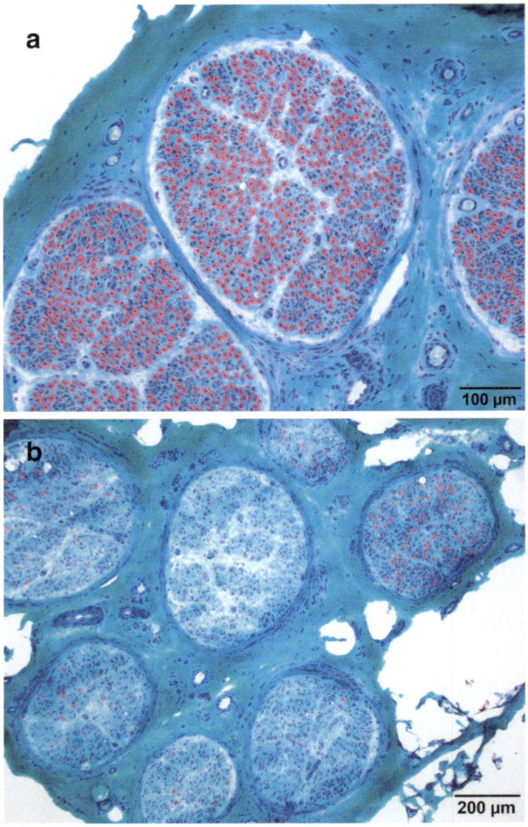

Fig. 2.18 Gomori trichrome stain highlights nerve myelin sheath in red. (**a**) Normal nerve. (**b**) A nerve with prominent differential fascicular loss of myelinated axons suggestive of a vascular etiology

Immunostains

Standard immunohistochemical (IHC) stains can be performed on FFPE never tissue to characterize inflammatory infiltrates, to highlight individual nerve or vascular components, and to classify neoplastic cells. Here we describe some commonly utilized IHCs and there utilities. ***CD45*** (leukocyte common antigen) stains all white blood cells and is commonly used to highlight any inflammatory cells. ***CD3*** is a common T cell marker that stains both helper T cells (***CD4*** positive) and cytotoxic T cells (***CD8*** positive). ***CD20*** is a B cell marker. ***CD68*** stains macrophages. ***CD31*** and ***CD34*** are an endothelial cell markers that help highlight blood vessels. ***Smooth muscle antigen (SMA)*** stains smooth muscle cells and helps to highlight vessel wall alterations in vasculitis cases. Regarding nerve components, ***neurofilament protein (NFP)*** and ***PGP9.5*** stains axons. ***Neural cell adhesion molecule (NCAM)*** is a marker for non-myelinating Schwann cells that highlights Remak bundles (unmyelinated fibers). ***Myelin basic protein*** and $\boldsymbol{P_0}$ stain myelin sheath. ***S100*** is a more general Schwann cell marker but is usually used in the context of neoplasms (i.e. Schwannoma, neurofibroma) rather than non-neoplastic nerve biopsies. ***Epithelial***

membrane antigen (EMA) stains perineurium. Finally, when amyloid is found, ***transthyretin, kappa,*** and ***lambda*** light chain immunostains can help further classify some cases into hereditary and acquired amyloidosis subtypes.

References

1. Sommer C, Brandner S, Dyck PJ, Magy L, Mellgren SI, Morbin M, et al. 147th ENMC international workshop: guideline on processing and evaluation of sural nerve biopsies, 15–17 December 2006, Naarden, The Netherlands. Neuromuscul Disord NMD. 2008;18(1):90–6.
2. Vital C, Vital A, Canron MH, Jaffre A, Viallard JF, Ragnaud JM, et al. Combined nerve and muscle biopsy in the diagnosis of vasculitic neuropathy. A 16-year retrospective study of 202 cases. J Peripher Nerv Syst JPNS. 2006;11(1):20–9.
3. Dyck PJ, Dyck PJB, Klein CJ, Low P, Amrami K, Engelstad J, et al. Companion to peripheral neuropathy E-book: illustrated cases and new developments: Elsevier Health Sciences; Philadelphia, PA. 2010. p. 3–23.
4. Jennette JC, Falk RJ, Bacon PA, Basu N, Cid MC, Ferrario F, et al. 2012 revised international Chapel Hill consensus conference nomenclature of vasculitides. Arthritis Rheum. 2013;65(1):1–11.
5. Collins MP, Hadden RD. The nonsystemic vasculitic neuropathies. Nat Rev Neurol. 2017;13(5):302–16.
6. Collins MP, Dyck PJ, Gronseth GS, Guillevin L, Hadden RD, Heuss D, et al. Peripheral nerve society guideline on the classification, diagnosis, investigation, and immunosuppressive therapy of non-systemic vasculitic neuropathy: executive summary. J Peripher Nerv Syst JPNS. 2010;15(3):176–84.
7. Ohkoshi N, Mizusawa H, Oguni E, Shoji S. Sural nerve biopsy in vasculitic neuropathies: morphometric analysis of the caliber of involved vessels. J Med. 1996;27(3–4):153–70.
8. Sugiura M, Koike H, Iijima M, Mori K, Hattori N, Katsuno M, et al. Clinicopathologic features of nonsystemic vasculitic neuropathy and microscopic polyangiitis-associated neuropathy: a comparative study. J Neurol Sci. 2006;241(1–2):31–7.
9. Dyck PJ, Benstead TJ, Conn DL, Stevens JC, Windebank AJ, Low PA. Nonsystemic vasculitic neuropathy. Brain J Neurol. 1987;110(Pt 4):843–53.
10. Heath D, Smith P. The electron microscopy of "fibrinoid necrosis" in pulmonary arteries. Thorax. 1978;33(5):579–95.
11. Amano S. Vascular changes in the brain of spontaneously hypertensive rats: hyaline and fibrinoid degeneration. J Pathol. 1977;121(2):119–28.
12. Pitcock JA, Johnson JG, Hatch FE, Acchiardo S, Muirhead EE, Brown PS. Malignant hypertension in blacks. Malignant intrarenal arterial disease as observed by light and electron microscopy. Hum Pathol. 1976;7(3):333–46.
13. Rosenblum WI. Fibrinoid necrosis of small brain arteries and arterioles and miliary aneurysms as causes of hypertensive hemorrhage: a critical reappraisal. Acta Neuropathol. 2008;116(4):361–9.
14. Renkawek K, Majkowska-Wierzbicka J, Krajewski S. Necrotic changes of the spinal cord with immune-complex-mediated disseminated vasculitis in a case of atypical allergic encephalomyelitis. J Neurol. 1985;232(6):368–73.
15. Rizzuto N, Morbin M, Cavallaro T, Ferrari S, Fallahi M, Galiazzo Rizzuto S. Focal lesions area feature of chronic inflammatory demyelinating polyneuropathy (CIDP). Acta Neuropathol. 1998;96(6):603–9.
16. Piccione EA, Engelstad J, Dyck PJ, Mauermann ML, Dispenzieri A, Dyck PJ. Nerve pathologic features differentiate POEMS syndrome from CIDP. Acta Neuropathol Commun. 2016;4(1):116.

17. Schutz G, Schroder JM. Number and size of epineurial blood vessels in normal and diseased human sural nerves. Cell Tissue Res. 1997;290(1):31–7.
18. Mawrin C, Schutz G, Schroder JM. Correlation between the number of epineurial and endoneurial blood vessels in diseased human sural nerves. Acta Neuropathol. 2001;102(4):364–72.
19. Yell PC, Burns DK, Dittmar EG, White CL 3rd, Cai C. Diffuse microvascular C5b-9 deposition is a common feature in muscle and nerve biopsies from diabetic patients. Acta Neuropathol Commun. 2018;6(1):11.
20. Ubogu EE. Inflammatory neuropathies: pathology, molecular markers and targets for specific therapeutic intervention. Acta Neuropathol. 2015;130(4):445–68.
21. Vallat JM, Leboutet MJ, Hugon J, Loubet A, Lubeau M, Fressinaud C. Acute pure sensory paraneoplastic neuropathy with perivascular endoneurial inflammation: ultrastructural study of capillary walls. Neurology. 1986;36(10):1395–9.
22. Manousakis G, Koch J, Sommerville RB, El-Dokla A, Harms MB, Al-Lozi MT, et al. Multifocal radiculoneuropathy during ipilimumab treatment of melanoma. Muscle Nerve. 2013;48(3):440–4.
23. Chimelli L, Freitas M, Nascimento O. Value of nerve biopsy in the diagnosis and follow-up of leprosy: the role of vascular lesions and usefulness of nerve studies in the detection of persistent bacilli. J Neurol. 1997;244(5):318–23.
24. Bosboom WM, Van den Berg LH, De Boer L, Van Son MJ, Veldman H, Franssen H, et al. The diagnostic value of sural nerve T cells in chronic inflammatory demyelinating polyneuropathy. Neurology. 1999;53(4):837–45.
25. Global leprosy update, 2016: accelerating reduction of disease burden. Releve epidemiologique hebdomadaire. 2017;92(35):501–19.
26. Bourque CN, Anderson BA, Martin del Campo C, Sima AA. Sensorimotor perineuritis--an autoimmune disease? Can J Neurol Sci. 1985;12(2):129–33.
27. Simmons Z, Albers JW, Sima AA. Case-of-the-month: perineuritis presenting as mononeuritis multiplex. Muscle Nerve. 1992;15(5):630–5.
28. Konishi T, Saida K, Ohnishi A, Nishitani H. Perineuritis in mononeuritis multiplex with cryoglobulinemia. Muscle Nerve. 1982;5(2):173–7.
29. Ricoy JR, Cabello A, Rodriguez J, Tellez I. Neuropathological studies on the toxic syndrome related to adulterated rapeseed oil in Spain. Brain J Neurol. 1983;106 (. Pt 4:817–35.
30. Said G, Lacroix C, Plante-Bordeneuve V, Le Page L, Pico F, Presles O, et al. Nerve granulomas and vasculitis in sarcoid peripheral neuropathy: a clinicopathological study of 11 patients. Brain J Neurol. 2002;125(Pt 2):264–75.
31. Dyck PJ, Engelstad J, Norell J, Dyck PJ. Microvasculitis in non-diabetic lumbosacral radiculoplexus neuropathy (LSRPN): similarity to the diabetic variety (DLSRPN). J Neuropathol Exp Neurol. 2000;59(6):525–38.
32. Lee SS, Yoon TY. Sensory perineuritis presented as a mononeuritis multiplex associated with livedo vasculitis. Clin Neurol Neurosurg. 2001;103(1):56–8.
33. Bradley JL, Thomas PK, King RH, Watkins PJ. A comparison of perineurial and vascular basal laminal changes in diabetic neuropathy. Acta Neuropathol. 1994;88(5):426–32.
34. King RH, Llewelyn JG, Thomas PK, Gilbey SG, Watkins PJ. Perineurial calcification. Neuropathol Appl Neurobiol. 1988;14(2):105–23.
35. Falk RH, Comenzo RL, Skinner M. The systemic amyloidoses. N Engl J Med. 1997;337(13):898–909.
36. Klein CJ, Vrana JA, Theis JD, Dyck PJ, Dyck PJ, Spinner RJ, et al. Mass spectrometric-based proteomic analysis of amyloid neuropathy type in nerve tissue. Arch Neurol. 2011;68(2):195–9.
37. Peter J, Dyck PJBD, Engelstad J. "Pathologic Alterations of Nerves". Peripheral neuropathy. 4th ed: W.B. Saunders;Philadelphia, Pennsylvania. 2005.
38. Nukada H, Dyck PJ. Acute ischemia causes axonal stasis, swelling, attenuation, and secondary demyelination. Ann Neurol. 1987;22(3):311–8.
39. Berini SE, Spinner RJ, Jentoft ME, Engelstad JK, Staff NP, Suanprasert N, et al. Chronic meralgia paresthetica and neurectomy: a clinical pathologic study. Neurology. 2014;82(17):1551–5.

40. Uceyler N, Necula G, Wagemann E, Toyka KV, Sommer C. Endoneurial edema in sural nerve may indicate recent onset inflammatory neuropathy. Muscle Nerve. 2016;53(5):705–10.
41. Hanyu N, Ikeda S, Nakadai A, Yanagisawa N, Powell HC. Peripheral nerve pathological findings in familial amyloid polyneuropathy: a correlative study of proximal sciatic nerve and sural nerve lesions. Ann Neurol. 1989;25(4):340–50.
42. Myers RR, Powell HC, Shapiro HM, Costello ML, Lampert PW. Changes in endoneurial fluid pressure, permeability, and peripheral nerve ultrastructure in experimental lead neuropathy. Ann Neurol. 1980;8(4):392–401.
43. Koike H, Iijima M, Sugiura M, Mori K, Hattori N, Ito H, et al. Alcoholic neuropathy is clinicopathologically distinct from thiamine-deficiency neuropathy. Ann Neurol. 2003;54(1):19–29.
44. Vital C, Vital A, Deminiere C, Julien J, Lagueny A, Steck AJ. Myelin modifications in 8 cases of peripheral neuropathy with Waldenstrom's macroglobulinemia and anti-MAG activity. Ultrastruct Pathol. 1997;21(6):509–16.
45. Vital C, Gherardi R, Vital A, Kopp N, Pellissier JF, Soubrier M, et al. Uncompacted myelin lamellae in polyneuropathy, organomegaly, endocrinopathy, M-protein and skin changes syndrome. Ultrastructural study of peripheral nerve biopsy from 22 patients. Acta Neuropathol. 1994;87(3):302–7.
46. Ohnishi A, Hirano A. Uncompacted myelin lamellae in dysglobulinemic neuropathy. J Neurol Sci. 1981;51(1):131–40.
47. Vital C, Brechenmacher C, Reiffers J, Lagueny A, Massonnat R, Julien J, et al. Uncompacted myelin lamellae in two cases of peripheral neuropathy. Acta Neuropathol. 1983;60(3–4):252–6.
48. Yoshikawa H, Dyck PJ. Uncompacted inner myelin lamellae in inherited tendency to pressure palsy. J Neuropathol Exp Neurol. 1991;50(5):649–57.
49. Vital C, Vital A, Bouillot S, Favereaux A, Lagueny A, Ferrer X, et al. Uncompacted myelin lamellae in peripheral nerve biopsy. Ultrastruct Pathol. 2003;27(1):1–5.
50. Busard HL, Gabreels-Festen AA, van 't Hof MA, Renier WO, Gabreels FJ. Polyglucosan bodies in sural nerve biopsies. Acta Neuropathol. 1990;80(5):554–7.
51. Bergouignan FX, Vital C. Occurrence of Renaut's bodies in a peripheral nerve. Arch Pathol Lab Med. 1984;108(4):330–3.
52. Jefferson D, Neary D, Eames RA. Renaut body distribution at sites of human peripheral nerve entrapment. J Neurol Sci. 1981;49(1):19–29.
53. Luse SA. Electron microscopic studies of brain tumors. Neurology. 1960;10:881–905.
54. Tohgi H, Tabuchi M, Tomonaga M, Izumiyama N. Spindle-shaped, cross-banded structures in human peripheral nerves. Acta Neuropathol. 1977;40(1):51–4.
55. Lehmann J. Fibrous long-spacing collagen in the perineurium of human sural nerve. Clin Neuropathol. 1983;2(3):134–7.
56. Deprez M, de Groote CC, Gollogly L, Reznik M, Martin JJ. Clinical and neuropathological parameters affecting the diagnostic yield of nerve biopsy. Neuromuscul Disord NMD. 2000;10(2):92–8.

Chapter 3
Skin Biopsy with Cutaneous Nerve Fiber Evaluation

Lan Zhou

Introduction

The past two decades have seen the development and increasingly use of skin biopsy with intraepdiermal nerve fiber density (IENFD) evaluation. Skin biopsy has become the gold standard diagnostic test for small fiber neuropathy (SFN).

SFN is a common neuromuscular disorder which predominantly affects myelinated Aδ and unmyelinated C fibers. According to a Dutch study, the minimum prevalence of SFN is 52.95 per 100,000 population [1]. SFN can be associated with many medical conditions, including diabetes mellitus, connective tissue diseases, sarcoidosis, B12 deficiency, amyloidosis, monoclonal gammopathy, thyroid dysfunction, HIV infection, sodium channelopathy, and paraneoplastic syndrome, among others [2–5].

Small fibers consist of small somatic sensory fibers and autonomic C fibers, which mediate somatic sensory and autonomic functions. Small sensory fibers innervate skin to control the perception of pinprick and thermal stimuli. Autonomic C fibers innervate involuntary muscles, which include cardiac muscle and smooth muscle. Smooth muscle is present in the walls of blood vessel, gastrointestinal (GI) tract, and genitourinary (GU) tract, among others. Autonomic fibers also innervate some glands, including lacrimal gland, salivary gland, and sweat gland. They control cardiac muscle contractility, blood vessel constriction and dilatation, GI and GU motility, and gland functions. Patients with small somatic sensory fiber abnormalities commonly present with pain, burning, tingling, and numbness. Examination often shows allodynia, hyperalgesias, and reduced pinprick and thermal sensation in the affected areas. Motor strength, proprioception, and tendon reflexes are usually preserved, because these modalities are the functions of large nerve fibers. When autonomic fibers are affected, patients may experience dry eyes, dry mouth, ortho-

L. Zhou (✉)
Departments of Neurology and Pathology, Boston University Medical Center, Boston, MA, USA
e-mail: lanzhou@bu.edu

L. Zhou et al. (eds.), *A Case-Based Guide to Neuromuscular Pathology*,
https://doi.org/10.1007/978-3-030-25682-1_3

static dizziness, palpitations, tachycardia, bowel constipation, urinary retention, sexual dysfunction, sweating abnormalities, and red or white skin discoloration. Examination may show orthostatic hypotension or skin changes [2, 6].

Patients with SFN may predominantly present with pain, and examination findings can be limited. Since pain is subjective, which can be caused by neurological conditions other than SFN, such as radiculopathy and central nervous system (CNS) disorders, or by a variety of non-neurological conditions, such as musculoskeletal disorders and arthritis, a specific diagnostic test is needed for SFN. Routine nerve conduction study (NCS) and electromyography (EMG), a valuable test for evaluating large fiber neuropathy, is typically normal in SFN, because the conduction velocities of small sensory nerve fibers are too slow for their conduction responses to be captured on the screen of routine NCS. EMG evaluates the function of motor nerve fibers which are large fibers. Small sensory nerve fibers were difficult to evaluate before the development of skin biopsy with intraepidermal nerve fiber density (IENFD) evaluation in 1990s [7–9]. This test allows direct visualization and evaluation of small cutaneous nerve fibers. The test is useful with a high diagnostic efficiency for evaluating distal SFN [10–13]. It is more sensitive and less invasive than sural nerve biopsy with electron microscopic evaluation of small myelinated and unmyelinated axons [14–17]. It is also useful for diagnosing non-length-dependent SFN [18–23] and focal SFN [24–27].

Skin biopsy is an office procedure. It is easy to perform and minimally invasive. The procedure takes about 10–15 minutes [28]. It has become more and more widely used by treating neurologists to diagnose patients with SFN. A growing number of diagnostic cutaneous nerve laboratories have been established in tertiary care centers and commercial settings. A task force of the European Federation of Neurological Societies (EFNS) published the first guideline paper regarding the use of skin biopsy in diagnosing SFN in 2005 [29], and a joint task force of EFNS and the Peripheral Nerve Society (PNS) published the second guideline paper in 2010 [30]. This chapter will give a brief review of skin biopsy procedure, skin biopsy specimen processing, and small cutaneous nerve fiber evaluation.

Skin Biopsy Procedure

Two methods are used to biopsy skin for evaluating cutaneous innervation, the 3-mm punch biopsy [8] and the blister technique [31]. The blister technique only removes epidermis by placing a suction capsule over the skin without damaging dermal capillaries. Although it is less invasive, painless, and does not cause bleeding, it is not commonly used because it is time-consuming, does not allow evaluation of dermal innervation, and no normative reference value of IENFD is established using this technique [30]. The 3-mm punch biopsy is the standard method for sampling skin. The current technique was initially developed at the Karolinska Institute [9], and later standardized by the groups at the University of Minnesota [7] and the Johns Hopkins University [8].

The 3-mm punch biopsy is routinely done in one lower limb. The biopsy is taken from the distal leg, which is 7–10 cm above the lateral malleolus. Additional biopsies may be taken from the lateral distal thigh (7–10 cm above the knee) and the lateral proximal thigh (7–10 cm below the greater trochanter) for evaluating the severity and the pattern of SFN, length-dependent *vs.* non-length-dependent [18–20, 22]. Biopsies taken from other sites may be indicated if focal or unilateral small fiber impairment is suspected, such as complex regional pain syndrome, meralgia paresthetica, and diabetic truncal neuropathy [24–27]. If no normative values are established at these sites, the contralateral unaffected sites should also be biopsied for comparison.

The 3-mm punch skin biopsy is minimally invasive. It can be done by a trained neurologist in an outpatient clinic. It takes about 10–15 minutes. It is done under local anesthesia, and the only time a patient may feel pain is when the anesthetic solution is injected to numb the biopsy site. After a biopsy site is identified, it is cleansed with alcohol swabs and injected with 1% lidocaine with 1:100,000 epinephrine. The vasoconstrictive effect of epinephrine can help reduce the bleeding. A 3-mm (diameter) disposable circular punch is then placed on the skin perpendicular to the skin surface and slowly twisted down until the punch is 3–4 mm (2/3 of the metal part) in. The biopsy is removed with the forceps and surgical blade technique. It is very important that the epidermis should not be pinched because intraepidermal nerve fibers will be evaluated (Fig. 3.1). Bleeding is usually minimum and easy to control by applying firm pressure to the biopsy site. It may not be necessary for patients to hold anticoagulants, antiplatelet agents, or non-steroidal anti-inflammatory agents for the procedure. But the biopsy site may need prolonged pressure and placement of an absorbable gelatin sponge (gelfoam) for hemostasis. No sutures are needed. The biopsy site is usually healed within 7–10 days by granulation, which leaves a small circular scar that gradually resolves. The biopsy sites

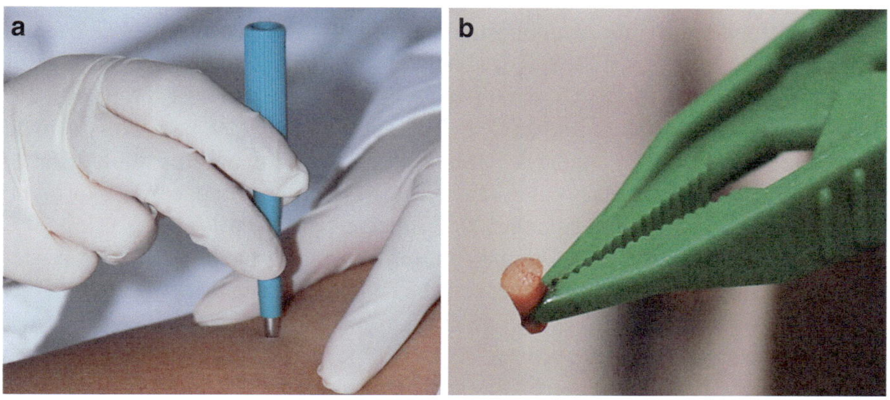

Fig. 3.1 3-mm punch skin biopsy for diagnosing small fiber neuropathy. (**a**) After cleaning the biopsy site, a 3-mm punch is placed on the site perpendicular to the skin surface and twisted down. (**b**) The skin biopsy should be picked up by a forceps to pinch the subcutaneous layer but not the top epidermis. (Reprinted by permission from Zhou [28])

should be covered with pressure gauzes after the biopsy is taken to prevent bleeding. The patient may start to take shower the day after the biopsy, remove the gauzes after the shower, and cove the biopsy sites with regular Band-Aids. The Band-Aids are then changed every day after shower for 7 days. To prevent infection, the patient may not take bath or go swimming during these 7 days. The 3-mm punch biopsy is safe. No serious side effects have been encountered by the author or reported in the literatures. The estimated frequency of non-serious side effects, including mild infection and excessive bleeding, is 1.9:1000 [30]. Mild infection at the biopsy site can be controlled by topical antibiotics, such as over-the-counter Neosporin, and bleeding can be controlled by prolonged pressure to the biopsy site without sutures.

Skin Biopsy Specimen Processing

The biopsy specimen should be placed into a tube filled with special fixative solution immediately after the biopsy is taken. The tube should be labeled with the patient's identification and the biopsy side and site. The normative values of small fiber densities at different sites are different [11, 12]. The normative values are also influenced by age and gender [32]. Therefore, these pieces of information should be clearly provided to pathologists. The specimens should be submitted to a cutaneous nerve laboratory, not a routine reference laboratory, as a special technique is used for processing. It is very important to contact a specialized cutaneous nerve laboratory regarding the fixative and specimen handling before planning a biopsy.

Immunohistochemical assays are used to detect an antigen expressed by nerve axons to visualize cutaneous nerve fibers for morphometric and morphological evaluation. Two methods of immunostaining have been used, the bright-field immunohistochemistry [8] and the immunofluorescence with [7] or without [9, 33] confocal microscopy. Since most diagnostic cutaneous nerve laboratories use the bright-field immunohistochemistry, this immunostaining method is briefly reviewed here.

After a skin biopsy is removed, it should be fixed immediately in fixative solution for approximately 24 hours. Two types of fixatives can be used, 2% paraformaldehyde-lysine-periodate (2% PLP) and Zamboni (2% paraformaldehyde and picric acid). Formalin, which is commonly used by routine histopathology laboratories, should be avoided because it may cause fragmented appearance of nerve fibers [11]. The skin specimen is then cryoprotected for at least 6 hours using 20% glycerol in 0.1 M Sorrensons phosphate buffer. After freezing, the specimen is sectioned at 50 μm. The wavy nerve fibers can be better viewed in thick 50-μm sections than in routine 5-μm sections. About 45–55 skin sections can be obtained from each specimen. Four non-adjacent sections from each specimen are chosen for immunostaining, and the rest can be stored in antifreeze solution (30% ethylene glycol) at −20°C for future use when needed.

Immunostaining is done manually under a dissecting microscope using free-floating skin sections and 96-well plates (Fig. 3.2). The primary antibody used in our lab for the immunostaining is a polyclonal antibody against protein gene product 9.5 (PGP9.5). PGP9.5 is an ubiquitin carboxyl-terminal hydrolase [34], which is a neuronal cytoplasmic marker. It is found in all types of efferent and afferent nerve

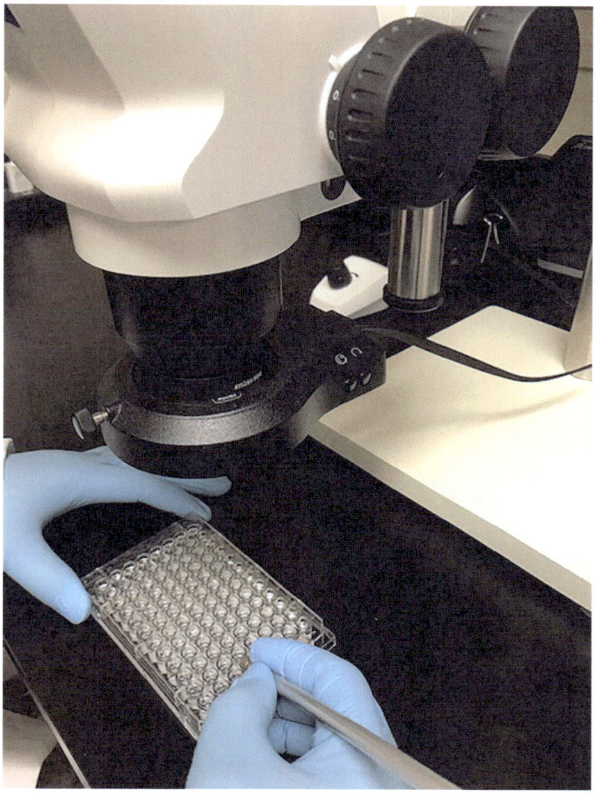

Fig. 3.2 Skin biopsy specimen processing. PGP9.5 immunostaining is done manually under a dissecting microscope using free-floating skin sections and 96-well plates

axons [35, 36], so it is a useful pan-axonal marker to highlight all the nerve fibers. After the primary antibody incubation, sections are incubated with a biotin-conjugated secondary antibody which binds to the primary antibody. This is followed by incubation with avidin-conjugated horseradish peroxidase, and avidin can bind to biotin. The immunostaining signal is then developed using an SG kit (blue chromogen/peroxidase substrate) which produces a blue-gray reaction product [8].

Small Cutaneous Nerve Fiber Evaluation

Intraepidermal Nerve Fiber Density Evaluation

Skin consists of three layers which are firmly attached to one another: the outer epidermis, the deeper dermis, and the subcutaneous layer. The cutaneous innervation was initially thought to mainly consist of a plexus of nerve fibers in the reticular dermis and a more superficial plexus of nerve fibers in the papillary dermis parallel to the skin surface. Rich innervation of epidermis was not demonstrated until late

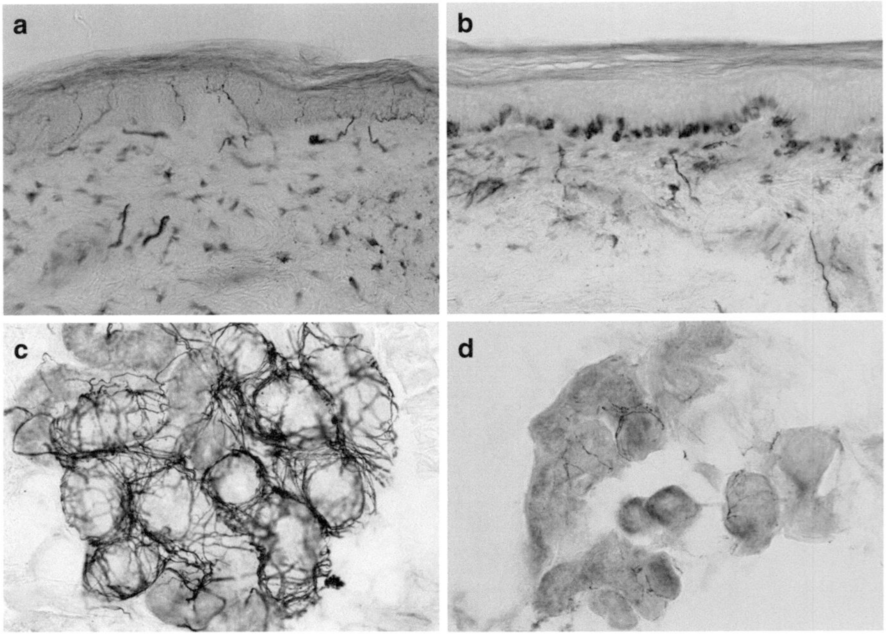

Fig. 3.3 Cutaneous innervation and denervation. (**a**) The epidermis is well-innervated by intraepidermal nerve fibers (arrows). (**b**) The epidermis is devoid of intraepidermal nerve fibers. (**c**) The sweat glands are well-innervated by sudomotor autonomic fibers. (**d**) The sweat glands are largely denervated

1980s and early 1990s by immunostaining using PGP9.5 antibodies [7, 9, 37]. The intraepidermal unmyelinated C fibers originate from sensory nerves as they express substance P and calcitonin gene-related peptide (CGRP) [38, 39]. In addition, these fibers arise entirely from dorsal root ganglions (DRG) as they disappear from skin after experimental dorsal root ganglionectomy, but not after dorsal rhizotomy, ventral rhizotomy, or sympathectomy [40]. Before reaching the epidermis, the unmyelinated C fibers are arranged in Remak bundles which also consist of non-myelinating Schwann cells. Axons exchange among Remak bundles as they pass from DRG to skin [41]. The Remak bundles lose their Schwann cells, and the S-100 staining signal of Schwann cells ends at the dermal-epidermal junction [8]. The unmyelinated C fibers ascend vertically through the epidermis between adjacent keratinocytes as free nerve endings [42] (Fig. 3.3).

Intraepidermal nerve fibers are quantified using a light microscope with 40x objective. A counting rule has been established [43] and recommended to use by EFNS/PNS [29, 30]. Briefly, the nerve fibers that cross the dermal-epidermal junction into the epidermis are counted. The nerve fibers that do not cross the dermal-epidermal junction are not counted. If a nerve fiber branches within epidermis, count as one fiber. If a nerve fiber branches below or within the dermal-epidermal junction, count as two fibers. According to the EFNS/PNS guideline, the nerve fragments within epidermis that do not cross the dermal-epidermal junction are not counted due to the concern that these fragments may be the extension of adjacent fibers on the same skin section that are visualized to cross the dermal-epidermal junction and already counted. Counting these fragments may result in overcounting. However, the original fibers that cross the dermal-epidermal junction may not be shown on the same section due to the wavy nature of the nerve fibers, so excluding these fragments may result in undercounting. Some cutaneous nerve laboratories do count these individual fibers that are within epidermis but without crossing the dermal-epidermal junction [8, 12, 20, 44, 45].

The diagnosis of SFN is made based on the reduction of IENFD. To calculate the linear density of IENF, the length of the epidermal surface is measured [30]. The IENFD is expressed as the number of IENF per length of section (IENF/mm). An alternative "ocular" method has been described and used [46–48], in which special sections are chosen for immunostaining with the assumption that the length of the epidermal surface of these sections is close to 3 mm. So the IENFD is calculated simply by dividing the number of IENF by 3. It has been shown that the IENFD obtained by this "ocular" method significantly correlate with the IENFD obtained from the quantification by measuring the length of the epidermal surface [46]. Further studies are deemed warranted to establish the reliability of the "ocular" method [29].

IENFD measurement is highly reproducible. Reproducibility is the highest when four sections from each biopsy specimen are counted [44]. After reviewers are trained to use the same counting rule, the interobserver and intraoberserver reliabilities are high [8, 12, 44, 49, 50]. There is no significant difference in IENFD when skin sections are stained by different cutaneous nerve laboratories as long as an identical methodology is used by these laboratories to process skin specimens and measure IENFD [44].

The technique of 3-mm punch biopsy with IENFD evaluation using the PGP9.5 immunostaining was standardized and first utilized to evaluate patients with SFN by University of Minnesota [7] and Johns Hopkins University [8]. In 1995, the Johns Hopkins group published the method of the bright-field PGP9.5 immunostaining and IENFD quantification [8]. The majority of the diagnostic cutaneous nerve laboratories adopted this method. By using this method, the Johns Hopkins group showed that the IENFD at the distal leg was lower in patients with HIV-seropositive and HIV-seronegative sensory neuropathy than in normal controls. They subsequently developed normative reference ranges at the distal leg and proximal thigh in 98 healthy subjects with age ranging from 13–82 years [12]. They showed a significantly higher IENFD in the youngest age decile (10–19 years) [11, 12]. By using the cut-off derived from the fifth percentile of the normative range at the distal leg to evaluate 20 patients with sensory neuropathy, they showed that the technique had a diagnostic efficiency of 88%. The high diagnostic efficiency of this technique was also demonstrated by other laboratories [10, 13]. By studying the cutaneous innervation at 5 sites, including distal leg, proximal calf, distal thigh, proximal thigh, and trunk in 10 healthy controls (ages 23–75 years), the Johns Hopkins group showed a normal rostral-to-caudal gradient of IENFD with a linear relationship to the distance from the spine [11]. IENFD at a proximal site was higher than that at a distal site. The IENFD at the proximal thigh was higher than that at the distal leg by about 60% [12].

Several laboratories studied normative reference values at the distal leg and found a decline of the IENFD with age [17, 46, 48–52]. A multicenter study developed the normative values of IENFD at the distal leg by evaluating 550 healthy subjects recruited from eight cutaneous nerve laboratories in Europe, USA, and Asia [32]. The study confirmed the age-related decline of IENFD. IENFD was also found to be influenced by gender but not height or weight. The study developed worldwide age- and sex-adjusted IENFD normative values for clinical use. However, the sensitivity, specificity, and diagnostic efficiency have not been fully determined. Our recent small-scale study suggested that the IENFD at the distal leg appeared influenced by the ethnicity, as the diagnostic sensitivity of using the worldwide age- and sex-adjusted normative reference values was lower in Chinses Americans than in non-Chinese Americans who had pure small fiber sensory neuropathy based on the clinical and electrodiagnostic evaluations [53]. Future large-scale studies are needed to fully address the ethnic differences in IENFD at the distal leg. The normative values may need to be adjusted in certain ethnic groups to improve the diagnostic sensitivity.

Intraepidermal Nerve Fiber Morphology Evaluation

IENFD can be normal at the early stage of SFN, which makes the disease difficult to diagnose because the skin biopsy diagnosis of SFN is based on the reduction of IENFD. However, in this setting, skin biopsy often shows prominent morphological changes of small fibers, including swellings, increased branching and fragmentation, and tortuous appearance (Fig. 3.4) [11, 14, 16, 47, 54–56]. Two studies investigated the diagnostic implication of IENF swellings in SFN [16, 47]. Both found a higher prevalence of IENF swellings at the distal leg in neuropathy patients than in healthy controls. Increased IENF swellings at the distal leg correlated with impaired heat-pain threshold, development of symptomatic neuropathy, and progression of neuropathy. In patients with small fiber sensory symptoms but normal IENFD, the presence of the large swellings of intraepidermal C fibers was found to be able to identify those who subsequently developed epidermal denervation [54]. Therefore, the abnormal morphological changes, especially the large swellings of intraepidermal nerve fibers, may represent small fiber degeneration. If these changes are prominent but IENFD are still normal, a repeat biopsy in 12 months may detect the reduction of IENFD and reach a final diagnosis of SFN.

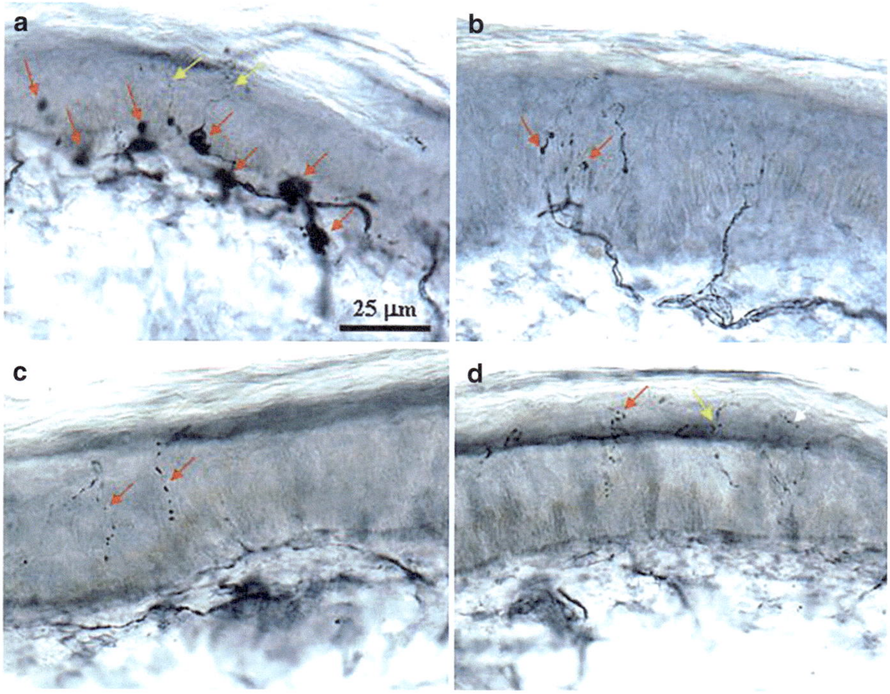

Fig. 3.4 Abnormal morphological changes of intraepidermal nerve fibers. (**a**) Abundant nerve fiber swellings of varying size (red arrows) are noted in epidermis, papillary dermis, and dermal-epidermal junction. (**b**) Many small IENF swellings are seen (red arrows). (**c**) Intraepidermal fibers are fragmented (red arrows) as compared to continuous fibers in **a** (yellow arrows). (**d**) Tortuous (red arrow), branched (yellow arrow), and horizontal (white arrow) fibers are present. (Reprinted with permission from Zhou et al. [45])

Cutaneous Autonomic Nerve Fiber Evaluation

There are several types of autonomic C fibers in the dermis that innervate blood vessel wall (vasomotor fibers), sweat gland (sudomotor fibers), and arrector pilorum smooth muscle (pilomotor fibers) (Fig. 3.5). A few reports have described the reduction of dermal autonomic fiber densities in patients with idiopathic SFN [57] or SFN and dysautonomia associated with diabetes [58], multiple system atrophy [59], and CADASIL [60]. Several studies have attempted to establish standard and reproducible methods to quantify dermal autonomic nerve fiber densities [58, 61–63] to facilitate clinical evaluation and research of autonomic dysfunction associated with SFN. Gibbons et al. have developed an automated method to quantify sudomotor fibers, and the sudomotor fiber density correlates well with the Neuropathy Impairment Score in the Lower Limb (NIS-LL) and the symptoms of reduced sweat production [62, 63]. Some cutaneous nerve laboratories include the measurements of sudomotor fiber densities in their skin biopsy reports. It remains to be determined

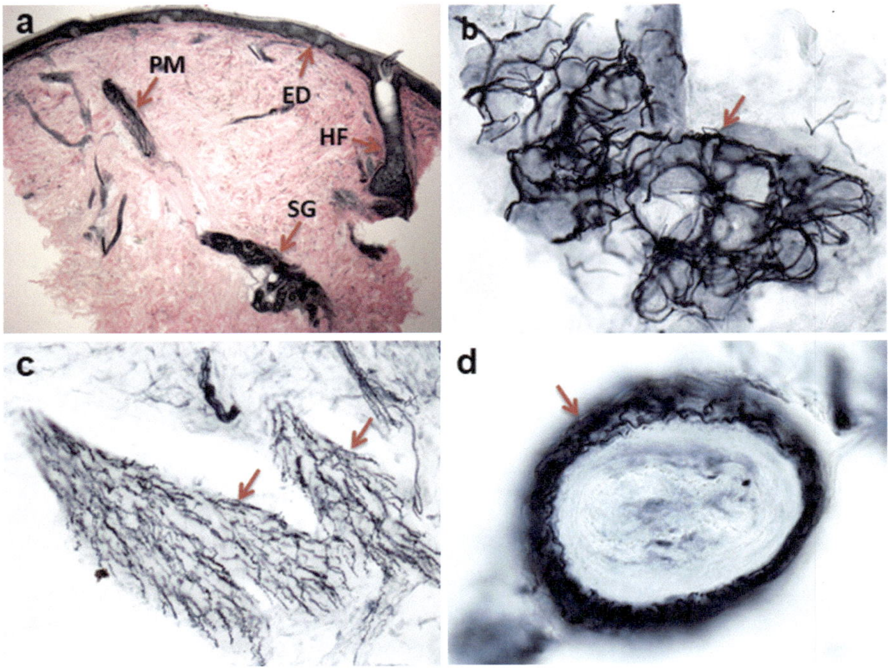

Fig. 3.5 Cutaneous autonomic nerve fibers. (**a**) A skin section immunostained with PGP9.5 shows the top layer of epidermis (ED), and hair follicle (HF), sweat glands (SG), and arrector pili smooth muscle (PM) in the dermis. (**b**) Dermal sudomotor autonomic fibers innervating sweat glands (arrow). (**c**) Dermal pilomotor autonomic fibers innervating arrectores pili muscle (arrows). (**d**) Dermal vasomotor autonomic fibers innervating a blood vessel (arrow)

whether the sudomotor fiber density correlates with the sudomotor function gauged by quantitative sudomotor axon reflex testing (QSART). Nolano et al. have developed a method to quantify pilomotor nerve fiber density (PNFD), and by using this method they have found that the PNFD is significantly reduced in diabetic patients as compared with normal controls. However, PNFD does not correlate with IENFD or total neuropathy score [58]. Future studies are needed to refine the measurements of dermal autonomic fibers and to fully determine the diagnostic utility of detecting dermal autonomic denervation [3, 30].

Treating neurologists who evaluate patients with SFN commonly ask whether they should order skin biopsy, QSART, cardiovascular autonomic testing or all of these tests, and which test has the highest diagnostic yield. The decision should be made based on the patient's symptoms. Skin biopsy, QSART, and cardiovascular autonomic testing evaluate different types of small fibers with different functions. Skin biopsy is mainly used to evaluate the number and morphology of somatic intraepidermal sensory fibers. QSART is to evaluate the functions of sudomotor autonomic fibers. Cardiovascular autonomic testing is to evaluate the functions of cardiovascular autonomic fibers. If a patient mainly presents with sensory symptoms, such as pain, burning, tingling, and numbness, skin biopsy should be ordered for evaluation. If a patient also has sweating abnormalities, QSART should be added. If a patient presents with orthostatic dizziness, palpitations, tachycardia, near-syncope, or syncope, cardiovascular autonomic testing should be ordered for evaluation. SFN that is associated with diabetes, sarcoidosis, Sjogren syndrome, or amyloidosis often manifests both somatic sensory symptoms and autonomic dysfunction. In these settings, skin biopsy, QSART, and cardiovascular autonomic testing can be complementary, and the diagnostic sensitivity can be improved if used together [64, 65].

Limited Usefulness of Skin Biopsy in Evaluation of SFN Etiologies

In addition to the PGP9.5 immunostaining, hematoxylin and eosin staining (HE) and Congo red staining are routinely done by most cutaneous nerve laboratories to evaluate for possible vasculitis and amyloidosis. Since skin biopsy for neuropathy is not a lesion biopsy, the likelihood of finding these abnormalities is extremely low, although amyloid deposition has been reported on skin biopsies taken for evaluation of SFN from patients with amyloidosis [66, 67]. Overall, the usefulness of skin biopsy in evaluation of SFN etiologies is very limited. The test is mainly used to diagnose SFN.

References

1. Peters MJ, Bakkers M, Merkies IS, Hoeijmakers JG, van Raak EP, Faber CG. Incidence and prevalence of small-fiber neuropathy: a survey in the Netherlands. Neurology. 2013;81(15):1356–60.
2. Tavee J, Zhou L. Small fiber neuropathy: a burning problem. Cleve Clin J Med. 2009;76(5):297–305.
3. Cazzato D, Lauria G. Small fibre neuropathy. Curr Opin Neurol. 2017;30(5):490–9.
4. Chan AC, Wilder-Smith EP. Small fiber neuropathy: getting bigger! Muscle Nerve. 2016;53(5):671–82.
5. Gibbons CH. Small fiber neuropathies. Continuum (Minneap Minn). 2014;20(5 Peripheral Nervous System Disorders):1398–412.
6. Lacomis D. Small-fiber neuropathy. Muscle Nerve. 2002;26(2):173–88.
7. Kennedy WR, Wendelschafer-Crabb G. The innervation of human epidermis. J Neurol Sci. 1993;115(2):184–90.
8. McCarthy BG, Hsieh ST, Stocks A, Hauer P, Macko C, Cornblath DR, et al. Cutaneous innervation in sensory neuropathies: evaluation by skin biopsy. Neurology. 1995;45(10):1848–55.
9. Wang L, Hilliges M, Jernberg T, Wiegleb-Edstrom D, Johansson O. Protein gene product 9.5-immunoreactive nerve fibres and cells in human skin. Cell Tissue Res. 1990;261(1):25–33.
10. Devigili G, Tugnoli V, Penza P, Camozzi F, Lombardi R, Melli G, et al. The diagnostic criteria for small fibre neuropathy: from symptoms to neuropathology. Brain. 2008;131.(Pt 7:1912–25.
11. Lauria G, Holland N, Hauer P, Cornblath DR, Griffin JW, McArthur JC. Epidermal innervation: changes with aging, topographic location, and in sensory neuropathy. J Neurol Sci. 1999;164(2):172–8.

12. McArthur JC, Stocks EA, Hauer P, Cornblath DR, Griffin JW. Epidermal nerve fiber density: normative reference range and diagnostic efficiency. Arch Neurol. 1998;55(12):1513–20.
13. Vlckova-Moravcova E, Bednarik J, Dusek L, Toyka KV, Sommer C. Diagnostic validity of epidermal nerve fiber densities in painful sensory neuropathies. Muscle Nerve. 2008;37(1):50–60.
14. Herrmann DN, Griffin JW, Hauer P, Cornblath DR, McArthur JC. Epidermal nerve fiber density and sural nerve morphometry in peripheral neuropathies. Neurology. 1999;53(8):1634–40.
15. Holland NR, Crawford TO, Hauer P, Cornblath DR, Griffin JW, McArthur JC. Small-fiber sensory neuropathies: clinical course and neuropathology of idiopathic cases. Ann Neurol. 1998;44(1):47–59.
16. Lauria G, Morbin M, Lombardi R, Borgna M, Mazzoleni G, Sghirlanzoni A, et al. Axonal swellings predict the degeneration of epidermal nerve fibers in painful neuropathies. Neurology. 2003;61(5):631–6.
17. Periquet MI, Novak V, Collins MP, Nagaraja HN, Erdem S, Nash SM, et al. Painful sensory neuropathy: prospective evaluation using skin biopsy. Neurology. 1999;53(8):1641–7.
18. Gemignani F, Giovanelli M, Vitetta F, Santilli D, Bellanova MF, Brindani F, et al. Non-length dependent small fiber neuropathy. A prospective case series. J Peripher Nerv Syst. 2010;15(1):57–62.
19. Gorson KC, Herrmann DN, Thiagarajan R, Brannagan TH, Chin RL, Kinsella LJ, et al. Non-length dependent small fibre neuropathy/ganglionopathy. J Neurol Neurosurg Psychiatry. 2008;79(2):163–9.
20. Khan S, Zhou L. Characterization of non-length-dependent small-fiber sensory neuropathy. Muscle Nerve. 2012;45(1):86–91.
21. Lauria G, Sghirlanzoni A, Lombardi R, Pareyson D. Epidermal nerve fiber density in sensory ganglionopathies: clinical and neurophysiologic correlations. Muscle Nerve. 2001;24(8):1034–9.
22. Provitera V, Gibbons CH, Wendelschafer-Crabb G, Donadio V, Vitale DF, Loavenbruck A, et al. The role of skin biopsy in differentiating small-fiber neuropathy from ganglionopathy. Eur J Neurol. 2018;25(6):848–53.
23. Chai J, Herrmann DN, Stanton M, Barbano RL, Logigian EL. Painful small-fiber neuropathy in Sjogren syndrome. Neurology. 2005;65(6):925–7.
24. Chemali KR, Zhou L. Small fiber degeneration in post-stroke complex regional pain syndrome I. Neurology. 2007;69(3):316–7.
25. Wongmek A, Shin S, Zhou L. Skin biopsy in assessing meralgia paresthetica. Muscle Nerve. 2016;53(4):641–3.
26. Lauria G, McArthur JC, Hauer PE, Griffin JW, Cornblath DR. Neuropathological alterations in diabetic truncal neuropathy: evaluation by skin biopsy. J Neurol Neurosurg Psychiatry. 1998;65(5):762–6.
27. Oaklander AL, Rissmiller JG, Gelman LB, Zheng L, Chang Y, Gott R. Evidence of focal small-fiber axonal degeneration in complex regional pain syndrome-I (reflex sympathetic dystrophy). Pain. 2006;120(3):235–43.
28. Zhou L. Skin Biopsy. In: Katirji B, Kaminski H, Ruff R, editors. Neuromuscular disorders in clinical practice. New York: Springer; 2014.
29. Lauria G, Cornblath DR, Johansson O, McArthur JC, Mellgren SI, Nolano M, et al. EFNS guidelines on the use of skin biopsy in the diagnosis of peripheral neuropathy. Eur J Neurol. 2005;12(10):747–58.
30. Lauria G, Hsieh ST, Johansson O, Kennedy WR, Leger JM, Mellgren SI, et al. European Federation of Neurological Societies/Peripheral Nerve Society guideline on the use of skin biopsy in the diagnosis of small fiber neuropathy. Report of a joint task force of the European Federation of Neurological Societies and the Peripheral Nerve Society. Eur J Neurol. 2010;17(7):903–12, e44–9.
31. Kennedy WR, Nolano M, Wendelschafer-Crabb G, Johnson TL, Tamura E. A skin blister method to study epidermal nerves in peripheral nerve disease. Muscle Nerve. 1999;22(3):360–71.

32. Lauria G, Bakkers M, Schmitz C, Lombardi R, Penza P, Devigili G, et al. Intraepidermal nerve fiber density at the distal leg: a worldwide normative reference study. J Peripher Nerv Syst. 2010;15(3):202–7.
33. Provitera V, Gibbons CH, Wendelschafer-Crabb G, Donadio V, Vitale DF, Stancanelli A, et al. A multi-center, multinational age- and gender-adjusted normative dataset for immunofluorescent intraepidermal nerve fiber density at the distal leg. Eur J Neurol. 2016;23(2):333–8.
34. Wilkinson KD, Lee KM, Deshpande S, Duerksen-Hughes P, Boss JM, Pohl J. The neuron-specific protein PGP 9.5 is a ubiquitin carboxyl-terminal hydrolase. Science. 1989;246(4930):670–3.
35. Gulbenkian S, Wharton J, Polak JM. The visualisation of cardiovascular innervation in the guinea pig using an antiserum to protein gene product 9.5 (PGP 9.5). J Auton Nerv Syst. 1987;18(3):235–47.
36. Lundberg LM, Alm P, Wharton J, Polak JM. Protein gene product 9.5 (PGP 9.5). A new neuronal marker visualizing the whole uterine innervation and pregnancy-induced and developmental changes in the guinea pig. Histochemistry. 1988;90(1):9–17.
37. Dalsgaard CJ, Rydh M, Haegerstrand A. Cutaneous innervation in man visualized with protein gene product 9.5 (PGP 9.5) antibodies. Histochemistry. 1989;92(5):385–90.
38. Bloom SR, Polak JM. The Prosser-White Oration 1981. Regulatory peptides and the skin. Clin Exp Dermatol. 1983;8(1):3–18.
39. Dalsgaard CJ, Jonsson CE, Hokfelt T, Cuello AC. Localization of substance P-immunoreactive nerve fibers in the human digital skin. Experientia. 1983;39(9):1018–20.
40. Li Y, Hsieh ST, Chien HF, Zhang X, McArthur JC, Griffin JW. Sensory and motor denervation influence epidermal thickness in rat foot glabrous skin. Exp Neurol. 1997;147(2):452–62.
41. Griffin JW, McArthur JC, Polydefkis M. Assessment of cutaneous innervation by skin biopsies. Curr Opin Neurol. 2001;14(5):655–9.
42. Hsieh ST, Choi S, Lin WM, Chang YC, McArthur JC, Griffin JW. Epidermal denervation and its effects on keratinocytes and Langerhans cells. J Neurocytol. 1996;25(9):513–24.
43. Kennedy WRMJ, Polydefkis MJ, Wendelschafer G, editors. Pathology and quantification of cutaneous innervation. Philadelphia: Elsevier Saunders; 2005.
44. Smith AG, Howard JR, Kroll R, Ramachandran P, Hauer P, Singleton JR, et al. The reliability of skin biopsy with measurement of intraepidermal nerve fiber density. J Neurol Sci. 2005;228(1):65–9.
45. Zhou L, Kitch DW, Evans SR, Hauer P, Raman S, Ebenezer GJ, et al. Correlates of epidermal nerve fiber densities in HIV-associated distal sensory polyneuropathy. Neurology. 2007;68(24):2113–9.
46. Chien HF, Tseng TJ, Lin WM, Yang CC, Chang YC, Chen RC, et al. Quantitative pathology of cutaneous nerve terminal degeneration in the human skin. Acta Neuropathol. 2001;102(5):455–61.
47. Herrmann DN, McDermott MP, Henderson D, Chen L, Akowuah K, Schifitto G. Epidermal nerve fiber density, axonal swellings and QST as predictors of HIV distal sensory neuropathy. Muscle Nerve. 2004;29(3):420–7.
48. Pan CL, Lin YH, Lin WM, Tai TY, Hsieh ST. Degeneration of nociceptive nerve terminals in human peripheral neuropathy. Neuroreport. 2001;12(4):787–92.
49. Bakkers M, Merkies IS, Lauria G, Devigili G, Penza P, Lombardi R, et al. Intraepidermal nerve fiber density and its application in sarcoidosis. Neurology. 2009;73(14):1142–8.
50. Goransson LG, Mellgren SI, Lindal S, Omdal R. The effect of age and gender on epidermal nerve fiber density. Neurology. 2004;62(5):774–7.
51. Chang YC, Lin WM, Hsieh ST. Effects of aging on human skin innervation. Neuroreport. 2004;15(1):149–53.
52. Umapathi T, Tan WL, Tan NC, Chan YH. Determinants of epidermal nerve fiber density in normal individuals. Muscle Nerve. 2006;33(6):742–6.
53. Jin P, Cheng L, Chen M, Zhou L. Low sensitivity of skin biopsy in diagnosing small fiber neuropathy in Chinese Americans. J Clin Neuromuscul Dis. 2018;20(1):1–6.

54. Gibbons CH, Griffin JW, Polydefkis M, Bonyhay I, Brown A, Hauer PE, et al. The utility of skin biopsy for prediction of progression in suspected small fiber neuropathy. Neurology. 2006;66(2):256–8.
55. Scott LJ, Griffin JW, Luciano C, Barton NW, Banerjee T, Crawford T, et al. Quantitative analysis of epidermal innervation in Fabry disease. Neurology. 1999;52(6):1249–54.
56. Smith AG, Ramachandran P, Tripp S, Singleton JR. Epidermal nerve innervation in impaired glucose tolerance and diabetes-associated neuropathy. Neurology. 2001;57(9):1701–4.
57. Dabby R, Vaknine H, Gilad R, Djaldetti R, Sadeh M. Evaluation of cutaneous autonomic innervation in idiopathic sensory small-fiber neuropathy. J Peripher Nerv Syst. 2007;12(2):98–101.
58. Nolano M, Provitera V, Caporaso G, Stancanelli A, Vitale DF, Santoro L. Quantification of pilomotor nerves: a new tool to evaluate autonomic involvement in diabetes. Neurology. 2010;75(12):1089–97.
59. Provitera V, Nolano M, Caporaso G, Stancanelli A, Manganelli F, Iodice R, et al. Postganglionic sudomotor denervation in patients with multiple system atrophy. Neurology. 2014;82(24):2223–9.
60. Nolano M, Provitera V, Donadio V, Caporaso G, Stancanelli A, Califano F, et al. Cutaneous sensory and autonomic denervation in CADASIL. Neurology. 2016;86(11):1039–44.
61. Donadio V, Nolano M, Provitera V, Stancanelli A, Lullo F, Liguori R, et al. Skin sympathetic adrenergic innervation: an immunofluorescence confocal study. Ann Neurol. 2006;59(2):376–81.
62. Gibbons CH, Illigens BM, Wang N, Freeman R. Quantification of sweat gland innervation: a clinical-pathologic correlation. Neurology. 2009;72(17):1479–86.
63. Gibbons CH, Illigens BM, Wang N, Freeman R. Quantification of sudomotor innervation: a comparison of three methods. Muscle Nerve. 2010;42(1):112–9.
64. Tavee JO, Karwa K, Ahmed Z, Thompson N, Parambil J, Culver DA. Sarcoidosis-associated small fiber neuropathy in a large cohort: clinical aspects and response to IVIG and anti-TNF alpha treatment. Respir Med. 2017;126:135–8.
65. Thaisetthawatkul P, Fernandes Filho JA, Herrmann DN. Contribution of QSART to the diagnosis of small fiber neuropathy. Muscle Nerve. 2013;48(6):883–8.
66. Ebenezer GJ, Liu Y, Judge DP, Cunningham K, Truelove S, Carter ND, et al. Cutaneous nerve biomarkers in transthyretin familial amyloid polyneuropathy. Ann Neurol. 2017;82(1):44–56.
67. Visser AC, Klein CJ. Wild-type TTR neuropathy with cardiomyopathy presenting with burning feet. Neurology. 2017;88(11):1101–2.

Part II
Myopathy Cases

Chapter 4
A 20-Year-Old Man with Acute Multi-organ Failure and Rhabdomyolysis

Lan Zhou and Susan C. Shin

History

A 20-year-old man with no significant past medical history was admitted to intensive care unit (ICU) for fulminant hepatic failure and encephalopathy. The night prior to the admission, the patient went to a nightclub with his girlfriend, where he ingested an unknown amount of "Molly" (purified derivative of 3,4-Methylenedioxy-methamphetamine (MDMA)). Later that evening the patient was noted to become confused and agitated, and he was brought to the emergency room from the night club. Upon arrival, the patient was hypertensive (BP: 218/168 mmHg), tachycardic (HR: 190 beats/minute), febrile (T: 109° F), rigid, diaphoretic and encephalopathic. He was intubated due to poor mental status and for airway protection. He was found to have fulminant liver failure, disseminated intravascular coagulation, and renal failure. He developed clinical seizures, and head CT and brain MRI revealed numerous subcortical punctate hemorrhages. A few days after the admission, he was found to have dark-color urine.

Physical Examination

The patient was not evaluated by a neurology team. According to the notes by ICU physicians, the patient's fever gradually resolved and there was no infection found. He was intubated and sedated. Cranial nerves were unremarkable with equal round and

L. Zhou (✉)
Departments of Neurology and Pathology, Boston University Medical Center, Boston, MA, USA
e-mail: lanzhou@bu.edu

S. C. Shin
Department of Neurology, Icahn School of Medicine at Mount Sinai, New York, NY, USA

L. Zhou et al. (eds.), *A Case-Based Guide to Neuromuscular Pathology*,
https://doi.org/10.1007/978-3-030-25682-1_4

reactive pupils. Corneal and gag reflexes were present. Spontaneous breathing was present. Muscle tone was diffusely reduced, but all extremities withdrew to nailbed pressure. Reflexes were 2+ and symmetric. Toes were downgoing bilaterally.

Investigations

Laboratory studies revealed ALT 4885 U/L (1–53 U/L), AST 3128 U/L (1–50 U/L), total bilirubin 6.1 mg/dL (0.1–1.2 mg/dL), LDH 2452 U/L (100–220 U/L), creatinine 5.17 mg/DL (0.7–1.2 MG/DL), and TSH 5.74 uIU/ML (0.34–5.6 uIU/ML). Serum creatine kinase (CK) level rapidly and markedly increased to 156,728 U/L (30–200 U/L) on day 12 post-admission. A right gastrocnemius muscle biopsy was performed on the following day when CK was 214,792 U/L.

Muscle Biopsy Findings

The right gastrocnemius muscle biopsy (Fig. 4.1) shows rare atrophic fibers and one regenerating fiber, which is non-specific and insignificant. There is no evidence of muscle necrosis or inflammation.

Final Diagnosis

Normal gastrocnemius muscle biopsy despite clinical rhabdomyolysis

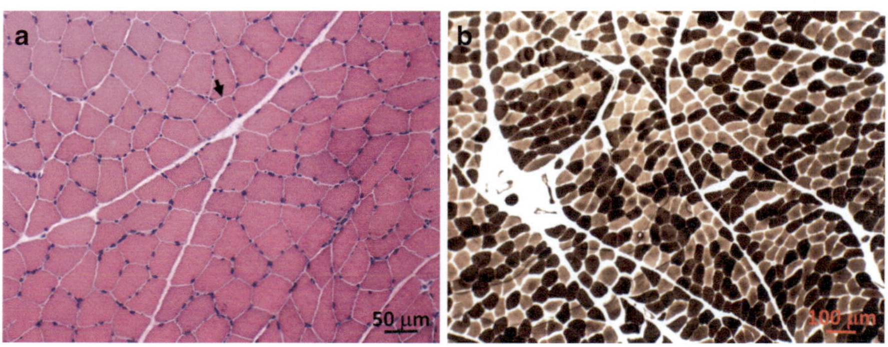

Fig. 4.1 (**a**) HE stain shows a rare atrophic fiber (arrow) but no myofiber necrosis or inflammation. (**b**) ATPase pH 9.4 stain shows normal fiber type distribution with no vacuolar changes to suggest myosin loss

Patient Follow-up

The CK level gradually returned to normal within 4 weeks. His multi-organ failure gradually resolved in 2 months. He was discharged from acute rehab in 3 months. He made a slow recovery over a course of 1 year.

Discussion

This is a striking case of rhabdomyolysis with an exceedingly high serum CK elevation but a normal muscle biopsy. It raises three management quesitons. (1) Was the muscle biopsy indicated? (2) Was it the right time to do a muscle biopsy? (3) Was it the right muscle selected for biopsy?

Rhabdomyolysis is defined as an acute muscle illness with marked serum CK elevation [1]. It results from acute necrosis of skeletal muscle with leakage of muscle constituents into blood circulation. It is a serious condition which can, but not always, cause myoglobinuria and acute renal failure, and even death [1–3]. According to a study of 475 inpatient cases with rhabdomyolysis [2], 60% were multifactorial. A detailed etiology analysis revealed that 46% cases were caused by exogenous toxins, 9% by trauma, 8% by neuroleptic malignant syndrome, 7% by seizures, and 7% idiopathic. About 10% of the cases were caused by underlying myopathies, including idiopathic inflammatory myopathies (27/475), metabolic myopathies (10/475), viral myositis (5/475), muscular dystrophies (3/475), and sarcoid myopathy (2/475). The most common cause of rhabdomyolysis is the exposure to exogenous toxins, including alcohol, illicit drugs, and prescribed medications with myotoxicity, such as antipsychotics, statins, selective serotonin reuptake inhibitors (SSRIs), Zidovudine, and Colchicine, among others. The purpose of a muscle biopsy in this setting is to determine whether the patient has an underlying myopathy that may require a specific treatment. Rhabdomyolysis itself does not need a muscle biopsy to confirm. In regard to the case presented here, the patient was known to suffer from the MDMA toxicity. MDMA is an amphetamine derivative. It is a popular recreational drug for adolescents and young adults who have misbelieve that the drug is safe. MDMA has unpredictable toxicity which can be life-threatening and fatal. Acute toxicity is caused by its sympathomimetic effects and serotonin syndrome, which can manifest hyperpyrexia, hypertension, encephalopathy, cerebral hemorrhage, hyponatremia, seizures, multi-organ failure, muscle rigidity and rhabdomyolysis [4] as seen in this case. The cause of rhabdomyolysis in this case is clear, which is the acute MDMA toxicity, given the history of presentation and the lack of a past medical history. Therefore, a muscle biopsy is not indicated, especially in the acute setting.

In general, a muscle biopsy should not be done at the peak of CK elevation during rhabdomyolysis, because the biopsy at this time point is most likely to show massive myofiber necrosis which can obscure the pathology of underlying myopathy.

Muscle biopsy is not needed in the majority of the rhabdomyolysis cases, as an inciting cause other than a primary myopathy can be identified and controlled in these cases. If a primary myopathy is of concern, a muscle biopsy should be done after the resolution of rhabdomyolysis, which may take a few weeks [5]. A muscle biopsy should be considered if CK level does not return to normal in the absence of a known cause, which may suggest an underlying primary myopathy, or if rhabdomyolysis is recurrent, which is commonly seen in metabolic myopathies. Patients with metabolic myopathies often report exercise intolerance, and rhabdomyolysis is usually triggered by strenuous physical activity.

It is surprising that the muscle biopsy in this case was unrevealing even the biopsy was done on the day when the patient's CK level was exceedingly high (>200,000 U/L). The importance of choosing a right muscle for biopsy cannot be overemphasized. Muscles are not equally affected by a disease process. While the majority of myopathies predominantly affect proximal limb muscles, a few preferentially affect distal limb, trunk, or facial muscles. The yield of a muscle biopsy is not 100%, and sampling error occurs frequently. In order to minimize the sampling error and increase the yield of a muscle biopsy, it is crucial to target a muscle for biopsy. Muscle selection can be challenging and should be done by treating neurologist not surgeon. The selection should be based on the pattern of clinical weakness, electromyography (EMG) findings, and/or muscle imaging findings [5, 6]. In a chronic myopathy, one should choose a muscle which is weak but not severely weak (MRC >3) for biopsy. If a muscle is severely weak and atrophic, the biopsy may show end-stage fibrofatty tissue replacement with limited number of myofibers available for evaluation, which is non-diagnostic. If a myopathy is acute or subacute when muscle chronic changes have not developed, one may choose a more severely affected muscle for biopsy to catch primary muscle pathology. Since the majority of myopathies predominantly affect proximal limb muscles, deltoid, biceps, and quadriceps muscles are most commonly chosen for biopsy, and these muscles have sufficient norms established for comparison with respect to myofiber size and fiber type percentages [7, 8]. If a myopathy predominantly affects distal limb muscles, tibialis anterior and gastrocnemius muscles may be selected for biopsy if they are affected. EMG is very useful not only to diagnose and characterize a myopathy but also to help select a muscle for biopsy. One should not choose a muscle that had recent injection, trauma, or needle EMG examination for biopsy to avoid confounding "needle myopathy" [9]. Since muscle involvement is often symmetrical in a myopathy, needle EMG of limb muscles is usually done on one side, and the muscle for biopsy is selected from the other side. It is worth mentioning that EMG can be normal in a mild myopathy, and some myopathies may have focal or asymmetrical limb muscle involvement. In these settings, skeletal muscle MRI and ultrasound can be useful in targeting a radiologically affected muscle or muscle area for biopsy.

Pearls

1. Understanding muscle biopsy indications is important to avoid unnecessary biopsy.
2. Choosing a right muscle for biopsy is critical, as muscle disease does not affect every muscle equally. Muscle selection should be carefully done by treating neurologist not surgeon, and should be based on clinical weakness, EMG findings, and/or muscle imaging findings.
3. The purpose of a muscle biopsy in a patient with rhabdomyolysis is to determine whether there is an underlying primary myopathy that may require specific management.
4. The most common cause of rhabdomyolysis is exogenous toxin exposure. An underlying primary myopathy is only found in 10% of inpatient cases of rhabdomyolysis. Therefore, the majority of patients with rhabdomyolysis do not need muscle biopsy.
5. A muscle biopsy should be considered in a patient with rhabdomyolysis if CK level does not return to normal without a known cause, which may suggest the presence of an underlying primary myopathy, or if rhabdomyolysis is recurrent, which is commonly seen in metabolic myopathies. A muscle biopsy should be done after rhabdomyolysis is resolved; it should not be done in the acute phase of rhabdomyolysis.

References

1. Gabow PA, Kaehny WD, Kelleher SP. The spectrum of rhabdomyolysis. Medicine (Baltimore). 1982;61(3):141–52.
2. Melli G, Chaudhry V, Cornblath DR. Rhabdomyolysis: an evaluation of 475 hospitalized patients. Medicine (Baltimore). 2005;84(6):377–85.
3. Ward MM. Factors predictive of acute renal failure in rhabdomyolysis. Arch Intern Med. 1988;148(7):1553–7.
4. Davies N, English W, Grundlingh J. MDMA toxicity: management of acute and life-threatening presentations. Br J Nurs. 2018;27(11):616–22.
5. Nance JR, Mammen AL. Diagnostic evaluation of rhabdomyolysis. Muscle Nerve. 2015;51(6):793–810.
6. Dubowitz V, Sewry CA, Oldfors A. The procedure of muscle biopsy. In: Muscle biopsy: a practical approach. 4th ed: China: Saunders/Elsevier; 2013. p. 2–15.
7. Schiaffino S, Reggiani C. Fiber types in mammalian skeletal muscles. Physiol Rev. 2011;91(4):1447–531.
8. Staron RS, Hagerman FC, Hikida RS, Murray TF, Hostler DP, Crill MT, et al. Fiber type composition of the vastus lateralis muscle of young men and women. J Histochem Cytochem. 2000;48(5):623–9.
9. Engel WK. Focal myopathic changes produced by electromyographic and hypodermic needles. "Needle myopathy. Arch Neurol. 1967;16(5):509–11.

Chapter 5
A 45-Year-Old Woman with Proximal Limb Weakness and Skin Peeling on Fingertips

Lan Zhou, Susan C. Shin, and Chunyu Cai

History

A 45-year-old Caucasian woman presented to our neuromuscular clinic for evaluation of muscle stiffness and weakness. Seven months prior to the presentation, she developed stiffness and cramps in her hands and wrists. She saw a rheumatologist and did not receive a specific diagnosis. The symptoms partially resolved after taking a non-steroidal anti-inflammatory agent. She then developed stiffness in the muscles that surrounded her knees, especially in her hamstrings, which prevented her from doing yoga or squats. The symptom was worse in the morning and better after exercise. She subsequently experienced weakness getting out of a chair and walking up stairs. She also developed intermittent mild muscle pain around the shoulders and in the thighs. She returned to her rheumatologist who ordered serum creatine kinase (CK) level which came back markedly elevated at 13,000 U/L. She also saw a neurologist; the repeat CK level was 19,000 U/L. She denied pigmenturia or rigorous exercise prior to getting the CK checked. She underwent a left quadriceps muscle biopsy at a local hospital, which reportedly showed "a necrotizing myopathy consistent with rhabdomyolysis". She only took 3 days of steroids before the muscle

L. Zhou (✉)
Departments of Neurology and Pathology, Boston University Medical Center, Boston, MA, USA
e-mail: lanzhou@bu.edu

S. C. Shin
Department of Neurology, Icahn School of Medicine at Mount Sinai, New York, NY, USA
e-mail: susan.shin@mssm.edu

C. Cai
Department of Pathology, University of Texas Southwestern Medical Center, Dallas, TX, USA
e-mail: chunyu.cai@UTSouthwestern.edu

L. Zhou et al. (eds.), *A Case-Based Guide to Neuromuscular Pathology*,
https://doi.org/10.1007/978-3-030-25682-1_5

biopsy, which helped a little. She denied chill, fever, weight loss, or breathing abnormalities. She denied febrile illness, myotoxic drug exposure, or foreign travel. She had no significant past medical history, and was on no medications. Family history was significant for hypothyroidism in her sister. She was an office worker.

Physical Examination

General examination was notable for the skin peeling at her fingertips and dupuytren's contracture involving the left digit 3. There was no skin rash. Cardiopulmonary examination was normal. Neurologic examination showed normal mental status, cranial nerve functions, sensation, coordination, and gait. Motor examination showed normal muscle tone, normal muscle bulk, and weakness in the bilateral deltoid (MRC 4+/5), infraspinatus (5−/5), and iliopsoas (4/5) muscles. Deep tendon reflexes were 2+ throughout. Toes were downgoing bilaterally.

Investigations

Serum CK level was 8,017 U/L. Complete blood count (CBC) and comprehensive metabolic panel were normal. Antinuclear antibodies (ANA), anti-extractable nuclear antigen antibodies (ENA), and rheumatoid factor were negative. Myositis antibody panel showed a positive anti-Jo-1 autoantibody. TSH and vitamin D levels were normal. Nerve conduction study (NCS) was normal. Needle electromyography (EMG) showed an irritable myopathy. A left deltoid muscle biopsy was performed.

Muscle Biopsy Findings

The left deltoid muscle biopsy (Fig. 5.1) showed an inflammatory myopathy with preferential perifascicular myofiber necrosis (Fig. 5.1a). The inflammation was predominantly perimysial, with focal extension into endomysium (Fig. 5.1b). The alkaline phosphatase reactivity was increased in perimysial connective tissue, indicating connective tissue damage (Fig. 5.1c). Perifascicular atrophy was present in several fascicles, which was more noticeable in the ATPase stains (Fig. 5.1d). There was no COX-deficient fiber. The findings are consistent with an inflammatory myopathy and compatible with antisynthetase syndrome (ASS).

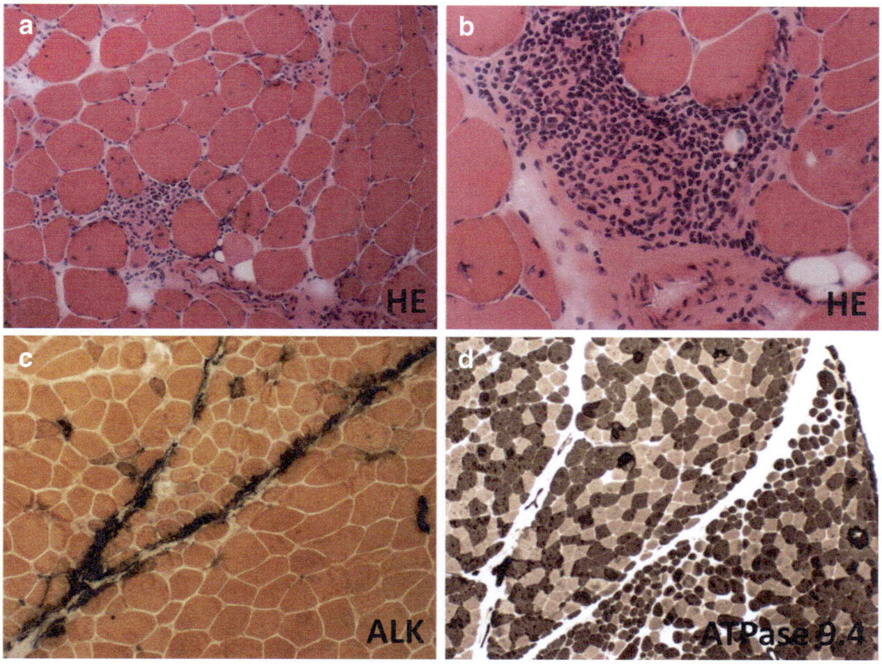

Fig. 5.1 Hematoxylin and eosin stain (HE) shows active myopathy with a large collection of lymphocytic infiltrates in perimysium and surrounding a perimysial blood vessel. Alkaline phosphatase stain (ALK) shows abnormal reactivity in scattered regenerating fibers and perimysium. APTase pH 9.4 stain (ATPase 9.4) shows 3 adjacent fascicles with perifascicular atrophy

Additional Investigation After the Muscle Biopsy Diagnosis

Given the biopsy findings and the presence of anti-Jo-1 autoantibody, the patient had computed tomography (CT) of chest, which showed patchy ground glass opacities, minimal reticulation, bronchiectasis, and mild honeycombing at the bilateral lung bases. Minimal ground glass opacities were also noted in the lingula. The findings are consistent with interstitial lung disease (ILD). CT of abdomen and pelvis was unremarkable. The age- and gender-appropriated cancer screening was unrevealing. During the follow up visit, she reported intermittent left hand coldness and cyanosis. Angiography revealed left brachial artery occlusion. Transesophageal echocardiogram (TEE) did not reveal any cardioembolic source.

Final Diagnosis

Antisynthetase Syndrome

Patient Follow-up

The patient was treated with Prednisone 40 mg once daily. She underwent left axillary-to-radial bypass using a non-reversed left greater saphenous vein harvested from the left leg. She was also treated with Coumadin. Her limb weakness and skin peeling at the fingertips (mechanic's hand) resolved 2 months after starting steroids. The symptoms of intermittent coldness and cyanosis of the left hand also resolved. She remained symptom free from her ILD standpoint. Chest CT abnormalities improved. The dose of prednisone was gradually tapered down to 20 mg daily. She tolerated the steroids well. She did not want to take a chronic immunosuppressive agent to spare the steroids use. She continued to do well 4 years after the initiation of the steroids treatment.

Discussion

The classification of idiopathic inflammatory myopathies (IIM) has been continuously evolving owing to the advances in the characterization of muscle inflammatory cell infiltrates, muscle pathology phenotypes, and autoantibody associations [1–12]. Based on the clinical presentation, muscle pathological features, and serological findings, IIM are currently classified into 5 distinct subtypes which include inclusion body myositis (IBM), polymyositis (PM), dermatomyositis (DM), immune-mediated necrotizing myopathy (IMNM), and antisynthetase syndrome (ASS) [1, 10, 13]. The percentage of each subtype varies in different study cohorts [9, 14]. IMNM is the most common subtype in the large Japanese (177/460, 38.5%) [14] and French (91/260, 35.0%) [9] cohorts. This is followed by IBM in the Japanese cohort (73/460, 15.9%) and French cohort (77/260, 29.6%). DM and ASS account for 12.2% and 11.1%, respectively, in the Japanese cohort, and 20.0% and 15.4%, respectively, in the French cohort. PM is rare, accounting for 4.1% in the Japanese cohort but none in the French cohort [9, 14], as most of the PM cases fall into IMNM or ASS after these 2 subtypes have been added to the IIM classification list [9]. In addition, PM associated with connective tissue diseases is often called "overlap myositis" rather than PM. Besides IIM, inflammatory myopathies also include rare eosinophilic fasciitis, focal myositis, and sarcoid granulomatous myositis [1].

Autoantibodies play an important role in shaping the current classification of IIM [1]. They correlate with the severity of muscle disease, extra-muscular manifestations, muscle pathology phenotypes, cancer risk, and treatment response [9, 14]. There are 16 myositis-specific autoantibodies associated with IIM, 8 with ASS, 5 with DM, 2 with IMNM, and 1 with IBM. The myositis-specific autoantibodies associated with ASS target aminoacyl-tRNA synthetases, including histidyl (Jo-1), threnyl (PL-7), alanyl (PL-12), isoleucyl (OJ), glycyl (EJ), asparaginyl (KS), phenylalanyl (ZO), and tyrosyl (YRS/HA) tRNA synthetases [15]. The 5 myositis-specific autoantibodies associated with DM target complex nucleosome remodeling histone deacetylase (Mi-2), melanoma differentiation-associated gene 5 (MDA5), small ubiquitin-like modifier activating enzyme (SAE), nuclear matrix protein 2

(NXP2), and transcription intermediary factor 1γ (TIF-1γ). The two myositis-specific autoantibodies associated with IMNM target signal recognition particle (SRP) and anti-3-hydroxy-3-methyglutaryl-coenzyme A reductase (HMGCR). Anti-NT5C1A antibody is associated with IBM, but it can also be present in Sjogren's syndrome and systemic lupus erythematosus (SLE). Myositis-associated antibodies include ANA, anti-Ro/SSA, anti-PM-Scl, anti-Ku, and anti-U2 snRNP.

IIM, except for IBM which is discussed in a separate chapter in this book, are autoimmune myopathies that manifest subacute, progressive, proximal limb weakness. While DM can affect both children and adults, PM, IMNM, and ASS predominantly affect adults. These subtypes also differ in the muscle disease severity, extra-muscular manifestations, serum autoantibody association, muscle biopsy features, and treatment response. In general, the muscle disease is mild in ASS but relatively severe in IMNM, especially in SRP-myopathy and statin-naïve HMGCR-myopathy which are discussed in a separate chapter. DM has a wide spectrum, which can be mild or refractory. Serum CK level is usually markedly elevated in IMNM and ASS, less elevated in PM and DM, and can be normal in DM. EMG typically shows an irritable myopathy. Extra-muscular manifestations are a feature of DM and ASS, less commonly seen in autoantibody-negative IMNM, and rare in autoantibody-positive IMNM. Typical skin lesions seen in DM include Gottron papules in finger knuckles, heliotrope erythema in eyelids, and rash in cheek, chest, shoulders, upper arms, and thighs. The presence of anti-MAD-5 autoantibody is associated with severe ILD, skin ulcers, and arthritis but mild muscle weakness. Calcinosis is mainly seen in juvenile DM and associated with anti-NXP-2 autoantibody. The presence of anti-TIF-1γ autoantibody is associated with a high risk of developing malignancies.

ASS is characterized by the presence of anti-tRNA synthetase autoantibodies, myositis, ILD, non-erosive arthritis, mechanic's hands, and Raynaud's phenomenon [8, 16]. The diagnostic criteria of ASS was developed in 2010 [17] and revised in 2011 [18]. To be diagnosed with ASS, one must have an anti-tRNA synthetase autoantibody and meet two major or one major and two minor criteria. The major criteria include ILD and myositis. The minor criteria include arthritis, Raynaud's phenomenon, and mechanic's hands. Therefore, the diagnosis of ASS requires clinical, serological, radiological, and pathological evaluation which may include serum CK and myositis antibody panel, NCS/EMG, high resolution computed tomography (HRCT) of chest, and muscle or lung biopsy. Our patient had anti-Jo-1 antibody and presented with myositis, arthralgia, mechanic's hands, and ILD, typical for ASS. In addition, our patient also had vasculopathy with left brachial artery occlusion. Vasculopathy is a known extra-muscular manifestation in dermatomyositis [19]; it has also been reportedly in association with ASS [20].

ASS has a female predominance with a mean age at onset of 60.2 years in one study cohort [21]. The most common manifestation in ASS is ILD with a prevalence of 86%, followed by myositis (73%) and arthritis (60%) [22]. Mechanic's hands with hyperkeratosis and scaling are common but often subtle. ILD is associated with the high morbidity and mortality of the disease. The cancer risk in ASS is low. Anti-Jo-1 autoantibody is by far the most common autoantibody in ASS. Anti-PL-7, anti-PL-12, anti-OJ, and anti-EJ autoantibodies are less common. Other autoantibodies are rare. While anti-Jo-1, anti-EJ, and anti-PL-7 autoantibodies are most often associated with myositis, anti-PL-12 autoantibody is often associated with amyopathic DM or ILD [23].

Muscle biopsy is useful to support the diagnosis of ASS myositis and to rule out other muscle diseases. The characteristic muscle pathological changes seen in ASS myositis are damages to both myofibers and perimysial connective tissue. Inflammation, when present, is most commonly perivascular in the perimysium (Figs. 5.1b and 5.2A1 and B1) that can extend into nearby endomysium. However, cases of predominantly endomysial inflammation with lymphocyte rimming viable myofibers are present (Fig. 5.2C1). Acute myofiber damages (i.e. necrotic fibers, myophagocytic fibers, regenerating fibers) can be scattered throughout but more frequent in the perifascicular region (Fig. 5.2A1). The preferential involvement of perimysial fibers is often more evident on the MHC1 and C5b-9 immunostains. MHC1 may show diffuse or patchy upregulation in myofibers, with perifascicular accentuation (Fig. 5.2A2, B2, and C2). C5b-9 shows strong sarcoplasmic reactivity in necrotic fibers (Fig. 5.2A3 black arrows), and sarcolemmal reactivity in viable but abnormal perifascicluar myofibers (Fig. 5.2A3 red arrows). True perifascicular atrophy with uniform small atrophic fibers (Fig. 5.1d) is uncommon in ASS myositis. Rather, the presence of frequent small regenerating fibers (highlighted by alkaline phosphatase stain, Fig. 5.2A4 arrows) interspersed by normal sized myofibers in the perifascicular region may give the appearance of patchy, uneven perifascicular atrophy (Fig. 5.2A1). Chronic myopathic changes (i.e. split fibers, hypertrophic fibers, interstitial fibrosis) are usually absent. The perimysial connective tissue damage is often widespread, best viewed in alkaline phosphatase stain (Figs. 5.1c, 5.2A4 and B4). Perimysial capillary abnormalities, including endothelial tubuloreticular inclusions (Fig. 5.2A5, arrow) and capillary C5b-9 deposition (Fig. 5.2A3, yellow arrows) are also common findings, although usually less pronounced than those in dermatomyositis. Intranuclear actin aggregate (Fig. 5.2B5, arrow) has been reported as a specific finding in ASS myositis [24].

Dermatomyositis shares many common pathological features with ASS myositis, including perifascicular atrophy, capillary C5b-9 deposition, endothelial tubuloreticular inclusions, and MHC1 upregulation in perifascicular fibers. ASS myositis usually has more widespread connective tissue damage evident on the alkaline phosphatase stain. Perifascicular atrophy in ASS is often irregular or patchy, composed of necrotic and regenerating fibers, with retained COX expression. DM, on the other hand, usually has uniform perifascicular atrophy that spans the full length of a fascicle (Fig. 5.3a, b). Perimysial connective tissue damage is minimal (Fig. 5.3c). The perifascicular atrophic fibers show zonal loss of COX reactivity and relatively retained SDH reactivity (Fig. 5.3d) [25], which is a useful distinctive feature [26]. MHC1 upregulation is usually restricted to perifascicular fibers rather than the diffuse upregulation with perifascicular accentuation seen in ASS myositis (Figs. 5.3e and 5.2A2, B2, and C2). Capillary C5b-9 deposition (Fig. 5.3f) and endothelial tubuloreticular inclusions are more abundant than ASS myositis.

Overlap myositis secondary to a systemic autoimmune disease such as lupus, systemic sclerosis, or Sjogren's syndrome may also demonstrate inflammatory myositis with perimysial connective tissue damage. The muscle biopsy in this setting often demonstrates pan-fascicular rather than perifascicular involvement (Fig. 5.4a). Regenerating fibers (Fig. 5.4b) and necrotic fibers (Fig. 5.4c) are ran-

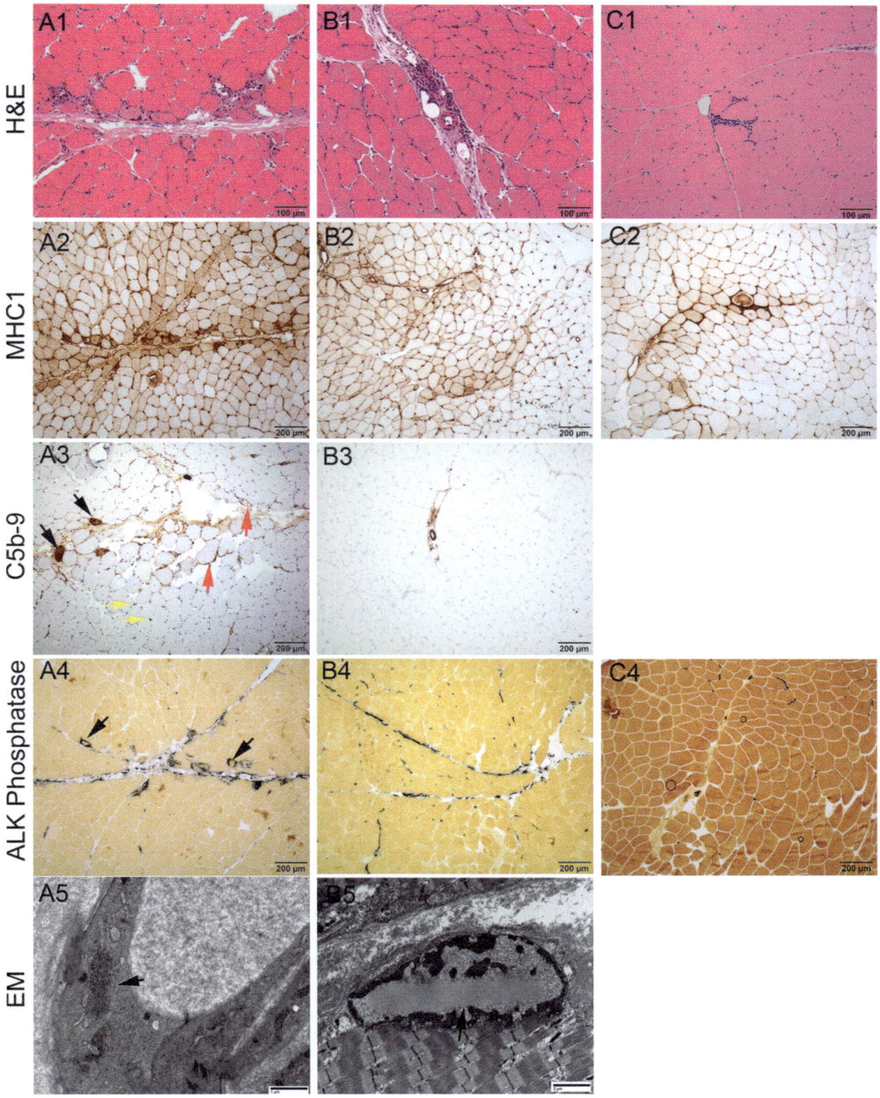

Fig. 5.2 Columns A-C represent three different patient's muscle biopsies, all with myopathy and confirmed presence of serum anti-Jo-1 autoantibody. Case A shows perifascicular necrotizing myopathy (**A1**) and diffuse MHC1 upregulation with perifascicular accentuation (**A2**). C5b-9 immunostain highlights necrotic fibers (**A3**, black arrows), sarcolemmal stain of some viable perifascicular fibers (**A3**, red arrows) and capillary reactivity (**A3**, yellow arrows). Alkaline phosphatase stain shows increased perimysial connective tissue reactivity and regenerating fibers (**A4**, black arrows). EM shows rare endothelial tubuloreticular inclusions (**A5**). Case B shows focal perivascular inflammation (**B1**) and patchy perifascicular myofiber MHC1 upregulation (**B2**). There is no significant myofiber necrosis (**B3**). Alkaline phosphatase stain shows increased perimysial connective tissue reactivity (**B4**). EM shows intranuclear actin aggregate (**B5**, arrow). Case C shows focal endomysial lymphocytic inflammation that rims a myofiber (**C1**). MHC1 immunostain shows patchy upregulation near the lymphocytic infiltrate and perimysium (**C2**). There is no significant myofiber necrosis or connective tissue alkaline phosphatase activity (**C4**)

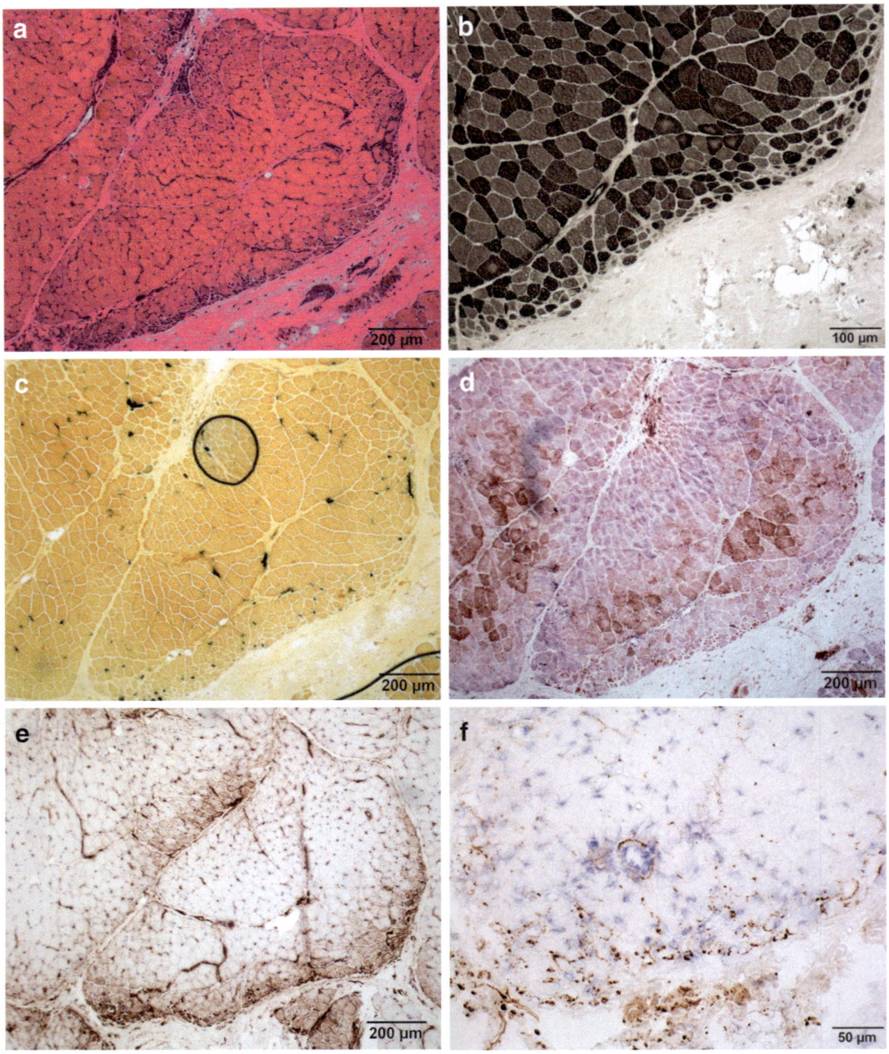

Fig. 5.3 Quadriceps muscle biopsy from an 8-year-old girl with dermatomyositis. (**a**) H&E shows uniform perifascicular atrophy with no skipping areas. (**b**) ATPase 9.4 highlights perifascicular atrophy and type 2 fiber atrophy. (**c**) Alkaline phosphatase shows no perimysial connective tissue damage or regenerating fibers in the perifascicular myofibers. (**d**) COX/SDH combination stain shows zonal loss of COX reactivity (brown) in the perifascicular fibers and relatively retained SDH reactivity (blue). (**e**) MHC class I immunostain shows selective upregulation in perifascicular fibers but not the fibers in the center of the fascicle. (**f**) C5b-9 immunostain shows terminal complement complex deposition in capillaries. There is no significant myofiber necrosis

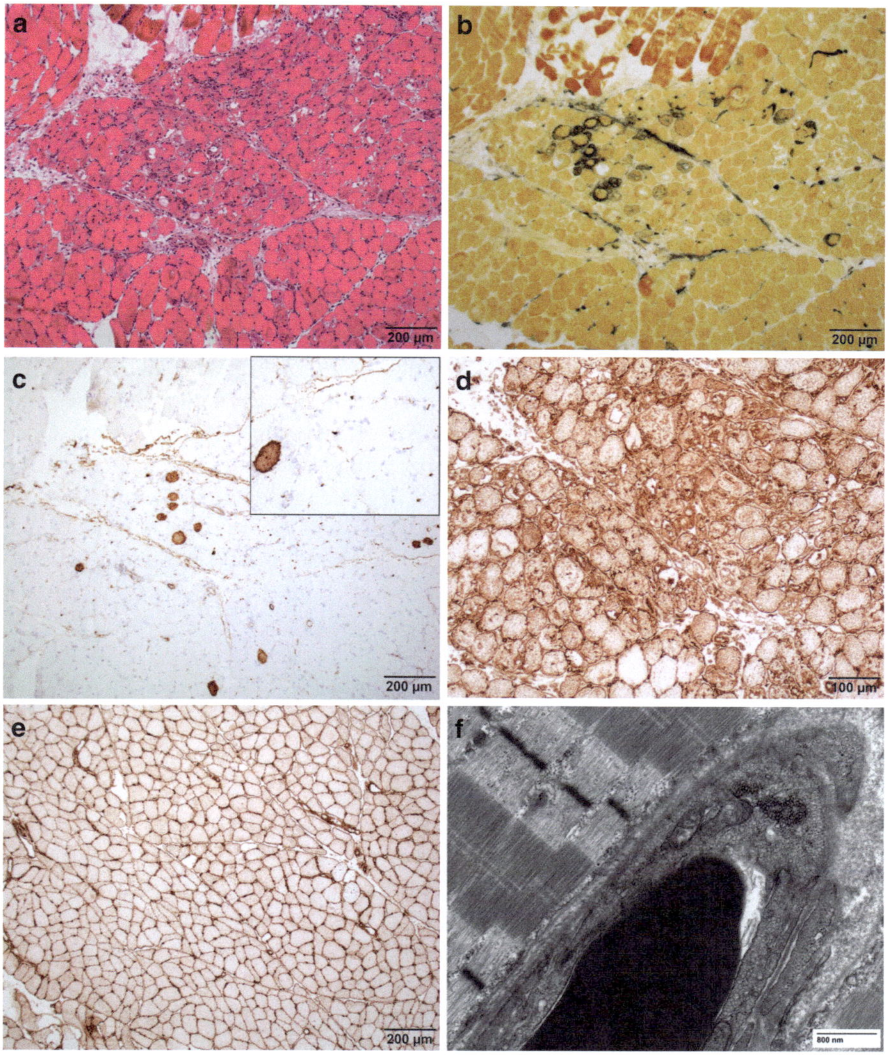

Fig. 5.4 Quadriceps muscle biopsy from a 35-year-old woman with lupus myositis. (**a**) H&E shows inflammatory myositis with pan-fascicular involvement. There is no perifascicular atrophy. (**b**) Alkaline phosphatase shows perimysial reactivity and frequent regenerating fibers. (**c**) C5b-9 immunostain shows frequent scattered necrotic fibers and capillary C5b-9 reactivity (inset). (**d**, **e**) MHC class I immunostain shows diffuse myofiber reactivity in both the myopathic region (**d**) and histologically normal region (**e**). (**f**) EM shows frequent endothelial tubuloreticular inclusions in capillaries

domly distributed. Capillary complement complex deposition is random (Fig. 5.4c). MHC1 is diffusely upregulated, even in histologically normal regions (Fig. 5.4d, e). Tubuloreticular inclusions (Fig. 5.4f) are frequently seen in patients with lupus, but rarely seen in patients with scleroderma or Sjogren's syndrome [27]. It should be noted that a wide range of overlapping pathology can be seen in ASS myositis, DM, and overlap myositis, and distinction is not always possible on the basis of pathology alone. Correlation with clinical symptomatology and serum autoantibody status is highly recommended.

Management of patients with ASS often requires multidisciplinary care provided by specialists in neurology, rheumatology, pulmonology, and rehabilitation. Corticosteroids is typically used as the first-line therapy, which can be used as monotherapy in mild cases. Additional immunosuppressive agents, such as azathioprine, mycophenolate mofeti, tacrolimus, rituximab, and cyclophosphamide, may be used for treating severe and refractory cases or as steroids-sparing agents. Once the disease symptoms improve and stabilize, immunosuppressive agents can be tapered. There are no research data, however, to guide the length of the immunosuppressive therapy or the rate of tapering. Myositis in ASS is usually mild, and it responds relatively well to immunosuppressive therapy [21] as seen in our patient.

Pearls

Clinical Pearls

1. IIM are currently classified into IBM, PM, DM, IMNM, and ASS with distinct clinical, serological, and muscle pathological features in each subtype.
2. Diagnostic evaluation of patients with IIM includes serum CK, myositis antibody panel, NCS/EMG, and muscle biopsy. High resolution chest CT is also important in evaluating patients with ASS.
3. ASS is characterized by the presence of anti-tRNA synthetase autoantibodies, myositis, ILD, arthritis, mechanic's hands, and Raynaud's phenomenon. The most common antisynthetase antibody detected in ASS is anti-Jo-1 autoantibody.
4. Muscle involvement in ASS manifests subacute, progressive, proximal limb weakness. Muscle weakness in ASS is usually mild and responds well to immunosuppression.
5. CK is often markedly elevated in ASS, EMG usually shows an irritable myopathy, and a muscle biopsy is useful to support the diagnosis and to rule out other muscle diseases.
6. Patients with ASS often require multidisciplinary care provided by neurologists, rheumatologists, pulmonologists, and physiatrists.

Pathology Pearls

1. The hallmarks of ASS myositis are perifascicular myofiber necrosis, perimysial connective tissue damage, and perivascular lymphocytic inflammation.
2. Muscle involvement is patchy in ASS. The presence of the above diagnostic features may be variable.
3. Diagnostic features on EM include myofiber intranuclear actin aggregates and capillary endothelial tubuloreticular inclusions. The former is reported to be specific for AAS myositis. The latter is usually less abundant and less well-formed than those seen in dermatomyositis.
4. Compared with dermatomyositis, ASS myositis often has more prominent perifascicular connective tissue damage and myofiber necrosis, less uniform perifascicular atrophy, and no zonal loss of COX reactivity in perifascicular fibers.

References

1. Allenbach Y, Benveniste O, Goebel HH, Stenzel W. Integrated classification of inflammatory myopathies. Neuropathol Appl Neurobiol. 2017;43(1):62–81.
2. Bohan A, Peter JB. Polymyositis and dermatomyositis (second of two parts). N Engl J Med. 1975;292(8):403–7.
3. Bucelli RC, Pestronk A. Immune myopathies with perimysial pathology: clinical and laboratory features. Neurol Neuroimmunol Neuroinflamm. 2018;5(2):e434.
4. Carpenter S, Karpati G, Heller I, Eisen A. Inclusion body myositis: a distinct variety of idiopathic inflammatory myopathy. Neurology. 1978;28(1):8–17.
5. Dalakas MC. Polymyositis, dermatomyositis and inclusion-body myositis. N Engl J Med. 1991;325(21):1487–98.
6. De Bleecker JL, De Paepe B, Aronica E, de Visser M, Group EMMBS, Amato A, et al. 205th ENMC International Workshop: pathology diagnosis of idiopathic inflammatory myopathies part II 28-30 March 2014, Naarden, The Netherlands. Neuromuscul Disord. 2015;25(3):268–72.
7. Hoogendijk JE, Amato AA, Lecky BR, Choy EH, Lundberg IE, Rose MR, et al. 119th ENMC international workshop: trial design in adult idiopathic inflammatory myopathies, with the exception of inclusion body myositis, 10–12 October 2003, Naarden, The Netherlands. Neuromuscul Disord. 2004;14(5):337–45.
8. Love LA, Leff RL, Fraser DD, Targoff IN, Dalakas M, Plotz PH, et al. A new approach to the classification of idiopathic inflammatory myopathy: myositis-specific autoantibodies define useful homogeneous patient groups. Medicine (Baltimore). 1991;70(6):360–74.
9. Mariampillai K, Granger B, Amelin D, Guiguet M, Hachulla E, Maurier F, et al. Development of a new classification system for idiopathic inflammatory myopathies based on clinical manifestations and myositis-specific autoantibodies. JAMA Neurol. 2018;75(12):1528–37.
10. McGrath ER, Doughty CT, Amato AA. Autoimmune myopathies: updates on evaluation and treatment. Neurotherapeutics. 2018;15(4):976–94.
11. Pestronk A. Acquired immune and inflammatory myopathies: pathologic classification. Curr Opin Rheumatol. 2011;23(6):595–604.
12. Troyanov Y, Targoff IN, Tremblay JL, Goulet JR, Raymond Y, Senecal JL. Novel classification of idiopathic inflammatory myopathies based on overlap syndrome features and autoantibodies: analysis of 100 French Canadian patients. Medicine (Baltimore). 2005;84(4):231–49.

13. Schmidt J. Current classification and management of inflammatory myopathies. J Neuromuscul Dis. 2018;5(2):109–29.
14. Suzuki S, Uruha A, Suzuki N, Nishino I. Integrated diagnosis project for inflammatory myopathies: an association between autoantibodies and muscle pathology. Autoimmun Rev. 2017;16(7):693–700.
15. Satoh M, Tanaka S, Ceribelli A, Calise SJ, Chan EK. A comprehensive overview on myositis-specific antibodies: new and old biomarkers in idiopathic inflammatory myopathy. Clin Rev Allergy Immunol. 2017;52(1):1–19.
16. Witt LJ, Curran JJ, Strek ME. The diagnosis and treatment of antisynthetase syndrome. Clin Pulm Med. 2016;23(5):218–26.
17. Connors GR, Christopher-Stine L, Oddis CV, Danoff SK. Interstitial lung disease associated with the idiopathic inflammatory myopathies: what progress has been made in the past 35 years? Chest. 2010;138(6):1464–74.
18. Solomon J, Swigris JJ, Brown KK. Myositis-related interstitial lung disease and antisynthetase syndrome. J Bras Pneumol. 2011;37(1):100–9.
19. Papadopoulou C, McCann LJ. The vasculopathy of juvenile dermatomyositis. Front Pediatr. 2018;6:284.
20. Wang CH, Wang NC, Lin TY, Chen CH. Anti-Jo-1 myositis and the antiphospholipid syndrome showing right ventricular thrombus: a novel overlap syndrome with atypical presentation. Mod Rheumatol. 2014;24(5):865–8.
21. Noguchi E, Uruha A, Suzuki S, Hamanaka K, Ohnuki Y, Tsugawa J, et al. Skeletal muscle involvement in antisynthetase syndrome. JAMA Neurol. 2017;74(8):992–9.
22. Hervier B, Meyer A, Dieval C, Uzunhan Y, Devilliers H, Launay D, et al. Pulmonary hypertension in antisynthetase syndrome (ASS): prevalence, aetiology and survival. Eur Respir J. 2013;42(5):1271–82.
23. Hamaguchi Y, Fujimoto M, Matsushita T, Kaji K, Komura K, Hasegawa M, et al. Common and distinct clinical features in adult patients with anti-aminoacyl-tRNA synthetase antibodies: heterogeneity within the syndrome. PLoS One. 2013;8(4):e60442.
24. Stenzel W, Preusse C, Allenbach Y, Pehl D, Junckerstorff R, Heppner FL, et al. Nuclear actin aggregation is a hallmark of anti-synthetase syndrome-induced dysimmune myopathy. Neurology. 2015;84(13):1346–54.
25. Alhatou MI, Sladky JT, Bagasra O, Glass JD. Mitochondrial abnormalities in dermatomyositis: characteristic pattern of neuropathology. J Mol Histol. 2004;35(6):615–9.
26. Cai C, Anthony DC, Pytel P. A pattern-based approach to the interpretation of skeletal muscle biopsies. Mod Pathol. 2019;32(4):462–83.
27. Bronner IM, Hoogendijk JE, Veldman H, Ramkema M, van den Bergh Weerman MA, Rozemuller AJ, et al. Tubuloreticular structures in different types of myositis: implications for pathogenesis. Ultrastruct Pathol. 2008;32(4):123–6.

Chapter 6
A 75-Year-Old Man with Slowly Progressive Leg and Hand Weakness

Lan Zhou and Chunyu Cai

History

A 75-year-old Caucasian man was referred to our neuromuscular clinic for evaluation of leg and hand weakness. Eight years prior to the presentation, he developed mild leg weakness with difficulty getting out of a car. The weakness had slowly progressed, and he also noticed difficulty climbing stairs and picking up his feet. Five years later after bilateral knee replacement, he had to use a cane to walk. After another year, he had to use a walker and then a wheelchair. He also developed progressive, left greater than right, hand weakness with difficulty making a fist. He denied double vision, droopy eyelids, or difficulty in chewing, swallowing, or breathing. He denied muscle fasciculations but admitted to mild muscle atrophy in the thighs. There was no pain or numbness. He had been on lovastatin for 5 years, which was discontinued by his cardiologist 1 year prior to the presentation with no improvement of his limb weakness. He was evaluated by a local neurologist. Nerve conduction study (NCS) and electromyography (EMG) reportedly showed an axonal sensorimotor polyneuropathy. Cervical, thoracic, and lumbosacral spine magnetic resonance imaging (MRI) studies without contrast reportedly showed multi-level mild spine degenerative changes with no spinal cord or nerve root compression. Lumbosacral spine MRI also revealed bilateral psoas muscle atrophy. He was referred to our clinic for further evaluation. He had a past medical history of hypertension, hyperlipidemia,

L. Zhou (✉)
Departments of Neurology and Pathology, Boston University Medical Center, Boston, MA, USA
e-mail: lanzhou@bu.edu

C. Cai
Department of Pathology, University of Texas Southwestern Medical Center, Dallas, TX, USA
e-mail: chunyu.cai@UTSouthwestern.edu

L. Zhou et al. (eds.), *A Case-Based Guide to Neuromuscular Pathology*,
https://doi.org/10.1007/978-3-030-25682-1_6

diabetes mellitus, and osteoarthritis. His medications included aspirin, lisinopril, hydrochlorothiazide, spironolactone, glipizide, metformin, omeprazole, and acetaminophen. His family history was positive for hypertension and diabetes but negative for muscle or nerve diseases. He did not drink alcohol or smoke cigarettes. He was a retired information technology supervisor.

Physical Examination

General examination was unremarkable. There was no spine tenderness. Neurologic examination showed normal mental status and cranial nerve functions. Motor examination revealed normal muscle tone, mild atrophy in the left forearm flexors and bilateral quadriceps, and weakness in the left finger flexors (MRC 4−/5), right index finger flexor (4+/5), bilateral finger extensors (4+/5), hip flexors (4−/5), knee extensors (3/5), knee flexors (4+/5), and foot and toe dorsiflexors (right: 4+/5; left: 3/5). Neck extensors and flexors were strong. There was no muscle fasciculation, scapular winging, or spine scoliosis. Pinprick sensation was reduced from the toes to mid-calves and from the fingers to mid-forearms. Vibratory sensation was reduced at the toes. Joint position sense was intact. Deep tendon reflexes were 1+ at the biceps, triceps, and brachioradialis, and absent at the knees and ankles. Toes were downgoing bilaterally. He was unable to walk due to the lower limb weakness.

Investigations

Serum creatine kinase (CK) level was normal at 226 U/L. Aldolase level was also normal at 2.5 U/L (normal <7.7). Complete blood count (CBC), comprehensive metabolic panel (CMP), thyroid stimulating hormone (TSH), free T4, vitamin B12, serum immunofixation, and vitamin D levels were all normal. Antinuclear antibodies (ANA), anti-extractable nuclear antigen antibodies (ENA), and myositis antibody panel were all negative. Anti-cytosolic 5′-nucleotide 1A (cN1A; NT5C1A) and anti-3-hydroxy-3-methyglutaryl-coenzyme A reductase (HMGCR) autoantibodies were also negative. HbA1C was 7.8%. A repeat NCS showed a severe, length-dependent, sensorimotor, axonal polyneuropathy. Needle EMG of selected left limb muscles showed an irritable myopathy with abnormal spontaneous activities in the forms of fibrillation potentials and positive sharp waves, and early recruitment of motor units of small amplitudes and short durations in the biceps, triceps, flexor digitorum profundus (FDP), and vastus lateralis muscles. Needle EMG also showed mixed large and small motor unit potentials in the tibialis anterior muscle. A right vastus lateralis muscle biopsy was performed.

Muscle Biopsy Findings

The right vastus lateralis muscle biopsy (Fig. 6.1) showed a chronic active inflammatory myopathy with increased fiber size variation, a few necrotic and regenerating myofibers, patchy primary endomysial inflammation, several red rimmed sarcoplasmic vacuoles, abundant cytochrome c oxidase (COX)-deficient myofibers,

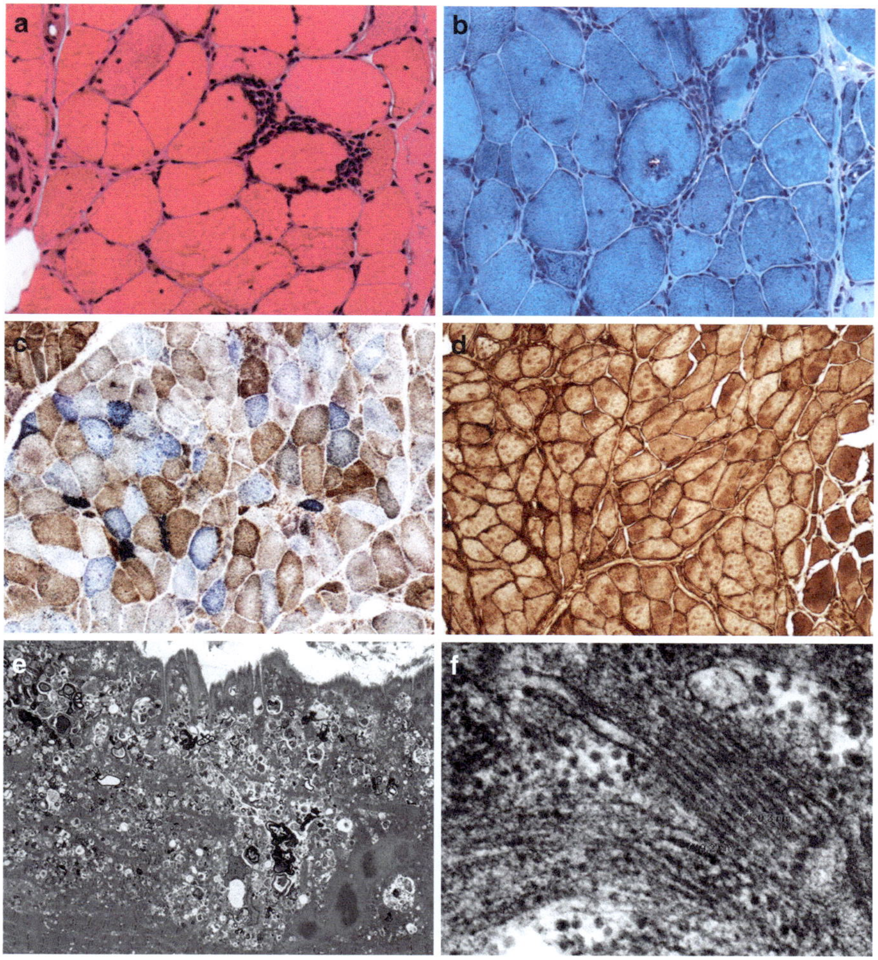

Fig. 6.1 Inclusion body myositis. Hematoxylin & eosin stain (**a**) shows lymphocytic invasion into viable myofibers. Gomori trichrome stain (**b**) shows a myofiber with sarcoplasmic red rimmed vacuole. COX/SDH stain (**c**) shows abundant COX-deficient myofibers (blue). MHC1 immunostain (**d**) shows diffuse sarcolemmal and sarcoplasmic upregulation of MHC1. EM (**e**: low power; **f**: high power) shows a vacuole containing abundant myeloid debris (**e**), and bundles of tubulofilamentous inclusions with individual filament measuring about 20 nm in diameter (**f**)

diffuse myofiber upregulation of class I major histocompatibility complex (MHC1), and increased endomysial connective tissue. Electron microscopy (EM) showed a few fibers containing small and large vacuoles consisting of myeloid debris, tubulo-filamentous inclusions with individual filament measuring about 20 nm in diameter, glycogen granules, and a few cytoplasmic bodies. The findings are characteristics of inclusion body myositis (IBM).

Final Diagnosis

Sporadic Inclusion Body Myositis.

Patient Follow-up

The diagnosis of IBM was discussed with the patient. He underwent physical therapy and occupational therapy. He had slow progression of his limb weakness over 2 years. His glycemic control improved after adjusting medications by his endocrinologist. His distal sensory deficits were stable.

Discussion

Sporadic inclusion body myositis (sIBM) is a type of idiopathic inflammatory myopathies (IIM) which also include polymyositis (PM), dermatomyositis (DM), antisynthetase syndrome (ASS), and immune-mediated necrotizing myopathy (IMNM) [1–3]. It is distinguished from the other types by its clinical weakness pattern, muscle biopsy features, autoantibody association, and resistance to immunosuppressive therapy. It is currently viewed as an inflammatory and degenerative muscle disease [4, 5].

The prevalence of sIBM varies in different populations and ethnic groups, ranging from 46 to 117 per million [6–8]. It is the second most common type of IIM, accounting for 15.9% (73/460) of IIM in a Japanese cohort [9] and 29.6% (77/260) in a French cohort [10]. The disease mainly affects men over age 50 years with the mean age of symptom onset ranging from 61–68 years. About 20% of the patients had a symptom onset in their 40s in one study cohort [11]. One of the current diagnostic criteria for sIBM is age at onset >45 years [12]. Young sIBM is more commonly seen in patients with HIV or HTLV infection, and sIBM is overrepresented in HIV-infected patients [13, 14].

The symptom onset of sIBM is usually insidious, and the progression is slow. The disease preferentially affects knee extensors and finger flexors. But the other limb muscles can be affected at an advanced stage. The initial symptom in a majority of the patients is caused by thigh muscle weakness with difficulty getting out of a car or climbing stairs and knee buckling when walking [15]. During the disease course, patients commonly develop finger flexor weakness with difficulty bending fingers to make a fist, and anterior distal leg muscle (tibialis anterior) weakness with difficulty picking up feet and resultant falls. The limb weakness is often asymmetrical as seen in our case. Difficulty swallowing (dysphagia) is not uncommon, which can cause weight loss and aspiration pneumonia, a major cause of mortality in sIBM. Respiratory weakness is mild and often asymptomatic. In rare cases of sIBM, patients present with head drop. Examination often shows limb weakness with asymmetry, more severely affecting knee extensors and finger flexors. Weakness may also be detected in ankle dorsiflexors, hip flexors, and finger extensors. Proximal upper limb weakness is uncommon and relatively mild if present. At a late stage, quadriceps and forearm muscle atrophy is prominent. Serum CK can be normal or mildly elevated, no greater than 15 times the upper limit of normal; it is rarely above 2000 U/L. EMG frequently shows fibrillation potentials and/or positive sharp waves, and mixed small and large motor unit potentials in the affected limb muscles [16]. Due to the late onset of the disease, asymmetrical limb weakness, common co-existing spine spondylosis and diabetes mellitus, normal or mildly elevated CK, and mixed large and small motor units on EMG, sIBM is often initially misdiagnosed with radiculopathy, neuropathy, or even motor neuron disease. A correct diagnosis can be delayed by several years [15] as seen in our case.

Anti-NT5C1A autoantibody was identified in sIBM in 2011 [17–19]. It helps not only explore the pathogenesis but also facilitate the diagnosis of sIBM. The test for detecting this autoantibody in serum is commercially available. This autoantibody test showed over 70% sensitivity and over 90% specificity for diagnosing sIBM [18, 20, 21]. It is highly specific for sIBM and rarely present in polymyositis, dermatomyositis, non-immune neuromuscular diseases, or non-neuromuscular autoimmune diseases such as systemic lupus erythematosus and Sjogren's syndrome [4]. The sensitivity and specificity of the test may vary due to different methods and cut-offs used by different laboratories. One study showed that female patients with sIBM were more likely to have a positive anti-NT5C1A autoantibody, and that sIBM patients with a positive anti-NT5C1A autoantibody were more likely to have dysphagia, facial weakness, respiratory muscle weakness, and severe leg weakness that requires assistive devices for ambulation [20]. The other studies did not find the association of this autoantibody with gender, age at onset, disease duration, weakness pattern, or prevalence of inflammation on muscle biopsy [18, 22]. It remains unclear whether the presence of this autoantibody influences muscle pathology, disease progression, or treatment response.

Muscle biopsy plays a key role in the diagnosis of sIBM, and the current diagnostic criteria for sIBM include both clinical and muscle biopsy features [12, 23]. Anti-NT5C1A autoantibody has not yet been incorporated into the diagnostic criteria. Muscle biopsy is particularly helpful at the early stage of the disease to avoid misdiagnosis or delay in making the correct diagnosis. We do see patients with isolated quadriceps weakness at the early stage of the disease, who subsequently develop finger flexor weakness after the muscle biopsy diagnosis of sIBM is made. It is important to select a muscle for biopsy to increase the diagnostic yield, as rimmed vacuoles, one of the key pathology features of sIBM, can be missed from muscle biopsies in 20% of patients with sIBM due to the sampling error [24]. The most commonly selected muscle for biopsy in sIBM is quadriceps. It should be noted that vastus lateralis and vastus medialis are affected sooner and greater than rectus femoris in sIBM, and rectus femoris can be relatively spared at the early stage of the disease [25]. Therefore, we usually biopsy vastus lateralis, and our biopsy yield is very high.

The characteristic features of sIBM on muscle biopsy include primary endomysial inflammation, mitochondrial abnormality, rimmed vacuoles and a background of chronic active myopathy. The inflammation is similar to polymyositis, dominated by T lymphocytes predominantly located in the endomysium that surround and invade viable myofibers, accompanied by diffuse MHC1 upregulation in myofibers. The mitochondria abnormality is reflected by the presence of substantially increased number of ragged red fibers on Gomori trichrome stain and COX-deficient fibers on COX or COX/SDH combined stains, far exceeding what is expected from the age related change. The vacuoles in sIBM contain red staining granules on Gomori trichrome and acid phosphatase stains, so called "red rimmed vacuoles". On EM, these red staining granules are composed of myeloid debris, also referred to as "myelinoid" or "lipidic" debris, due to their resemblance to myelin ovoids in peripheral nerve (Fig. 6.1e). The more characteristic inclusion is the tubulofilamentous inclusion, which is considered a form of amyloid and may show apple green bi-referengence on Congo red stain and bright fluorescence signal under fluorescence light through the red Rhodamine filter.

The diagnosis of sIBM is not difficult to make when all the diagnostic features are present on muscle biopsy. However, the presence of primary inflammation, MHC1 upregulation, and rimmed vacuoles are variable and may make the diagnosis challenging when absent. sIBM cases lacking rimmed vacuoles need to be differentiated from polymyositis with mitochondria abnormality and other inflammatory myopathies. In sIBM, the chronic myopathic changes (e.g. hypertrophied fibers, split fibers, interstitial fibrosis, and fatty tissue replacement) are usually much more prominent than in polymyositis. The presence of p62 and TDP43 positive protein aggregates in myofibers [26, 27] and a positive serum anti-NT5C1A antibody may help differentiate sIBM from polymyositis. The distinction is important as polymyositis with mitochondria abnormality may respond to methotrexate therapy [28].

Sporadic IBM patients who has been treated with corticosteroids may lack inflammation or MHC1 upregulation. These muscle biopsies show chronic myopathy with rimmed vacuoles that need to be differentiated from hereditary IBM (hIBM), myofibrillar myopathies, distal myopathies, limb girdle muscular dystrophies, and chronic denervation atrophy. Clinical history, family history, and weakness pattern are critical in differentiating these disease entities. hIBM patients usually present younger with atypical weakness patterns. Patients with UDP-N-acetylglucosamine 2-epimerase/N-acetylmannosamine kinase (GNE) mutations (hIBM2) typically show quadriceps-sparing muscle weakness [29]. Patients with myosin heavy chain 2 (MYH2) mutations (hIBM3) present with joint contracture, ophthalmoplegia, and weakness. Patients with valosin-containing protein (VCP) mutations present with the complex of IBM, Paget's disease of bone, and frontal temporal dementia (h-IBMPFD); some may also have features of amyotrophic lateral sclerosis or Charcot-Marie-Tooth disease. Muscle biopsies show prominent neurogenic features in addition to IBM [30]. Muscle biopsies in patients with desmin mutations (hIBM1) usually show myofibrillar myopathy with more prominent protein aggregates than rimmed vacuoles. Patients with oculopharyngeal muscular dystrophy (OPMD) caused by the PABPN1 mutation present with ptosis and dysphagia in addition to proximal limb weakness. Muscle biopsy (Fig. 6.2) shows inclusion body myopathy that lacks inflammation. The number of COX-deficient fibers may or may not be increased. The presence of intranuclear filamentous inclusions in a low percentage of myofibers is a distinguishing feature of the disease (Fig. 6.2e, f) [31]. In some cases with very chronic denervation atrophy, muscle biopsies may show marked fiber size variation, interstitial fibrosis and secondary myopathic changes that resemble a primary myopathy. Vacuoles can be present. These cases typically show fiber type grouping and lack substantial COX-deficient fibers.

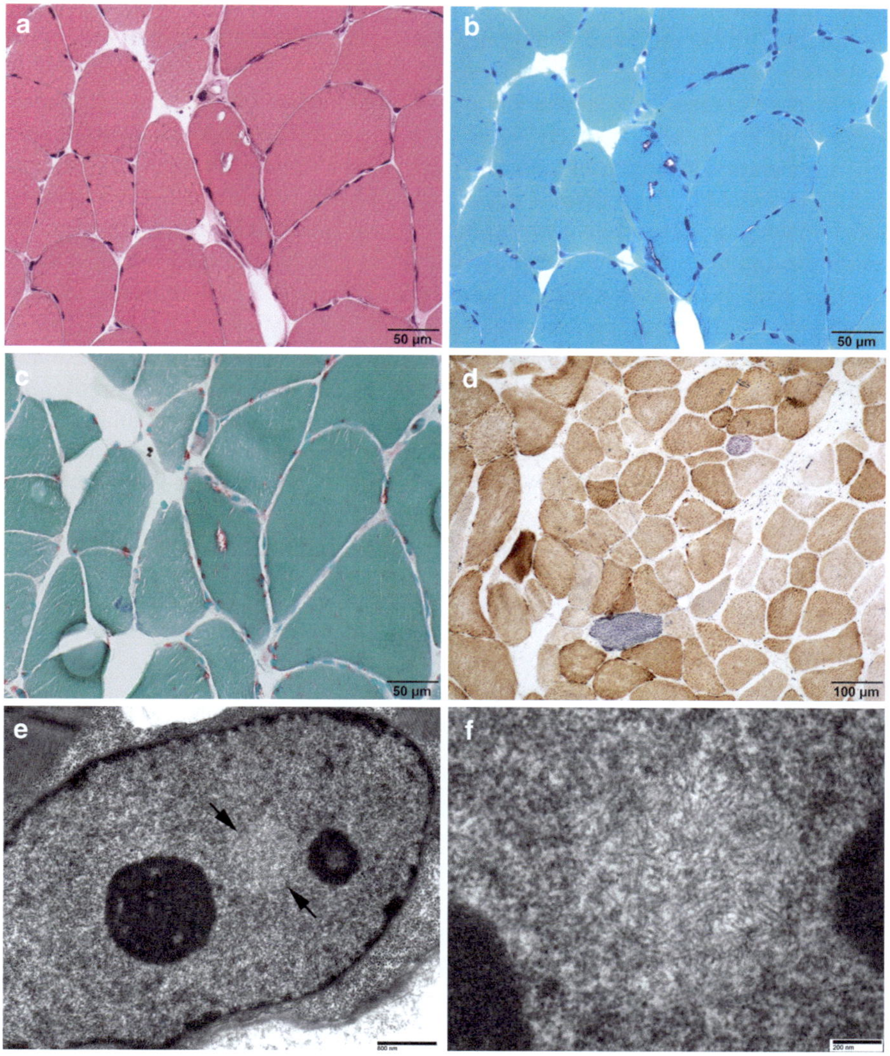

Fig. 6.2 A 90-year-old man with oculopharyngeal muscular dystrophy (OPMD). H&E stain (**a**) shows chronic myopathy with vacuoles. Gomori trichrome (**b**) and acid phosphatase (**c**) stains shows red granules in the vacuoles. COX/SDH stain (**d**) shows occasional COX deficient fibers, within the normal range for his age. Low (**e**, between arrows) and high (**f**) magnification images from EM shows intranuclear filamentous inclusions

Although sIBM is slowly progressive with a normal lifespan [32], the disease is debilitating with gradual loss of independent ambulation and hand dexterity. The mean time after the symptom onset for needing a cane is 7.5–10 years, and for needing a wheelchair is 13–15 years [11, 15, 32–34]. Aspiration pneumonia from dysphagia may cause premature mortality.

sIBM is resistant to immunosuppressive therapies that are routinely used for treating other types of IIM. There is no effective treatment for sIBM at this point. The management is mainly supportive. Rehabilitation is important to maximize function and prevent falls. Swallow evaluation and diet modification should be done in patients with dysphagia to prevent aspiration. Dysphagia may be treated transiently with pharyngoesophageal dilation or cricopharyngeal myotomy [35].

The development of effective therapy for sIBM relies on the thorough understanding of the disease pathogenesis. sIBM is currently viewed as an inflammatory and degenerative myopathy, as muscle biopsy shows both inflammatory and degenerative features [4, 5]. It remains unclear and debated whether sIBM is a primary inflammatory or degenerative myopathy. Several lines of evidence supports the autoimmunity in sIBM, which includes the whole-genome linkage to an HLA autoimmune haplotype, a circulating autoantibody, a marked T cell signature in gene expression profile, the presence of clonal highly differentiated cytotoxic CD8+ T cells in blood and muscle that are resistant to many immunotherapies, primary endomysial inflammation with cytotoxic CD8+ T cells surrounding and infiltrating normal-appearing myofibers, and diffuse myofiber MHC1 upregulation [4]. Evidence that supports a prominent degenerative pathogenesis includes sarcoplasmic rimmed vacuoles, myofiber protein aggregates, mitochondrial abnormality with excessive COX-deficient myofibers, and lack of a favorable response to immunosuppression. The therapy development has been targeting both inflammation and degeneration [4, 5].

Pearls

Clinical Pearls

1. sIBM is a type of IIM with unique weakness pattern, EMG findings, autoantibody association, muscle biopsy features, and resistance to immunosuppressive therapies.
2. sIBM is an insidious, late-onset, progressive myopathy that predominantly affects men above 50 years of age with preferential and asymmetrical involvement of knee extensors and finger flexors.
3. Young sIBM is more commonly seen in patients with HIV or HTLV infection. sIBM is overrepresented in HIV-infected patients. Viral infection status should be evaluated in patients with young-onset sIBM.

4. Serum CK is normal or mildly elevated (no greater than 15 times the upper limit of normal), and EMG often shows fibrillation potentials and/or positive sharp waves and mixed small and large motor unit potentials in affected muscles in sIBM.
5. Serum anti-NT5C1A autoantibody has over 70% sensitivity and over 90% specificity for sIBM. This autoantibody may be associated with increased likelihood of dysphagia, facial weakness, respiratory muscle weakness, and severe leg weakness requiring assistive devices for ambulation.
6. Muscle biopsy plays a key role in the diagnosis of sIBM. Vastus lateralis and vastus medialis are affected sooner and greater than rectus femoris in sIBM; choosing one of the vasti for biopsy may increase the diagnostic yield especially at the early stage of the disease.
7. Currently there is no effective therapy for sIBM. The management is mainly supportive to maximize function and prevent falls and aspiration.

Pathology Pearls

1. The characteristic muscle biopsy features of sIBM include primary endomysial inflammation, red rimmed vacuoles, excessive COX-deficient fibers, a few ragged red fibers, diffuse myofiber upregulation of MHC1, and a background of chronic active myopathy. These features may or may not all be present.
2. EM often shows sarcoplasmic vacuoles containing myeloid debris, glycogen granules, and characteristic tubulofilamentous inclusions with individual filament measuring 15–20 nm in diameter.

References

1. Allenbach Y, Benveniste O, Goebel HH, Stenzel W. Integrated classification of inflammatory myopathies. Neuropathol Appl Neurobiol. 2017;43(1):62–81.
2. McGrath ER, Doughty CT, Amato AA. Autoimmune myopathies: updates on evaluation and treatment. Neurotherapeutics. 2018;15(4):976–94.
3. Schmidt J. Current classification and Management of Inflammatory Myopathies. J Neuromuscul Dis. 2018;5(2):109–29.
4. Greenberg SA. Inclusion body myositis: clinical features and pathogenesis. Nat Rev Rheumatol. 2019;15:257–72.
5. Weihl CC, Mammen AL. Sporadic inclusion body myositis - a myodegenerative disease or an inflammatory myopathy. Neuropathol Appl Neurobiol. 2017;43(1):82–91.
6. Callan A, Capkun G, Vasanthaprasad V, Freitas R, Needham M. A systematic review and meta-analysis of prevalence studies of sporadic inclusion body myositis. J Neuromuscul Dis. 2017;4(2):127–37.
7. Keshishian A, Greenberg SA, Agashivala N, Baser O, Johnson K. Health care costs and comorbidities for patients with inclusion body myositis. Curr Med Res Opin. 2018;34(9):1679–85.

8. Lefter S, Hardiman O, Ryan AM. A population-based epidemiologic study of adult neuromuscular disease in the Republic of Ireland. Neurology. 2017;88(3):304–13.
9. Suzuki S, Uruha A, Suzuki N, Nishino I. Integrated Diagnosis Project for Inflammatory Myopathies: an association between autoantibodies and muscle pathology. Autoimmun Rev. 2017;16(7):693–700.
10. Mariampillai K, Granger B, Amelin D, Guiguet M, Hachulla E, Maurier F, et al. Development of a new classification system for idiopathic inflammatory myopathies based on clinical manifestations and myositis-specific autoantibodies. JAMA Neurol. 2018;75(12):1528–37.
11. Badrising UA, Maat-Schieman ML, van Houwelingen JC, van Doorn PA, van Duinen SG, van Engelen BG, et al. Inclusion body myositis. Clinical features and clinical course of the disease in 64 patients. J Neurol. 2005;252(12):1448–54.
12. Rose MR, Group EIW. 188th ENMC international workshop: inclusion body myositis, 2-4 December 2011, Naarden, The Netherlands. Neuromuscul Disord. 2013;23(12):1044–55.
13. Cupler EJ, Leon-Monzon M, Miller J, Semino-Mora C, Anderson TL, Dalakas MC. Inclusion body myositis in HIV-1 and HTLV-1 infected patients. Brain. 1996;119(Pt 6):1887–93.
14. Lloyd TE, Pinal-Fernandez I, Michelle EH, Christopher-Stine L, Pak K, Sacktor N, et al. Overlapping features of polymyositis and inclusion body myositis in HIV-infected patients. Neurology. 2017;88(15):1454–60.
15. Needham M, James I, Corbett A, Day T, Christiansen F, Phillips B, et al. Sporadic inclusion body myositis: phenotypic variability and influence of HLA-DR3 in a cohort of 57 Australian cases. J Neurol Neurosurg Psychiatry. 2008;79(9):1056–60.
16. Joy JL, Oh SJ, Baysal AI. Electrophysiological spectrum of inclusion body myositis. Muscle Nerve. 1990;13(10):949–51.
17. Salajegheh M, Lam T, Greenberg SA. Autoantibodies against a 43 KDa muscle protein in inclusion body myositis. PLoS One. 2011;6(5):e20266.
18. Larman HB, Salajegheh M, Nazareno R, Lam T, Sauld J, Steen H, et al. Cytosolic 5′-nucleotidase 1A autoimmunity in sporadic inclusion body myositis. Ann Neurol. 2013;73(3):408–18.
19. Pluk H, van Hoeve BJ, van Dooren SH, Stammen-Vogelzangs J, van der Heijden A, Schelhaas HJ, et al. Autoantibodies to cytosolic 5′-nucleotidase 1A in inclusion body myositis. Ann Neurol. 2013;73(3):397–407.
20. Goyal NA, Cash TM, Alam U, Enam S, Tierney P, Araujo N, et al. Seropositivity for NT5c1A antibody in sporadic inclusion body myositis predicts more severe motor, bulbar and respiratory involvement. J Neurol Neurosurg Psychiatry. 2016;87(4):373–8.
21. Greenberg SA. Cytoplasmic 5′-nucleotidase autoantibodies in inclusion body myositis: isotypes and diagnostic utility. Muscle Nerve. 2014;50(4):488–92.
22. Lloyd TE, Christopher-Stine L, Pinal-Fernandez I, Tiniakou E, Petri M, Baer A, et al. Cytosolic 5'-Nucleotidase 1A as a target of circulating autoantibodies in autoimmune diseases. Arthritis Care Res (Hoboken). 2016;68(1):66–71.
23. Lloyd TE, Mammen AL, Amato AA, Weiss MD, Needham M, Greenberg SA. Evaluation and construction of diagnostic criteria for inclusion body myositis. Neurology. 2014;83(5):426–33.
24. Chahin N, Engel AG. Correlation of muscle biopsy, clinical course, and outcome in PM and sporadic IBM. Neurology. 2008;70(6):418–24.
25. Phillips BA, Cala LA, Thickbroom GW, Melsom A, Zilko PJ, Mastaglia FL. Patterns of muscle involvement in inclusion body myositis: clinical and magnetic resonance imaging study. Muscle Nerve. 2001;24(11):1526–34.
26. Hiniker A, Daniels BH, Lee HS, Margeta M. Comparative utility of LC3, p62 and TDP-43 immunohistochemistry in differentiation of inclusion body myositis from polymyositis and related inflammatory myopathies. Acta Neuropathol Commun. 2013;1:29.
27. Temiz P, Weihl CC, Pestronk A. Inflammatory myopathies with mitochondrial pathology and protein aggregates. J Neurol Sci. 2009;278(1–2):25–9.
28. Levine TD, Pestronk A. Inflammatory myopathy with cytochrome oxidase negative muscle fibers: methotrexate treatment. Muscle Nerve. 1998;21(12):1724–8.

29. Vasconcelos OM, Raju R, Dalakas MC. GNE mutations in an American family with quadriceps-sparing IBM and lack of mutations in s-IBM. Neurology. 2002;59(11):1776–9.
30. Kazamel M, Sorenson EJ, McEvoy KM, Jones LK Jr, Leep-Hunderfund AN, Mauermann ML, et al. Clinical spectrum of valosin containing protein (VCP)-opathy. Muscle Nerve. 2016;54(1):94–9.
31. Blumen SC, Sadeh M, Korczyn AD, Rouche A, Nisipeanu P, Asherov A, et al. Intranuclear inclusions in oculopharyngeal muscular dystrophy among Bukhara Jews. Neurology. 1996;46(5):1324–8.
32. Benveniste O, Guiguet M, Freebody J, Dubourg O, Squier W, Maisonobe T, et al. Long-term observational study of sporadic inclusion body myositis. Brain. 2011;134.(Pt 11:3176–84.
33. Cortese A, Machado P, Morrow J, Dewar L, Hiscock A, Miller A, et al. Longitudinal observational study of sporadic inclusion body myositis: implications for clinical trials. Neuromuscul Disord. 2013;23(5):404–12.
34. Cox FM, Titulaer MJ, Sont JK, Wintzen AR, Verschuuren JJ, Badrising UA. A 12-year follow-up in sporadic inclusion body myositis: an end stage with major disabilities. Brain. 2011;134(Pt 11):3167–75.
35. Oh TH, Brumfield KA, Hoskin TL, Kasperbauer JL, Basford JR. Dysphagia in inclusion body myositis: clinical features, management, and clinical outcome. Am J Phys Med Rehabil. 2008;87(11):883–9.

Chapter 7
A 53-Year-Old Woman with Proximal Limb Weakness and Marked CK Elevation

Lan Zhou and Chunyu Cai

History

A 53-year-old Hispanic woman presented to our neuromuscular clinic for a second opinion on her inflammatory myopathy. Four years prior to the presentation, she began to notice bilateral leg weakness with difficulty climbing stairs. Shortly after, she also noticed upper arm weakness with difficulty lifting up her arms over her head. She saw a local rheumatologist and underwent a right vastus lateralis muscle biopsy. The biopsy reportedly showed acute myopathic changes with scanty interstitial inflammation, mild type 2 myofiber atrophy, and mild denervation atrophy. She was treated with prednisone 60 mg once daily which was gradually tapered to 15 mg once daily due to the side effects. She took methotrexate for a short period of time, and it was discontinued because of "a spot in the lung". She tried azathioprine 150 mg twice daily for 2 years, and it was discontinued due to the lack of effect. Upon presentation, she had been receiving monthly intravenous infusion of immunoglobulin (IVIg) for 1–1/2 years and taking oral mycophenylate 1000 mg twice daily for 4 months. She was also on prednisone 15 mg once daily. Despite these treatments, she had little improvement in her limb weakness. Serum creatine kinase (CK) level had been markedly elevated ranging from 2000s to 7000s U/L. She denied skin rash, joint pain, or respiratory symptoms. She reported frequent abdominal cramps after taking mycophenylate. Her past medical history was significant for hypertension, hyperlipidemia,

L. Zhou (✉)
Departments of Neurology and Pathology, Boston University Medical Center, Boston, MA, USA
e-mail: lanzhou@bu.edu

C. Cai
Department of Pathology, University of Texas Southwestern Medical Center, Dallas, TX, USA
e-mail: chunyu.cai@UTSouthwestern.edu

L. Zhou et al. (eds.), *A Case-Based Guide to Neuromuscular Pathology*,
https://doi.org/10.1007/978-3-030-25682-1_7

steroid-induced diabetes mellitus, and uterine fibroids. Her medications included prednisone, mycophenylate, monthly IVIg, pantoprazole, fosamax, calcium, vitamin D, insulin, and lisinopril. She did take a statin drug in the past, which was started after she developed muscle weakness, and the drug was discontinued 4 months later. Family history was positive for hypertension, diabetes mellitus, and a thyroid disease. She did not drink alcohol or smoke cigarettes. She was unemployed.

Physical Examination

General examination was unremarkable. There was no skin rash. Her mental status and cranial nerve functions were normal. Motor examination revealed normal muscle tone, normal muscle bulk, and weakness in the bilateral deltoid (MRC 4+/5), biceps (4−/5), triceps (4−/5), iliopsoas (3/5), and quadriceps (4+/5) muscles. Neck extensors and flexors were strong. She could not get up from a chair without her hands to push the chair. There was no scapular winging or calf hypertrophy. Sensation and coordination were normal. Deep tendon reflexes were diminished throughout. Toes were downgoing bilaterally. Her gait was steady but waddling.

Investigations

Serum CK level was 7,217 U/L. Aldolase level was 42.9 U/L (normal <7.7). Complete blood count (CBC) showed mild anemia. Comprehensive metabolic panel were normal. Antinuclear antibodies (ANA) and anti-extractable nuclear antigen antibodies (ENA) were negative. Myositis antibody panel showed a positive anti-signal recognition particle (SRP) autoantibody. Anti-3-hydroxy-3-methyglutaryl-coenzyme A reductase (HMGCR) autoantibody was negative. Paraneoplastic antibody panel was negative. TSH and vitamin D levels were normal. HbA1C was 7.0%. While waiting for the result of the myositis antibody panel, a left biceps muscle biopsy was performed.

Muscle Biopsy Findings

The left biceps muscle biopsy (Fig. 7.1) showed a chronic active inflammatory myopathy with abundant necrotic fibers infiltrated by macrophages (myophagocytosis), a few regenerating fibers, markedly increased fiber size variation, endomysial and perimysial fibrosis, and scattered myofibers with upregulation of class I major histocompatibility complex (MHC1). Immunostains for dystrophin epitopes, alpha-sarcoglycan, caveolin-3, and dysferlin revealed intact sarcolemmal reactivity, comparable to that present in sections stained for beta-spectrin reactivity. The findings are consistent with a severe immune-mediated necrotizing myopathy (IMNM).

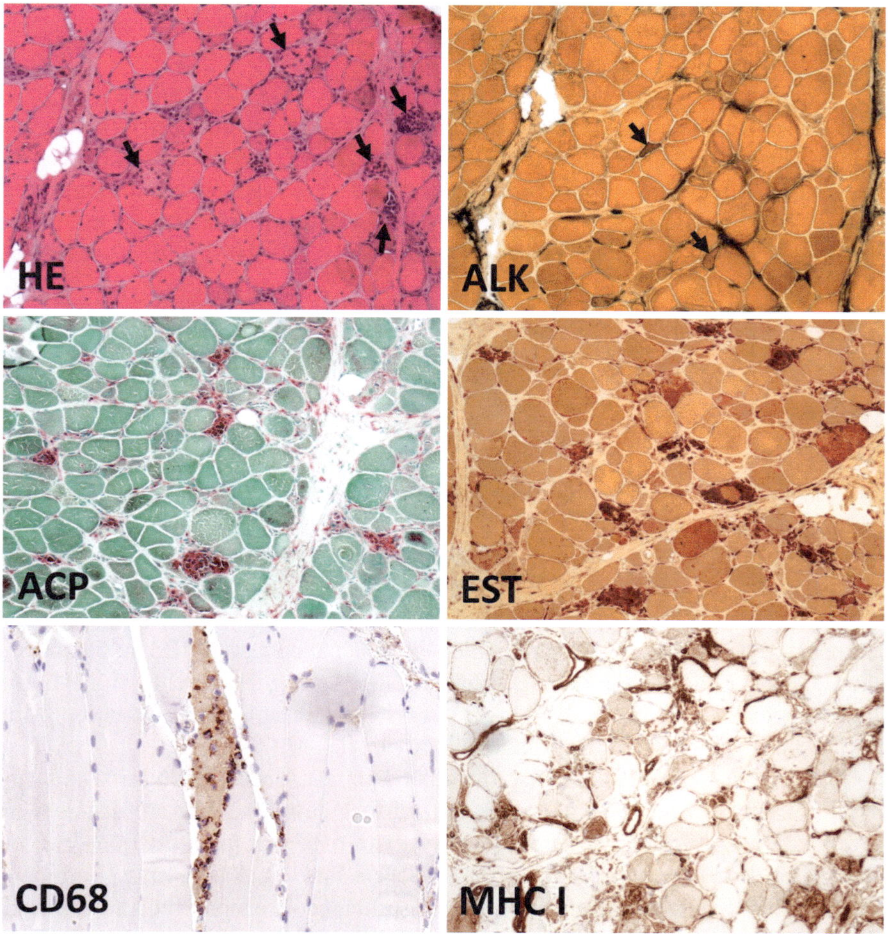

Fig. 7.1 Hematoxylin & eosin (HE) statin shows abundant necrotic fibers and myophagocytosis (arrows), increased fiber size variation with many polygonal atrophic fibers, and endomysial and perimysial fibrosis. Alkaline phosphatase (ALK) stain shows a few regenerating fibers (arrows) and patchy increase of perimysial reactivity indicating perimysium injury. Acid phosphatase (ACP) and esterase (EST) stains shows multiple foci of myophagocytosis with acid phosphatase and esterase reactive macrophages. CD68 immunostain (CD68) shows many CD68+ macrophages infiltrating a necrotic myofiber. MHC1 immunostain shows patchy sarcoplasmic upregulation of MHC1 in necrotic and many non-necrotic myofibers, in addition to the normal reactivity in perimysial and endomysial blood vessels

Final Diagnosis

Immune-mediated necrotizing myopathy associated with anti-SRP autoantibody (anti-SRP myopathy)

Patient Follow-up

The patient was treated with Rituximab. Her blood CD3-CD19+ B cell number went down from 357 to <1 cells/μL (normal: 110–570). She continued to take prednisone 15 mg once daily and receive IVIg treatment every 3 weeks. She also underwent physical therapy. Her weakness slowly improved. Eighteen months later, her follow-up examination showed resolution of the weakness in the deltoid and quadriceps muscles. The weakness in the bilateral iliopsoas (3+/5), biceps (4/5), and triceps (4/5) muscles slightly improved.

Discussion

IMNM, also known as necrotizing autoimmune myopathy (NAM), is a type of idiopathic inflammatory myopathy (IIM) [1, 2]. It is distinguished by its muscle biopsy features of myofiber necrosis with no or limited lymphocytic infiltrates [1–4]. The disease is categorized into three distinct clinical subtypes based on the autoantibody status: anti-SRP myopathy, anti-HMGCR myopathy, and autoantibody-negative (seronegative) IMNM [5]. A large study of 460 patients with IIM in Japan [6] showed that 177/460 (38.5%) patients had IMNM. Among the patients with IMNM, autoantibodies were detected in 115/177 (65%), with anti-SRP autoantibody in 69/177 (39%) and anti-HMGCR autoantibody in 46/177 (26%).

Although all subtypes of IMNM in adults manifest subacute, progressive, symmetric, proximal limb weakness and marked CK elevation, they are different in several aspects including weakness severity, extra-muscular manifestations, cancer association, and treatment response [5, 7]. Severe limb weakness, muscle atrophy, neck weakness, dysphagia, and respiratory insufficiency are more frequently seen in anti-SRP myopathy than in anti-HMGCR myopathy [6]. Extra-muscular manifestations, such as skin rash, arthritis, and Raynaud's phenomenon, are rare in both seropositive subtypes. The seronegative subtype shows frequent occurrence of connective tissue diseases and a high rate of extra-muscular disease activity [8]. Anti-HMGCR myopathy can be seen in patients with or without statin exposure [9], with the percentage of statin-induced anti-HMGCR myopathy ranging from 14% to 63% in different cohorts [3, 10–13]. Comparing with statin-induced anti-HMGCR myopathy, statin-naïve anti-HMGCR myopathy shows a younger age at onset, a more severe disease, and a worse prognosis [8, 14]. The risk of cancer is markedly increased in seronegative IMNM, slightly increased in anti-HMGCR myopathy, but not increased in anti-SRP myopathy. No specific type of cancer is predominate [15]. It has been reported that seronegative IMNM can be induced by programmed death-1 (PD-1) inhibitors that are used as cancer immunotherapy [16].

Although IMNM is mainly seen in adults, it can also be seen in children. It is worth noting that children with anti-SRP myopathy and anti-HMGCR myopathy may present with slowly progressive proximal weakness, mimicking a limb girdle muscular dystrophy [17, 18]. It is thus advocated that the autoantibodies should be tested in children who have a muscular dystrophy phenotype but no family history or a confirmative gene test result [5]. Children with anti-SRP myopathy and anti-HMGCR myopathy can respond favorably to immunosuppressive therapy if diagnosed and treated early [17–19].

Although anti-SRP and anti-HMGCR autoantibodies are highly specific for IMNM, a muscle biopsy is still needed to establish the diagnosis and to exclude other diagnoses, especially in patients with seronegative IMNM. Pathologically, the morphology of anti-SRP, anti-HMGCR and seronegative IMNM is similar. The muscle biopsy shows randomly scattered necrotic fibers at different stages of resolution (Fig. 7.2a), but only minimal or no lymphocytic inflammation. The muscle may show significant chronic myopathic changes such as myofiber hypertrophy, interstitial fibrosis, abnormal internal architecture (Fig. 7.2b), and even rimmed vacuoles (Fig. 7.2c). Perimysial connective tissue damage, indicated by abnormal alkaline phosphatase reactivity, is usually absent but may be focally present in cases with abundant necrotic fibers (Fig. 7.2d). C5b-9 immunostain shows strong sarcoplasmic reactivity in necrotic fibers (Fig. 7.2e black arrow) and membranous staining on scattered viable myofibers (Fig. 7.2e blue arrow). Class I major histocompatibility complex expression is upregulated in individually scattered myofibers (Fig. 7.2f). In mild cases, rare necrotic/regenerating fibers (Fig. 7.3a) and scattered myofibers with MHC1 upregulation (Fig. 7.3b) may be the only abnormal findings. The amount of necrotic fibers on muscle biopsy does not always correlate with serum CK or autoantibody levels (Fig. 7.3).

Cases with chronic active myopathic changes need to be differentiated from inclusion body myositis (IBM) and muscular dystrophies. Features of IBM that are usually absent in IMNM include primary lymphocytic invasion into viable myofiber, substantially increased COX-deficient myofibers, and diffuse MHC1 upregulation in myofibers. Muscular dystrophies usually contain much more pronounced chronic changes and fibrofatty replacement than active necrosis. Clinically, IMNM is usually easy to differentiate from IBM and muscular dystrophy. The IMNM cases that contain only acute myopathic damages need to be differentiated from rhabdomyolysis secondary to myotoxins or a metabolic myopathy. The necrotic fibers in both IMNM and rhabdomyolysis are randomly scattered. The monophasic nature of rhabdomyolysis is usually evident by the presence of abundant damaged fibers all at similar stage of necrosis or regeneration, while IMNM typically shows more temporal heterogeneity. The presence or absence of mitochondria, glycogen or lipid accumulation should be carefully examined in such cases to evaluate for metabolic myopathies.

The management of IMNM consists of aggressive immunosuppressive therapy, cancer screening in patients with seronegative IMNM and anti-HMGCR myopathy, and rehabilitation. There are no clinical trials to guide the treatment of different subtypes of IMNM. To avoid long-term disability from muscle atrophy and fatty replacement, immunosuppressive therapy should be initiated early and aggressively. Patients with IMNM often require more than one immunosuppressive agents. Corticosteroids plus methotrexate is the common initial treatment regimen. Other chronic immunosuppressive agents that can be used include azathioprine, mycophenylate, tarcrolimus, cyclosporine, and cyclophosphamide. Patients with anti-SRP myopathy and statin-naïve anti-HMGCR myopathy are

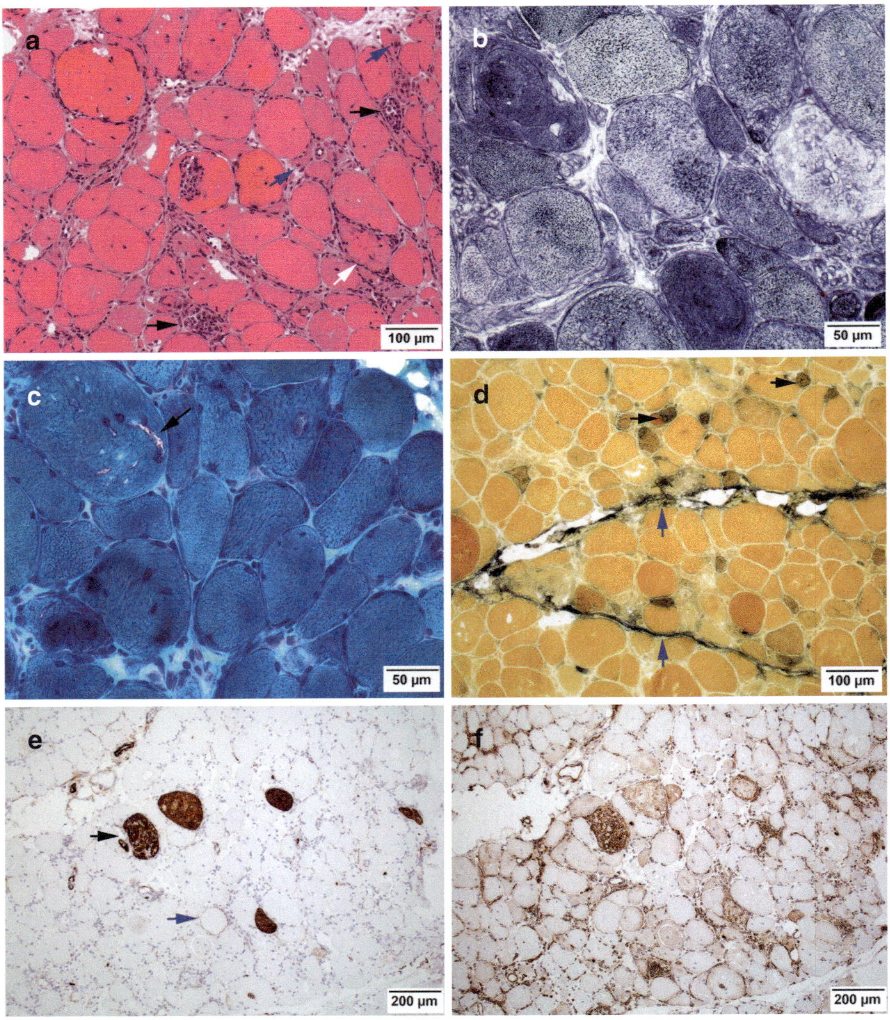

Fig. 7.2 Biopsy from a 49-year-old man with progressive muscle weakness, CK over 7,000 U/L, and a positive anti-HMGCR autoantibody. (**a**) H&E shows abundant acutely necrotic fibers (white arrow), myophagocytic fibers (black arrows), and regenerating fibers (blue arrows). There is marked fiber size variation and interstitial fibrosis. (**b**) NADH-TR stain shows markedly abnormal internal architecture as a result of chronic myopathy. (**c**) Gomori trichrome stain highlights rare rimmed vacuoles (arrow). (**d**) Alkaline phosphatase stain shows abundant regenerating fibers (black arrows) and patchy increase of perimysial reactivity indicating perimysium injury (blue arrows). (**e**) C5b-9 immunostain stain shows strong sarcoplasmic reactivity in necrotic fibers (black arrow) and sarcolemmal reactivity (blue arrows) in some viable myofibers. (**f**) MHC1 immunostain shows scattered rather than diffuse myofiber upregulation

often refractory to the treatment as seen in our case, and rituximab should be considered early in the disease course. IVIg is recommended and may be used as monotherapy for statin-induced anti-HMGCR myopathy especially in those who have contraindications to the use of steroids [20]. It is recommended that patients

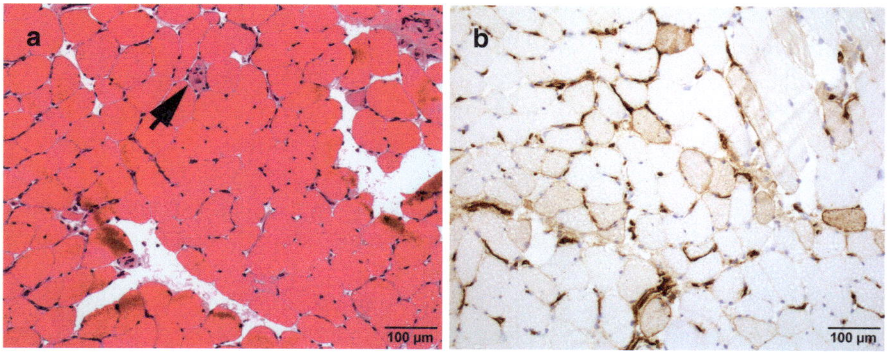

Fig. 7.3 Biopsy from a 58-year-old woman with progressive muscle weakness, CK in a range of 7,000–9,000 U/L, and a positive anti-HMGCR autoantibody. (**a**) H&E shows only a rare necrotic fiber (arrow). (**b**) MHC1 immunostain shows scattered viable fibers with MHC1 upregulation

with seronegative IMNM and anti-HMGCR myopathy undergo computed tomography (CT) of chest, abdomen, and pelvis, and age- and gender-appropriate cancer screening [5]. Rehabilitation is important to prevent disuse atrophy and to improve functionality.

Pearls

Clinical Pearls

1. IMNM has three distinct subtypes: anti-SRP myopathy, anti-HMGCR myopathy, and seronegative IMNM.
2. Patients with IMNM manifest progressive proximal limb weakness and marked CK elevation. The disease is more severe in anti-SRP myopathy and statin-naïve anti-HMGCR myopathy.
3. Extra-muscular manifestations are rare in the seropositive subtypes but more frequent in the seronegative subtype.
4. Although anti-SRP and anti-HMGCR autoantibodies are highly specific for IMNM, a muscle biopsy is still needed to establish the diagnosis of IMNM and to exclude other diagnoses, especially in patients with seronegative IMNM.
5. The risk of cancer is markedly increased in seronegative IMNM, slightly increased in anti-HMGCR myopathy, but not increased in anti-SRP myopathy.
6. The management of IMNM consists of aggressive immunosuppressive therapy, cancer screening in patients with seronegative IMNM and anti-HMGCR myopathy, and rehabilitation.
7. Children with anti-SRP myopathy and anti-HMGCR myopathy may resemble a limb girdle muscular dystrophy; they often have a favorable response to immunosuppressive therapy if diagnosed and treated early.

Pathology Pearls

1. The characteristic muscle biopsy findings in IMNM are randomly scattered necrotic fibers at different stages of resolution, and absence of significant inflammation. MHC1 myofiber expression is individually scattered, rather than diffuse or patchy.
2. The amount of myofiber damage on muscle biopsy does not always correlate with serum CK level, autoantibody concentration, or clinical severity.
3. IMNM may have significant chronic myopathic changes that histologically resemble inclusion body myositis or muscular dystrophy on biopsy.
4. IMNM differs from rhabdomyolysis by temporal heterogeneity of myofiber damage. However, distinction cannot always be made solely based on histology.

References

1. De Bleecker JL, De Paepe B, Aronica E, de Visser M, Group EMMBS, Amato A, et al. 205th ENMC International Workshop: pathology diagnosis of idiopathic inflammatory myopathies part II 28-30 March 2014, Naarden, The Netherlands. Neuromuscul Disord. 2015;25(3):268–72.
2. Hoogendijk JE, Amato AA, Lecky BR, Choy EH, Lundberg IE, Rose MR, et al. 119th ENMC international workshop: trial design in adult idiopathic inflammatory myopathies, with the exception of inclusion body myositis, 10-12 October 2003, Naarden, The Netherlands. Neuromuscul Disord. 2004;14(5):337–45.
3. Alshehri A, Choksi R, Bucelli R, Pestronk A. Myopathy with anti-HMGCR antibodies: perimysium and myofiber pathology. Neurol Neuroimmunol Neuroinflamm. 2015;2(4):e124.
4. Chung T, Christopher-Stine L, Paik JJ, Corse A, Mammen AL. The composition of cellular infiltrates in anti-HMG-CoA reductase-associated myopathy. Muscle Nerve. 2015;52(2):189–95.
5. Pinal-Fernandez I, Casal-Dominguez M, Mammen AL. Immune-mediated necrotizing myopathy. Curr Rheumatol Rep. 2018;20(4):21.
6. Watanabe Y, Uruha A, Suzuki S, Nakahara J, Hamanaka K, Takayama K, et al. Clinical features and prognosis in anti-SRP and anti-HMGCR necrotising myopathy. J Neurol Neurosurg Psychiatry. 2016;87(10):1038–44.
7. Allenbach Y, Mammen AL, Benveniste O, Stenzel W, Immune-Mediated Necrotizing Myopathies Working Group. 224th ENMC International Workshop:: Clinico-sero-pathological classification of immune-mediated necrotizing myopathies Zandvoort, The Netherlands, 14–16 October 2016. Neuromuscul Disord. 2018;28(1):87–99.
8. Lim J, Rietveld A, De Bleecker JL, Badrising UA, Saris CGJ, van der Kooi AJ, et al. Seronegative patients form a distinctive subgroup of immune-mediated necrotizing myopathy. Neurol Neuroimmunol Neuroinflamm. 2019;6(1):e513.
9. Mohassel P, Mammen AL. Anti-HMGCR myopathy. J Neuromuscul Dis. 2018;5(1):11–20.
10. Allenbach Y, Drouot L, Rigolet A, Charuel JL, Jouen F, Romero NB, et al. Anti-HMGCR autoantibodies in European patients with autoimmune necrotizing myopathies: inconstant exposure to statin. Medicine (Baltimore). 2014;93(3):150–7.

11. Christopher-Stine L, Casciola-Rosen LA, Hong G, Chung T, Corse AM, Mammen AL. A novel autoantibody recognizing 200-kd and 100-kd proteins is associated with an immune-mediated necrotizing myopathy. Arthritis Rheum. 2010;62(9):2757–66.
12. Ge Y, Lu X, Peng Q, Shu X, Wang G. Clinical characteristics of anti-3-hydroxy-3-methylglutaryl coenzyme A reductase antibodies in Chinese patients with idiopathic inflammatory myopathies. PLoS One. 2015;10(10):e0141616.
13. Watanabe Y, Suzuki S, Nishimura H, Murata KY, Kurashige T, Ikawa M, et al. Statins and myotoxic effects associated with anti-3-hydroxy-3-methylglutaryl-coenzyme A reductase autoantibodies: an observational study in Japan. Medicine (Baltimore). 2015;94(4):e416.
14. Tiniakou E, Pinal-Fernandez I, Lloyd TE, Albayda J, Paik J, Werner JL, et al. More severe disease and slower recovery in younger patients with anti-3-hydroxy-3-methylglutaryl-coenzyme A reductase-associated autoimmune myopathy. Rheumatology (Oxford). 2017;56(5):787–94.
15. Allenbach Y, Keraen J, Bouvier AM, Jooste V, Champtiaux N, Hervier B, et al. High risk of cancer in autoimmune necrotizing myopathies: usefulness of myositis specific antibody. Brain. 2016;139.(Pt 8:2131–5.
16. Liewluck T, Kao JC, Mauermann ML. PD-1 inhibitor-associated myopathies: emerging immune-mediated myopathies. J Immunother. 2018;41(4):208–11.
17. Mohassel P, Landon-Cardinal O, Foley AR, Donkervoort S, Pak KS, Wahl C, et al. Anti-HMGCR myopathy may resemble limb-girdle muscular dystrophy. Neurol Neuroimmunol Neuroinflamm. 2019;6(1):e523.
18. Zhao Y, Liu X, Zhang W, Yuan Y. Childhood autoimmune necrotizing myopathy with anti-signal recognition particle antibodies. Muscle Nerve. 2017;56(6):1181–7.
19. Liang WC, Uruha A, Suzuki S, Murakami N, Takeshita E, Chen WZ, et al. Pediatric necrotizing myopathy associated with anti-3-hydroxy-3-methylglutaryl-coenzyme A reductase antibodies. Rheumatology (Oxford). 2017;56(2):287–93.
20. Mammen AL, Tiniakou E. Intravenous immune globulin for statin-triggered autoimmune myopathy. N Engl J Med. 2015;373(17):1680–2.

Chapter 8
A 61-Year-Old Woman with Progressive Distal Limb and Deltoid Muscle Weakness

Lan Zhou

History

A 61-year-old Caucasian woman developed mild right foot drop 1 year prior to the presentation. This was followed by left foot weakness, right finger drop, and then left finger drop. She also reported difficulty holding arms up lately. She could still get up from a chair and walk upstairs without difficulties. She reported muscle cramps in the posterior compartment of the distal legs, but no muscle atrophy or fasciculations. She denied double vision, blurry vision, droopy eyelids, or difficulty chewing, swallowing or breathing. There had been no pain or numbness. There had been no fatigue, weight loss, chill, fever, sinusitis, cough or skin lesions. She had a past medical history of migraine headaches and gastro-esophageal acid reflux disorder. She took Tylenol as needed and Pepcid. She had a family history of hypertension but no rheumatological diseases or muscle diseases. She did not smoke cigarettes or drink alcohol.

Physical Examination

Her general examination was unremarkable. Neurological examination showed normal mental status and cranial nerve functions. Muscle tone and bulks were normal in the upper and lower extremities. Weakness was detected in the bilateral deltoid (MRC: 4+/5), forearm pronators (4/5), wrist and finger extensors (2/5), intrinsic hand muscles (4−/5), and foot and toe dorsiflexors (4/5). She could get up from a chair without her hands to push. There was no

L. Zhou (✉)
Departments of Neurology and Pathology, Boston University Medical Center, Boston, MA, USA
e-mail: lanzhou@bu.edu

L. Zhou et al. (eds.), *A Case-Based Guide to Neuromuscular Pathology*,
https://doi.org/10.1007/978-3-030-25682-1_8

spine scoliosis, scapular wining, calf hypertrophy, or foot deformity. Sensory was intact to pinprick, vibratory sensation, and joint position. Deep tendon reflexes were 2+ throughout. Toes were downgoing bilaterally. Coordination testing was normal. Gait was steady, and she was able to walk on her toes but not heels.

Investigations

Serum creatine kinase (CK) level was mildly elevated at 344 IU/L (normal: 30–200). CBC, comprehensive metabolic panel, TSH, free T4, B12, HbA1C, ESR, ANA, ENA, rheumatoid factor, copper level, anti-GM1, GD1b, and GQ1b antibodies were all unremarkable. Nerve conduction study (NCS) was normal. Needle EMG of selected limb muscles showed abnormal spontaneous activities in the forms of fibrillation potentials and positive sharp waves, and early recruitment of small-amplitude and short-duration motor unit potentials in the deltoid, pronator tares, extensor digitorum communis, first dorsal interosseous, and tibialis anterior muscles. The findings were consistent with an irritable myopathy affecting distal > proximal and upper > lower limb muscles. A left deltoid muscle biopsy was performed.

Muscle Biopsy Findings

The left deltoid muscle biopsy revealed non-caseating granulomas (Fig. 8.1) with no acid-fast bacilli (AFB), Gomori methenamine silver (GMS) positive micro-organisms or polarizable materials. There were occasional scattered atrophic,

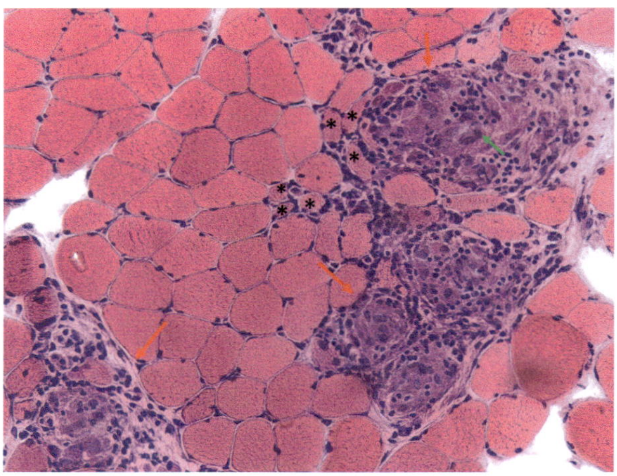

Fig. 8.1 Non-caseating granulomatous myositis. Muscle cross sections stained with hematoxylin & eosin (HE) show several endomysial and perimysial granulomas (red arrows) consisting of multinucleated giant cells (green arrow) and epithelioid cells which are mixed with lymphocytes. A few adjacent atrophic muscle fibers (∗) are present

degenerating, and regenerating fibers. There was no esterase-positive fiber, target or targetoid change, fiber type grouping or grouped atrophy to suggest a neurogenic process.

Additional Investigations After the Muscle Biopsy Diagnosis

The patient's serum angiotensin-converting enzyme (ACE) level was normal. Computerized tomography (CT) of the chest, abdomen, and pelvis was unremarkable.

Final Diagnosis

Isolated granulomatous myositis.

Patient Follow-up

The patient was started on Prednisone 60 mg once daily. She also underwent physical therapy. Two months after the treatment, she showed improvement in her muscle strength. The dose of Prednisone was gradually tapered down to 20 mg once daily. She tolerated the treatment well. One year after the treatment, she only showed mild stable weakness in the wrist and finger extensors (4/5) and intrinsic hand muscles (4+/5). She was subsequently followed by her local neurologist.

Discussion

Granulomatous myositis is a rare muscle biopsy diagnosis. In a large series of 2,985 muscle biopsies, only 12 (0.4%) showed granulomatous inflammation [1]. Although muscle granulomas have been reported in association with many medical conditions, including sarcoidosis, infections, Crohn disease, lymphoma, thymoma, graft-versus-host-disease, anti-PD-1 therapy and others, the condition can be present in isolation [1–12]. It is most commonly seen in association with systemic sarcoidosis followed by idiopathic with no causes identified [1, 13].

Muscle involvement is not uncommon in systemic sarcoidosis; however, it is mostly asymptomatic with muscle granulomas found in autopsy or random muscle biopsy [14]. Patients with symptomatic muscle involvement can present with palpable muscle nodules, acute myositis, or much more commonly chronic myopathy [5, 14, 15]. Chronic myopathy caused by sarcoidosis usually has symptom onset after 50 years of age with a female predominance. The disease manifests symmetrical, proximal, lower limb weakness. With time, some patients may develop weakness in the upper limbs and distal limb muscles, and some patients may also have dysphagia [5, 8, 16]. The clinical presentation of our patient is seemingly different. The initial symptoms in our patient were mainly distal with foot drop and finger and wrist drop. She developed mild weakness in the deltoid muscles late in the course. Her muscle involvement was more broad and severe in the upper limbs than in the lower limbs. This pattern is mostly seen in isolated granulomatous myositis [5, 8].

Due to the rarity of granulomatous myositis, there has been no large-scale comparison study to fully characterize the clinical features of sarcoid chronic myopathy and isolated granulomatous myositis. Only a few retrospective small series studies have been published [5, 8]. It is not entirely clear whether isolated granulomatous myositis is a distinct entity or a special presentation of sarcoidosis. At present, the diagnosis of isolated granulomatous myositis is made based on the clinical presentation, the presence of granulomatous myositis on muscle biopsy, and the absence of identifiable causes especially the symptoms and findings of systemic sarcoidosis. Sarcoidosis is an immune-mediated multiorgan disorder of unknown cause. It typically involves lungs, skin, lymph nodes, eyes, and parotid glands. Nervous system involvement is uncommon, and symptomatic muscle involvement is exceedingly rare [17, 18]. The diagnosis is established by imaging studies and tissue pathology. Given the common involvement of mediastinal lymph nodes and lungs, chest CT is important in the diagnostic evaluation. Serum ACE level can be elevated, but it is neither sensitive nor specific [19]. Gallium 67 scan is not as sensitive as fluorodeoxyglucose positron emission tomography (FDG-PET) in detecting occult systemic disease [20]. Our patient did not have any symptoms or signs to suggest systemic sarcoidosis. Her CT scan of the chest, abdomen, and pelvis did not reveal abnormalities in other organs, although she did not have gallium 67 scan or FDG-PET scan. Given her clinical presentation, granulomatous myositis shown on her muscle biopsy, and lack of symptoms, signs or CT findings of other organ involvement, the diagnosis for her was isolated granulomatous myositis.

It has been shown that isolated granulomatous myositis and sarcoid chronic myopathy are not different in age at onset, serum CK, EMG, or muscle biopsy findings [5, 8]. Both are late-onset, predominantly affecting people above 50 years of age. Both have normal or mildly elevated serum CK levels. EMG in both mostly shows irritable myopathic changes in the affected muscles. Muscle biopsies in both reveal non-caseating granulomas in endomysium or perimysium with epithelioid histiocytes mixed with T lymphocytes. Multinucleated giant cells may also be present. Our patient had all these features. Due to the late disease onset, prominent distal limb involvement, and additional proximal limb involvement at a late stage, isolated granulomatous myositis can mimic sporadic inclusion body myositis (sIBM) [21] or motor neuropathy. sIBM predominantly affects knee extensors and finger flexors. Our patient shows prominant wrist, finger and foot drop but no significant weakness in the finger flexors or knee extensors, which is atypical for sIBM. EMG is important for differentiating a myopathic condition from a neurogenic condition. Muscle biopsy is essential for establishing the diagnosis of granulomatous myositis. Muscle biopsy in sIBM usually does not show granulomas but shows a constellation of endomysial inflammation, red-rimmed vacuole, tubulofilamentous inclusions, and increased number of COX-deficient fibers. Our patient's muscle biopsy did not show these features.

There are no controlled studies to guide the treatment of isolated granulomatous myositis or sarcoid chronic myopathy. According to the anecdotal reports [5, 8], the first-line treatment is oral Prednisone, and the treatment response is mixed. Adding a chronic immunosuppressant or immune modulating therapy is usually ineffective. But in general, isolated granulomatous myositis is milder with little disability.

Pearls

Clinical Pearls

1. Granulomatous myositis is rare and can be associated with many medical conditions, most commonly systemic sarcoidosis followed by idiopathic with no causes identified.
2. Unlike sarcoid chronic myopathy which mainly affects proximal lower limb muscles, isolated granulomatous myositis predominantly affects distal limb muscles and upper limb muscles.
3. Both isolated granulomatous myositis and sarcoid chronic myopathy manifest late symptom onset, normal or mildly elevated serum CK level, irritable myopathy on EMG, and non-caseating granulomatous inflammation on muscle biopsy.
4. There are no controlled studies to guide the treatment of isolated granulomatous myositis or sarcoid chronic myopathy. Oral Prednisone is usually the first-line therapy which shows mixed treatment responses. Chronic immunosuppressive or immune modulating therapies are usually ineffective.
5. Comparing with sarcoid chronic myopathy, isolated granulomatous myositis is mild with little disability.

Pathology Pearls

1. Muscle biopsy is essential for establishing the diagnosis of granulomatous myositis.
2. Muscle biopsies in both isolated granulomatous myositis and sarcoid chronic myopathy show non-caseating granulomas in endomysium and/or perimysium consisting of epithelioid histiocytes and multinucleated giant cells mixed with T lymphocytes. Myopathic changes, including myofiber atrophy, degeneration, and regeneration, are usually mild.

References

1. Prayson RA. Granulomatous myositis. Clinicopathologic study of 12 cases. Am J Clin Pathol. 1999;112(1):63–8.
2. Chan LL, Chee TS, Thoo FL. Case report: MR features of granulomatous myositis. Clin Radiol. 1997;52(10):794–6.
3. Halverson PB, Lahiri S, Wojno WC, Sulaiman AR. Sporotrichal arthritis presenting as granulomatous myositis. Arthritis Rheum. 1985;28(12):1425–9.
4. Kaushik S, Flagg E, Wise CM, Hadfield G, McCarty JM. Granulomatous myositis: a manifestation of chronic graft-versus-host disease. Skelet Radiol. 2002;31(4):226–9.
5. Le Roux K, Streichenberger N, Vial C, Petiot P, Feasson L, Bouhour F, et al. Granulomatous myositis: a clinical study of thirteen cases. Muscle Nerve. 2007;35(2):171–7.
6. Menard DB, Haddad H, Blain JG, Beaudry R, Devroede G, Masse S. Granulomatous myositis and myopathy associated with crohn's colitis. N Engl J Med. 1976;295(15):818–9.
7. Min HS, Hyun CL, Paik JH, Jeon YK, Choi G, Park SH, et al. An autopsy case of aggressive CD30+ extra-nodal NK/T-cell lymphoma initially manifested with granulomatous myositis. Leuk Lymphoma. 2006;47(2):347–52.
8. Mozaffar T, Lopate G, Pestronk A. Clinical correlates of granulomas in muscle. J Neurol. 1998;245(8):519–24.
9. Nakamura Y, Kurihara N, Sato A, Nakamura M, Koyama K, Suzuki H, et al. Muscle sarcoidosis following malignant lymphoma: diagnosis by MR imaging. Skelet Radiol. 2002;31(12):702–5.
10. Herrmann DN, Blaivas M, Wald JJ, Feldman EL. Granulomatous myositis, primary biliary cirrhosis, pancytopenia, and thymoma. Muscle Nerve. 2000;23(7):1133–6.
11. Kojan S, Alothman A, Althani Z, Alshehri A, Mansour N, Khathaami A, et al. Granulomatous myositis associated with brucellosis: a case report and literature review. Muscle Nerve. 2012;45(2):290–3.
12. Uchio N, Taira K, Ikenaga C, Unuma A, Kadoya M, Kubota A, et al. Granulomatous myositis induced by anti-PD-1 monoclonal antibodies. Neurol Neuroimmunol Neuroinflamm. 2018;5(4):e464.
13. Prieto-Gonzalez S, Grau JM. Diagnosis and classification of granulomatous myositis. Autoimmun Rev. 2014;13(4–5):372–4.
14. Silverstein A, Siltzbach LE. Muscle involvement in sarcoidosis: Asymptomatic, myositis, and myopathy. Arch Neurol. 1969;21(3):235–41.
15. Douglas AC, Macleod JG, Matthews JD. Symptomatic sarcoidosis of skeletal muscle. J Neurol Neurosurg Psychiatry. 1973;36(6):1034–40.
16. Maeshima S, Koike H, Noda S, Noda T, Nakanishi H, Iijima M, et al. Clinicopathological features of sarcoidosis manifesting as generalized chronic myopathy. J Neurol. 2015;262(4):1035–45.
17. Tavee JO, Stern BJ. Neurosarcoidosis. Continuum (Minneap Minn). 2014;20(3 Neurology of Systemic Disease):545–59.
18. Lacomis D. Neurosarcoidosis. Curr Neuropharmacol. 2011;9(3):429–36.
19. Culver DA. Sarcoidosis. Immunol Allergy Clin North Am. 2012;32(4):487–511.
20. Keijsers RG, Grutters JC, Thomeer M, Du Bois RM, Van Buul MM, Lavalaye J, et al. Imaging the inflammatory activity of sarcoidosis: sensitivity and inter observer agreement of (67)Ga imaging and (18)F-FDG PET. Q J Nucl Med Mol Imaging. 2011;55(1):66–71.
21. Larue S, Maisonobe T, Benveniste O, Chapelon-Abric C, Lidove O, Papo T, et al. Distal muscle involvement in granulomatous myositis can mimic inclusion body myositis. J Neurol Neurosurg Psychiatry. 2011;82(6):674–7.

Chapter 9
A 63-Year-Old Woman with Debilitating Muscle Pain

Lan Zhou

History

A 63-year-old Caucasian woman presented with debilitating muscle pain. She developed a rapid onset of severe soreness in the muscles of buttocks and thighs with fatigue. Over the course of 3 weeks, the symptoms progressed to involve her upper arms. She had difficulty climbing stairs and washing her hair because of the pain. She had no spine pain, shooting limb pain, or numbness. She had no fever, weight loss, appetite loss, joint pain, skin rash, or urinary symptoms. She went to a local hospital emergency department, and was discharged with pain medications. Due to the progressive symptoms, she went to the local hospital emergency department again, and was admitted for evaluation. Her serum creatine kinase (CK) level, thyroid stimulating hormone, free T4, ANA, ENA, and rheumatoid factor were unremarkable. Cervical and lumbosacral spine MRIs with and without contrast showed mild multi-level degenerative changes. She was discharged without a clear diagnosis. One week later, she presented to our emergency department for the progressive symptoms that significantly affected her function. She could not walk long distance or function as a physician due to the severe pain and fatigue in her proximal limb muscles. She was admitted to our neurology service for evaluation and treatment. She had a past medical history of hypothyroidism and poliomyelitis with mild residual left foot weakness. She took levothyroxine for hypothyroidism. Her family history was positive for hypertension and thyroid dysfunction. She did not smoke cigarettes, drink alcohol, or use illicit drugs.

L. Zhou (✉)
Departments of Neurology and Pathology, Boston University Medical Center, Boston, MA, USA
e-mail: lanzhou@bu.edu

L. Zhou et al. (eds.), *A Case-Based Guide to Neuromuscular Pathology*,
https://doi.org/10.1007/978-3-030-25682-1_9

Physical Examination

Her vital signs were normal. She was distressed by the muscle pain. General examination was otherwise unremarkable. Neurological examination showed normal mental status, cranial nerve functions, sensation, and coordination. There was severe tenderness to palpation in the bilateral deltoid, biceps, gluteal, and quadriceps muscles. Strength was intact except for her known mild residual weakness in the left foot and toes from prior polio infection. Deep tendon reflexes were absent at the ankles and normal elsewhere. Her gait was antalgic and slow; she fatigued very quickly, requiring frequent rest.

Investigations

Blood tests showed mildly elevated CK level at 367 IU/L (normal 25–175) and aldolase level at 9.1 U/L (normal 1.5–8.1). C-reactive protein (CRP) and erythrocyte sedimentation rate (ESR) were markedly elevated at 124 mg/L (normal 0–5.0) and 79 mm/hr (normal 0–20), respectively. Antineutrophil cytoplasmic antibody (ANCA) titer was elevated at 1:160 (normal <1:20), and myeloperoxidase (MPO) antibody was positive at 186 U/mL (normal 0–19). Antibodies to proteinase 3 (PR3) and Jo-1 were negative. Urinalysis showed microscopic hematuria and proteinuria. Chest CT showed a very small lung nodule. Nerve conduction study (NCS) was normal. Electromyography (EMG) showed no abnormal spontaneous activity but subtle early recruitment of a few small motor unit potentials in the biceps and deltoid muscles, suggestive of a subtle non-irritable myopathy. A left deltoid muscle biopsy was performed for further evaluation.

Muscle Biopsy Findings

The muscle biopsy showed acute necrotizing vasculitis with transmural inflammation and fibrinoid necrosis of blood vessel walls involving several small- and medium-sized perimysial blood vessels (Fig. 9.1). There was no myopathic change or endomysial inflammation.

Final Diagnosis

ANCA-Associated Vasculitis

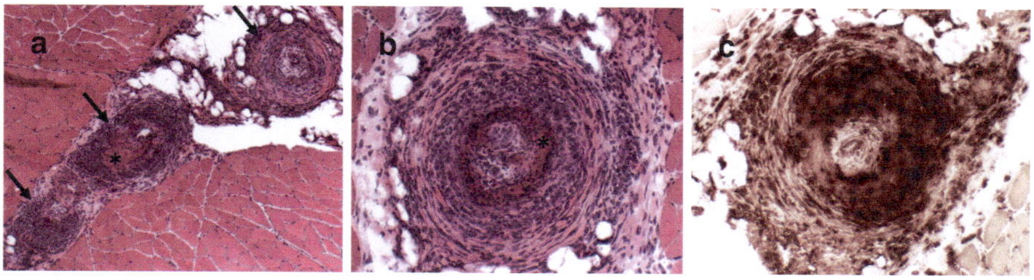

Fig. 9.1 H&E stain (**a** and **b**) shows transmural inflammation involving several perimysial blood vessels (arrows), destruction of blood vessel walls with deposition of fibrinoid material (asterisks), and occlusion of blood vessel lumen. Acid phosphatase stain (**c**) shows that some of the mononuclear inflammatory cells are acid phosphatase-positive macrophages

Patient Follow-up

The patient was treated with intravenous (IV) infusion of methylprednisolone 1 gram/day for 5 days. She showed marked improvement of her symptoms. After completing the course of IV steroids treatment, her muscle pain largely resolved and she was able to walk fast without fatigue. Due to the abnormalities revealed by urinalysis, she underwent a renal biopsy which showed crescentic glomerulonephritis. She was discharged on oral Prednisone and started on Rituximab by rheumatology. She was subsequently followed by rheumatology.

Discussion

ANCA are autoantibodies to neutrophilic granules and monocytic lysosomes [1]. There are two major types of ANCA, perinuclear ANCA (p-ANCA) and cytoplasmic ANCA (c-ANCA). The major antigens targeted by p-ANCA and c-ANCA are MPO and PR3, respectively. ANCA have been associated with three distinct vasculitides which involve inflammation of small-sized blood vessels: microscopic polyangiitis (MPA), granulomatosis with polyangiitis (GPA, previously known as Wegener granulomatosis), and eosinophilic granulomatosis with polyangiitis (EGPA; previously known as Churg-Strauss Syndrome) [2–6]. The majority of patients with MPA are positive for MPO antibody, patients with GPA are usually positive for PR3 antibody, and about 50% of patients with EGPA are positive for MPO antibody [4]. Our patient had MPA.

ANCA-associated vasculitis (AAV) affects both genders equally; most of the patients are Caucasians and Hispanics. MPA is the most common AAV in Asians with a similar annual incidence in Japan and United Kingdom [7]. The estimated prevalence of AAV is 46–184 per million [8]. AAV is a multisystem disease, mostly affecting kidney, lung, skin and nerve. Nervous system is frequently involved in AAV with peripheral neuropathy predominated in each type of AAV (9). Common presentations of peripheral nervous system involvement include mononeuritis multiplex, distal sensorimotor axonal polyneuropathy, and isolated cranial mononeuropathies [9, 10]. Muscle involvement is not as common as the nerve involvement. Patients with MPA are usually older with more severe renal disease along with skin rash and neuropathy [3]. Although myalgia is not uncommon in AAV, which have been reported in 48.2% patients with MPA [11], myalgia or muscle weakness as the predominant presentation without other systemic symptoms or neuropathies is exceedingly rare [12–14]. The clinical diagnosis can be delayed as seen in our case because of this rare entity. Our patient did not have objective weakness, CK was mildly elevated, and the EMG findings were very subtle. But the muscle biopsy showed fulminant necrotizing vasculitis. The severe myalgia is most likely due to muscle ischemia.

The diagnosis of AAV is established by findings of vasculitis on tissue biopsy and positive ANCA in serum. Muscle biopsy plays an important role in diagnosing AAV when muscle symptoms are prominent [12–14], and it may spare the need for a more invasive biopsy of an internal organ [15]. Tissue biopsy in MPA typically shows necrotizing vasculitis but no granulomatous inflammation as seen in GPA or EGPA. On muscle biopsy, the vasculitis mainly affects small- and medium-sized perimysial arterioles [12, 14, 16]. The pathological features of necrotizing vasculitis include transmural inflammation and fibrinoid necrosis of blood vessel walls. This frequently results in the occlusion of blood vessel lumen, causing tissue ischemia.

The pathogenesis of AAV is not entirely clear [5, 6]. MPO-ANCA has been shown to be pathogenic by the active transfer experiment in a murine model [17] and the passive transfer of the disease in a newborn from a mother with positive MPO-ANCA [18]. Evidence that supports a pathogenic role of PR3-ANCA is still lacking. Neutrophil priming, T cell disturbance, ANCA production, complement system activation, and high levels of circulating inflammatory cytokines have all been implicated in the pathogenesis of AAV, and they become the targets of therapy development [5].

Treatment of AAV consists of two phases: remission induction therapy and maintenance therapy [6]. The combination of corticosteroids and another immunosuppressive agent is used for inducing disease remission. Corticosteroids is the cornerstone of the therapy for AAV. The initial treatment can be oral prednisone 1 mg/kg/day or intravenous infusion of methylprednisolone 1 gram/day for 3–5 days followed by oral prednisone. The dose can be gradually tapered after 2–4 weeks of treatment to reduce the side effects. It can be used alone for mild AAV, but usually another immunosuppressive agent is needed especially for patients with GPA and severe MPA and EGPA. At present, cyclophosphamide and rituximab are two choices to combine with steroids for remission induction. Rituximab is as effective as and probably less toxic than cyclophosphamide with respect to the risks of infertility and late cancers [19–21]. It is a monoclonal anti-CD20 antibody depleting B cells with subsequent reduction of ANCA and B cell cytokines. It is used as 4 infusions of 375 mg/m^2 each given at 1-week intervals. Plasmapheresis may be used as a rescue treatment for severe cases of AAV [22–24]. Once clinical remission is achieved, maintenance therapy is critical to prevent disease relapses. The conventional immunosuppressive agents used for this purpose include azathioprine and methotrexate, and they are equally effective and safe [25, 26]. Mycophenolate mofetil showed a higher relapse rate than azathioprine [27]. Rituximab is another option for the maintenance therapy especially in patients following a corticosteroids-rituximab-based induction. It can be given at the point of the B-lymphocyte reconstitution based on the CD19+ CD20+ lymphocyte count and/or ANCA reappearance or significant titer increase [28], or at regular intervals every 6–12 months independent of the B-cell count or ANCA status [29–33]. The efficacy of using rituximab every 4 months as maintenance therapy for AAV has been undergoing evaluation by a large-scale study [34].

Pearls

Clinical Pearls

1. Acute, severe, and progressive myalgia should raise a suspicion for vasculitis, especially in the presence of markedly elevated ESR and CRP and positive ANCA. The pain is most likely caused by muscle ischemia.
2. Acute, severe, and progressive myalgia can be a predominant initial presentation of AAV. Biopsy of a symptomatic muscle is essential to establish a tissue diagnosis to initiate prompt treatment.
3. Treatment of AAV consists of induction therapy to induce disease remission by using corticosteroids plus rituximab or cyclophosphamide, and maintenance therapy to prevent disease relapses by using azathioprine, methotrexate, or rituximab.

Pathology Pearls

1. The hallmark of acute vasculitis is transmural inflammation and destruction of blood vessel walls with deposition of fibrinoid material (fibrinoid necrosis). It can cause blood vessel lumen occlusion and subsequent tissue ischemia.
2. Necrotizing vasculitis revealed by a muscle biopsy usually affects small- and medium-sized arterioles in perimysium.

References

1. Davies DJ, Moran JE, Niall JF, Ryan GB. Segmental necrotising glomerulonephritis with antineutrophil antibody: possible arbovirus aetiology? Br Med J (Clin Res Ed). 1982;285(6342):606.
2. Kallenberg CG. The diagnosis and classification of microscopic polyangiitis. J Autoimmun. 2014;48–49:90–3.

3. Yates M, Watts R. ANCA-associated vasculitis. Clin Med (Lond). 2017;17(1):60–4.
4. Jennette JC, Falk RJ, Bacon PA, Basu N, Cid MC, Ferrario F, et al. 2012 revised International Chapel Hill Consensus Conference Nomenclature of Vasculitides. Arthritis Rheum. 2013;65(1):1–11.
5. Nakazawa D, Masuda S, Tomaru U, Ishizu A. Pathogenesis and therapeutic interventions for ANCA-associated vasculitis. Nat Rev Rheumatol. 2018.
6. Pagnoux C. Updates in ANCA-associated vasculitis. Eur J Rheumatol. 2016;3(3):122–33.
7. Fujimoto S, Watts RA, Kobayashi S, Suzuki K, Jayne DR, Scott DG, et al. Comparison of the epidemiology of anti-neutrophil cytoplasmic antibody-associated vasculitis between Japan and the U.K. Rheumatology (Oxford). 2011;50(10):1916–20.
8. Watts RA, Mahr A, Mohammad AJ, Gatenby P, Basu N, Flores-Suarez LF. Classification, epidemiology and clinical subgrouping of antineutrophil cytoplasmic antibody (ANCA)-associated vasculitis. Nephrol Dial Transplant. 2015;30(Suppl 1):i14–22.
9. Zhang W, Zhou G, Shi Q, Zhang X, Zeng XF, Zhang FC. Clinical analysis of nervous system involvement in ANCA-associated systemic vasculitides. Clin Exp Rheumatol. 2009;27(1 Suppl 52):S65–9.
10. Koike H, Sobue G. Clinicopathological features of neuropathy in anti-neutrophil cytoplasmic antibody-associated vasculitis. Clin Exp Nephrol. 2013;17(5):683–5.
11. Guillevin L, Durand-Gasselin B, Cevallos R, Gayraud M, Lhote F, Callard P, et al. Microscopic polyangiitis: clinical and laboratory findings in eighty-five patients. Arthritis Rheum. 1999;42(3):421–30.
12. Birnbaum J, Danoff S, Askin FB, Stone JH. Microscopic polyangiitis presenting as a "pulmonary-muscle" syndrome: is subclinical alveolar hemorrhage the mechanism of pulmonary fibrosis? Arthritis Rheum. 2007;56(6):2065–71.
13. Kim MY, Bae SY, Lee M, Chung H, Lee J, Ahn JK, et al. A case of ANCA-associated vasculitis presenting with calf claudication. Rheumatol Int. 2012;32(9):2909–12.
14. Oiwa H, Kurashige T. Muscle weakness as a presenting symptom in ANCA-associated vasculitis. Eur J Rheumatol. 2018;5(2):139–41.
15. Hervier B, Durant C, Masseau A, Ponge T, Hamidou M, Mussini JM. Use of muscle biopsies for diagnosis of systemic vasculitides. J Rheumatol. 2011;38(3):470–4.
16. Bahou E, Zhou L. ANCA-associated vasculitis predominantly presenting with severe myalgias. Neurol Neuroimmunol Neuroinflamm. 2017;4(4):e365.
17. Xiao H, Heeringa P, Hu P, Liu Z, Zhao M, Aratani Y, et al. Antineutrophil cytoplasmic autoantibodies specific for myeloperoxidase cause glomerulonephritis and vasculitis in mice. J Clin Invest. 2002;110(7):955–63.
18. Bansal PJ, Tobin MC. Neonatal microscopic polyangiitis secondary to transfer of maternal myeloperoxidase-antineutrophil cytoplasmic antibody resulting in neonatal pulmonary hemorrhage and renal involvement. Ann Allergy Asthma Immunol. 2004;93(4):398–401.
19. Jones RB, Tervaert JW, Hauser T, Luqmani R, Morgan MD, Peh CA, et al. Rituximab versus cyclophosphamide in ANCA-associated renal vasculitis. N Engl J Med. 2010;363(3):211–20.
20. Specks U, Merkel PA, Seo P, Spiera R, Langford CA, Hoffman GS, et al. Efficacy of remission-induction regimens for ANCA-associated vasculitis. N Engl J Med. 2013;369(5):417–27.
21. Stone JH, Merkel PA, Spiera R, Seo P, Langford CA, Hoffman GS, et al. Rituximab versus cyclophosphamide for ANCA-associated vasculitis. N Engl J Med. 2010;363(3):221–32.
22. de Joode AA, Sanders JS, Smid WM, Stegeman CA. Plasmapheresis rescue therapy in progressive systemic ANCA-associated vasculitis: single-center results of stepwise escalation of immunosuppression. J Clin Apher. 2014;29(5):266–72.
23. Walsh M, Catapano F, Szpirt W, Thorlund K, Bruchfeld A, Guillevin L, et al. Plasma exchange for renal vasculitis and idiopathic rapidly progressive glomerulonephritis: a meta-analysis. Am J Kidney Dis. 2011;57(4):566–74.
24. Walsh M, Merkel PA, Peh CA, Szpirt W, Guillevin L, Pusey CD, et al. Plasma exchange and glucocorticoid dosing in the treatment of anti-neutrophil cytoplasm antibody associated vasculitis (PEXIVAS): protocol for a randomized controlled trial. Trials. 2013;14:73.

25. Jayne D, Rasmussen N, Andrassy K, Bacon P, Tervaert JW, Dadoniene J, et al. A randomized trial of maintenance therapy for vasculitis associated with antineutrophil cytoplasmic autoantibodies. N Engl J Med. 2003;349(1):36–44.
26. Pagnoux C, Mahr A, Hamidou MA, Boffa JJ, Ruivard M, Ducroix JP, et al. Azathioprine or methotrexate maintenance for ANCA-associated vasculitis. N Engl J Med. 2008;359(26):2790–803.
27. Hiemstra TF, Walsh M, Mahr A, Savage CO, de Groot K, Harper L, et al. Mycophenolate mofetil vs azathioprine for remission maintenance in antineutrophil cytoplasmic antibody-associated vasculitis: a randomized controlled trial. JAMA. 2010;304(21):2381–8.
28. Cartin-Ceba R, Golbin JM, Keogh KA, Peikert T, Sanchez-Menendez M, Ytterberg SR, et al. Rituximab for remission induction and maintenance in refractory granulomatosis with polyangiitis (Wegener's): ten-year experience at a single center. Arthritis Rheum. 2012;64(11):3770–8.
29. Besada E, Koldingsnes W, Nossent JC. Long-term efficacy and safety of pre-emptive maintenance therapy with rituximab in granulomatosis with polyangiitis: results from a single centre. Rheumatology (Oxford). 2013;52(11):2041–7.
30. Charles P, Neel A, Tieulie N, Hot A, Pugnet G, Decaux O, et al. Rituximab for induction and maintenance treatment of ANCA-associated vasculitides: a multicentre retrospective study on 80 patients. Rheumatology (Oxford). 2014;53(3):532–9.
31. Jones RB, Ferraro AJ, Chaudhry AN, Brogan P, Salama AD, Smith KG, et al. A multicenter survey of rituximab therapy for refractory antineutrophil cytoplasmic antibody-associated vasculitis. Arthritis Rheum. 2009;60(7):2156–68.
32. Roubaud-Baudron C, Pagnoux C, Meaux-Ruault N, Grasland A, Zoulim A, LE Guen J, et al. Rituximab maintenance therapy for granulomatosis with polyangiitis and microscopic polyangiitis. J Rheumatol. 2012;39(1):125–30.
33. Smith RM, Jones RB, Guerry MJ, Laurino S, Catapano F, Chaudhry A, et al. Rituximab for remission maintenance in relapsing antineutrophil cytoplasmic antibody-associated vasculitis. Arthritis Rheum. 2012;64(11):3760–9.
34. Gopaluni S, Smith RM, Lewin M, McAlear CA, Mynard K, Jones RB, et al. Rituximab versus azathioprine as therapy for maintenance of remission for anti-neutrophil cytoplasm antibody-associated vasculitis (RITAZAREM): study protocol for a randomized controlled trial. Trials. 2017;18(1):112.

Chapter 10
A 33-Year-Old Woman with Pain and Swelling in the Right Calf and Persistent Fever

Lan Zhou, Laura K. Stein, and Susan C. Shin

History

A 33-year-old woman presented with 3 weeks of pain and swelling in the right calf and persistent fever despite completing 10 days of oral antibiotics cephalexin for possible cellulitis. Lower extremity Doppler was negative for deep vein thrombosis. The patient was started on empiric broad-spectrum antibiotics with intravenous (IV) vancomycin and zosyn for presumed cellulitis. With ongoing fevers 1 week after the presentation, the antibiotics coverage was broadened and changed to Imipenem. The patient continued to have high-grade fevers, right calf pain and swelling despite being treated with broad spectrum IV antibiotics. She did not have cough or urinary pain. She had a past medical history of lupus on Prednisone 10 mg once daily and Plaquenil 200 mg once daily.

Physical Examination

The patient appeared ill with body temperature 100.8 °C. Heart rate, blood pressure, and breathing were normal. There was remarkable edema, skin red discoloration, and tenderness in the right calf. Mental status and cranial nerves were intact. There was no weakness or numbness, although the movement of the right distal leg and foot was limited due to the pain.

L. Zhou (✉)
Departments of Neurology and Pathology, Boston University Medical Center, Boston, MA, USA
e-mail: lanzhou@bu.edu

L. K. Stein · S. C. Shin
Department of Neurology, Icahn School of Medicine at Mount Sinai, New York, NY, USA

L. Zhou et al. (eds.), *A Case-Based Guide to Neuromuscular Pathology*,
https://doi.org/10.1007/978-3-030-25682-1_10

Investigations

Computer tomography (CT) scan of the right lower extremity demonstrated focal skin thickening along the posterior-lateral aspect of the mid-distal right calf, subcutaneous fat stranding, and inflammatory changes suggestive of cellulitis. Gallium scan was also suggestive of cellulitis localized to the medial proximal tibia below the knee. Right distal leg magnetic resonance imaging (MRI) demonstrated extensive signal abnormalities of the medial gastrocenemius and soleus muscles, and small crecentric fluid collections along these muscles. Due to the concern of a focal myositis, two weeks after the presentation, the patient underwent a right gastrocnemius biopsy and washout.

Muscle Biopsy Findings

The right gastrocnemius muscle biopsy revealed necrotizing granulomatous fasciitis and myositis with the presence of many acid-fast bacilli (AFB) positive micro-organisms (Fig. 10.1). Gram stain and Grocott's methenamine silver (GMS) stain showed no Gram positive or negative bacterial or fungal organisms (data not shown). The findings are consistent with mycobacterial infection.

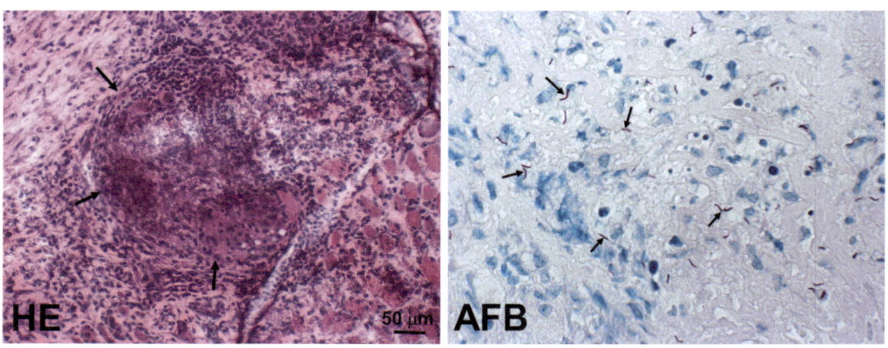

Fig. 10.1 Necrotizing granulomatous fasciitis and myositis with the presence of AFB positive micro-organisms. Muscle cross sections with hematoxylin and eosin (HE) and acid fact bacilli (AFB) stains show necrotizing granulomatous inflammation involving fascia and adjacent muscle tissue (HE, arrows) with the presence of many AFB positive bacteria in the necrotic tissue (AFB, arrows)

Final Diagnosis

Mycobacterial fasciitis and myositis

Patient Follow-up

The patient was isolated and started on rifampin, isoniazid, pyrazinamide, and ethambutol to cover mycobacterium tuberculosis (TB) infection. Approximately 1 week after the muscle biopsy, the patient developed right ankle and hip pain as well as cervical lymphadenopathy. CT scan of the neck showed necrotic internal jugular lymphadenopathy consistent with scrofula. CT of the chest, abdomen, and pelvis demonstrated multiple bibasilar pulmonary nodules, necrotic mesenteric lymph nodes, and fluid collections of the right iliacus and psoas muscles. The patient was subsequently found to have positive TB cultures in sputum, bone lesions, and cervical lymph nodes. She underwent drainage of multiple fluid collections. The patient's 6-month hospital course was complicated by drug rash, immune reconstitution syndrome, failure to thrive, worsening renal function and isoniazid-induced hepatotoxicity. Throughout the prolonged hospital course, she never demonstrated respiratory symptoms. She eventually showed significant improvement with the TB therapy and was discharged home with a plan to complete eleven total months of TB therapy.

Discussion

It is well known that patients with systemic lupus erythematosus are at increased risk for TB and other opportunistic infections because of the immunosuppression these patients require. Multiple studies have demonstrated that serious infections and extra-pulmonary manifestations are more common in this patient population [1, 2]. While approximately 3% of patients with TB have musculoskeletal involvement, the incidence of the even more uncommon manifestation of myositis is unknown [3]. It has been speculated that skeletal muscle is highly resistant to tuberculosis infection, based on its low oxygen and high lactate levels, as well as the lack of reticulo-endothelial tissue [4, 5].

Of the rare cases of TB myositis in the literature, it has been most commonly described in immunosuppressed patients, including those with systemic lupus erythematosus, rheumatoid arthritis, and HIV infection [3–5]. In each of the described cases of TB myositis, the diagnosis was made with fluid culture, and patients presented similarly with ongoing fever, pain, and swelling. To our best knowledge, this is the first reported case of TB fasciitis and myositis with the initially diagnosis suspected by muscle biopsy findings.

Granulomatous myositis is a rare muscle pathology diagnosis. It can be seen in association with sarcoidosis, infections, Churg-Strauss Syndrome, Crohn disease, and anti-PD1 therapy, among others [6–11]. Granuloma consists of epithelioid cells, multinucleated giant cells, lymphocytes and other inflammatory cells. Necrotizing granulomatous inflammation shows necrotic tissue with granular and cheese-like cellular debris in the areas with granulomas. It is mostly seen in mycobacterial and fungal infections. The necrotizing granulomatous fasciitis and myositis seen in our case is caused by TB infection.

Our case illustrates that febrile focal myositis should raise a strong clinical suspicion for infectious myositis. Infection work up should be done on muscle biopsy specimens. TB can infect muscle, and should be considered especially in immunocompromised patients even without pulmonary symptoms.

Pearls

Clinical Pearls

1. Although uncommon, TB can infect muscle in immunocompromised hosts. Disseminated mycobacterium tuberculosis infection may initially present with febrile focal myositis.
2. One should consider the possibility of TB as the etiologic infectious agent in an immunocompromised patient with febrile focal myositis even without pulmonary symptoms.

Pathology Pearls

1. Febrile focal myositis should raise a suspicion for infectious etiologies, and infection work up should be done on muscle biopsy specimens by special stains, including Gram, GMS, and AFB stains.
2. Necrotizing granulomatous myositis is mostly seen in mycobacterial and fungal infections, and AFB and GMS stains can help differentiate.

References

1. Hou CL, Tsai YC, Chen LC, Huang JL. Tuberculosis infection in patients with systemic lupus erythematosus: pulmonary and extra-pulmonary infection compared. Clin Rheumatol. 2008;27(5):557–63.

2. Tam LS, Li EK, Wong SM, Szeto CC. Risk factors and clinical features for tuberculosis among patients with systemic lupus erythematosus in Hong Kong. Scand J Rheumatol. 2002;31(5):296–300.
3. Migkos MP, Somarakis GA, Markatseli TE, Matthaiou M, Kosta P, Voulgari PV, et al. Tuberculous pyomyositis in a rheumatoid arthritis patient treated with anakinra. Clin Exp Rheumatol. 2015;33(5):734–6.
4. Khosla P, Aroaa N, Jain S. Tubercular pyomyositis in a case of rheumatoid arthritis being treated with infliximab. Int J Rheum Dis. 2010;13(1):82–5.
5. Trikha V, Varshney MK, Rastogi S. Isolated tuberculosis of the vastus lateralis muscle: a case report. Scand J Infect Dis. 2006;38(4):304–6.
6. Kaushik S, Flagg E, Wise CM, Hadfield G, McCarty JM. Granulomatous myositis: a manifestation of chronic graft-versus-host disease. Skelet Radiol. 2002;31(4):226–9.
7. Menard DB, Haddad H, Blain JG, Beaudry R, Devroede G, Masse S. Granulomatous myositis and myopathy associated with crohn's colitis. N Engl J Med. 1976;295(15):818–9.
8. Mozaffar T, Lopate G, Pestronk A. Clinical correlates of granulomas in muscle. J Neurol. 1998;245(8):519–24.
9. Vital A, Vital C, Viallard JF, Ragnaud JM, Canron MH, Lagueny A. Neuro-muscular biopsy in Churg-Strauss syndrome: 24 cases. J Neuropathol Exp Neurol. 2006;65(2):187–92.
10. Wolfe SM, Pinals RS, Aelion JA, Goodman RE. Myopathy in sarcoidosis: clinical and pathologic study of four cases and review of the literature. Semin Arthritis Rheum. 1987;16(4):300–6.
11. Uchio N, Taira K, Ikenaga C, Unuma A, Kadoya M, Kubota A, et al. Granulomatous myositis induced by anti-PD-1 monoclonal antibodies. Neurol Neuroimmunol Neuroinflamm. 2018;5(4):e464.

Chapter 11
A 28-Year-Old Woman with Proximal Limb Weakness and Scapular Winging

Rahul Abhyankar, Chunyu Cai, and Jaya R. Trivedi

History

A 28-year-old woman presented with a few years of progressive weakness. An avid athlete, she played softball in college but developed exercise fatigue and dyspnea on exertion. She had constant leg soreness that got worse post exercise. Over time, she developed difficulty going upstairs, carrying groceries, and picking up her nieces and nephews. She did not have dysphagia, diplopia, or ptosis. Her fraternal twin sister carried a clinical diagnosis of limb girdle muscular dystrophy of unknown type, but her parents and grandparents did not have limb weakness.

Physical Examination

Her general examination was unremarkable. On strength testing, she had symmetric proximal limb muscle weakness and mild scapular winging. Hip adductors were weaker than abductors. There was no facial weakness.

R. Abhyankar · J. R. Trivedi (✉)
Department of Neurology & Neurotherapeutics, University of Texas Southwestern Medical Center, Dallas, TX, USA
e-mail: jaya.trivedi@UTSouthwestern.edu

C. Cai
Department of Pathology, University of Texas Southwestern Medical Center, Dallas, TX, USA
e-mail: Chunyu.cai@utsouthwestern.edu

L. Zhou et al. (eds.), *A Case-Based Guide to Neuromuscular Pathology*,
https://doi.org/10.1007/978-3-030-25682-1_11

Investigations

CK level was mildly elevated 493 U/L (normal: < 200). ANA was negative. TSH and free T4 were normal. AST and ALT were mildly elevated but GGT was normal. She was initially evaluated by rheumatology, and NCS/EMG was not requested. MRI of the thighs showed moderate to severe atrophy and fatty infiltration of the hamstrings, adductor muscles, and gluteal muscles. A left quadriceps muscle biopsy was ordered.

Muscle Biopsy Findings

The left quadriceps muscle biopsy (Fig. 11.1) revealed mild chronic active myopathy with intact expression of dystrophin, alpha-sarcoglycan, alpha-dystroglycan, caveolin-3, dysferlin, and emerin. Immunostain for MHC Class I showed no abnormal myofiber upregulation.

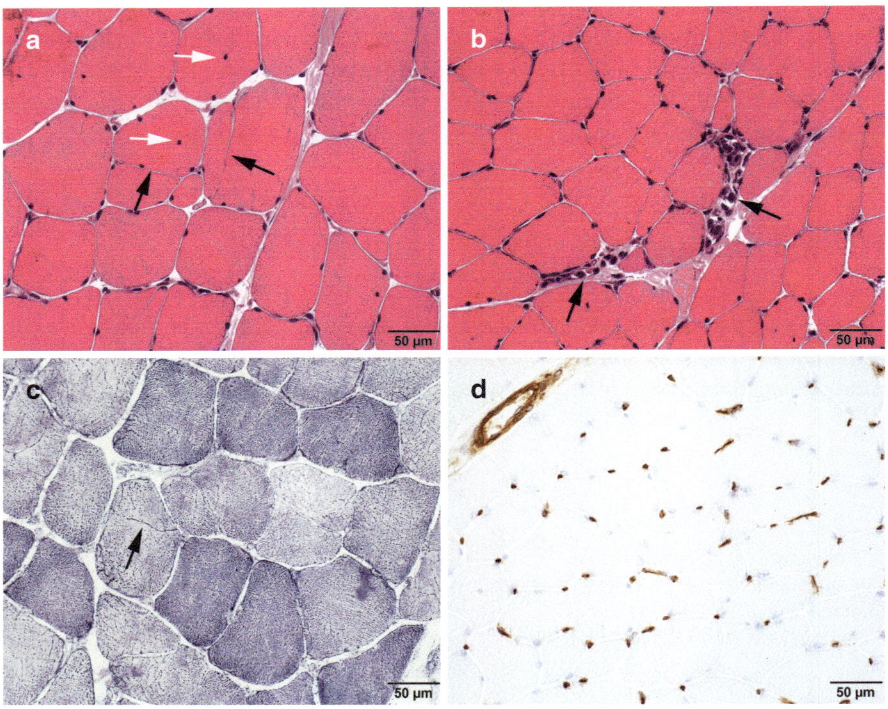

Fig. 11.1 Quadriceps muscle biopsy shows mild chronic active myopathy. (**a**), Chronic features include marked fiber size variation, split fibers (black arrows) and frequent internalized nuclei (white arrows). (**b**), Active features include occasional necrotic fibers (arrows) and absence of regenerating fibers. (**c**), NADH-TR stain highlights split fibers (arrow). No lobulated myofibers are seen in this biopsy. (**d**), MHC I stain shows a normal capillary staining pattern, there is no abnormal myofiber reactivity

Additional Investigation After Muscle Biopsy Diagnosis

The patient was referred to our neuromuscular clinic after obtaining the muscle biopsy diagnosis. Based on her history, family history, MRI, and muscle biopsy findings, a limb-girdle muscular dystrophy (LGMD) was suspected. Subsequent genetic testing revealed two variants in the *CAPN3* gene: c.1468C > T (p.R490W) and c.1063C > T (p.R355W), both of which have been reported as pathogenic mutations [1, 2].

Final Diagnosis

Limb girdle muscular dystrophy type 2A (LGMD2A).

Patient Follow-up

Patient underwent physical therapy for balance training and started using a cane for safe ambulation. At follow up, she complained of daily bouts of coughing, worse with lying flat. Transthoracic echocardiogram was normal. Spirometry showed FVC 89% predicted, MIP 54% predicted, and MEP 84% predicted. She was diagnosed with mild restrictive lung disease. One year after diagnosis, she gave birth to her first child without obstetric complication.

Discussion

The limb girdle muscular dystrophies (LGMD) are genetically heterogeneous, autosomally inherited, have a childhood to adult onset, and are characterized by progressive muscle weakness and wasting of the shoulder- and pelvic-girdle muscles [3]. LGMD is the fourth most common form of muscular dystrophy, with a prevalence of 1.63 per 100, 000 [4]. Autosomal dominant subtypes are denoted as LGMD1 and autosomal recessive subtypes are denoted as LGMD2. There are many subtypes of LGMD: 26 LGMD2 and 8 LGMD1. In general, LGMD2 is more common than LGMD1.

LGMD2A is most common in American and European countries, except in Denmark where LGMD2I is more common [3]. Its clinical presentation is variable with a wide range in onset from childhood to adulthood, but teenage onset is typical. Muscle weakness can start in the pelvic girdle (Leyden-Mobius variant) or the shoulder girdle (Erb variant). Young patients can present with asymptomatic hyper-CKemia or transient eosinophilic myositis [5]. Characteristic features include toe walking in early childhood, scapular winging, scoliosis, axial muscle weakness, joint contractures (especially of the Achilles tendon), and sparing of the facial muscles. The hamstrings, gluteal muscles, and hip adductors are often weak and atrophic. Cardiac function is distinctly normal. As the illness progresses over decades, ambulation is impaired and nearly half the patients become wheelchair dependent. Respiratory complication can be seen in some patients, but is not a salient feature of LGMD2A. There is some gender variability with women having less weakness compared to men [6].

LGMD2A is caused by mutations in the *CAPN3* gene found on chromosome 15, which encodes for calpain-3 [5]. Calpain-3 is a muscle specific protein involved in sarcomere remodeling. Though its exact function is unknown, calpain-3 helps target actin and myosin for proteasomal degradation via ubiquitination. It is highly active in both muscle catabolism and anabolism [7].

The differential diagnosis for LGMD2A is broad. It is often hard to clinically distinguish LGMD2A from other forms of autosomal recessive LGMD such as LGMD2B (dysferlinopathy), LGMD2C-2F (sarcoglycanopathies), LGMD2G (telethoninopathy), and LGMD2J (titinopathy), thereby necessitating a muscle biopsy and/or genetic analysis. Duchenne and Becker muscular dystrophy also have a clinical presentation identical to LGMD2A, but these disorders have prominent cardiac involvement and inheritance pattern is X-linked recessive. Emery-Dreifuss muscular dystrophy presents with joint contractures similar to LGMD2A, but cardiac involvement is more conspicuous. Facioscapulohumeral muscular dystrophy also presents with progressive proximal shoulder girdle weakness, but prominent facial weakness and autosomal dominant inheritance should distinguish this from LGMD2A. LGMD2A can also be confused for metabolic myopathy given exercise intolerance and myalgia. However, most cases of metabolic myopathy can be readily distinguished from limb girdle muscular dystrophy by muscle biopsy.

Serum CK is elevated 5-80× normal in LGMD2A and needle electromyography shows a myopathic pattern. Genetic testing confirms the diagnosis; however, it is not uncommon to detect variants of unknown significance in which case a muscle biopsy should be performed [5]. Since limb girdle muscular dystrophy is phenotypically diverse, a multigene panel is preferred over single gene testing. The 24 coding exons of *CAPN3* can be directly sequenced by next-generation exome sequencing whereas intron mutations can be identified by analysis of complementary DNA (cDNA) [5, 8, 9].

MRI may be a valuable tool for preliminary screening of LGMD2A and can enhance the efficiency of muscle biopsy and DNA analysis. MRI shows a characteristic pattern of muscle involvement: severe fatty infiltration in the long head of biceps femoris, semimembranosus, semitendinosus, and adductor muscles [6, 10] as seen in our patient.

Muscle biopsy can aid in diagnosis by confirming dystrophic changes in muscle and excluding other disease processes such as metabolic myopathies, immune mediated myopathies, or neurogenic etiologies. The hallmarks of dystrophic changes are chronic active myopathic changes with ongoing myofiber necrosis in a background of endomysial fibrosis and fatty replacement. Other less specific chronic changes include marked fiber size variation with presence of hypertrophic fibers, split fibers, and frequent internalized nuclei. These changes are reflective of the time course of the disease process rather than any particular disease. It is usually not possible to specifically classify a muscular dystrophy based on histology or enzyme histochemistry alone. Two helpful features have been reported in association with LGMD2A, including (1) markedly reduced regenerating fibers compared to other muscular dystrophies [5] and (2) eosinophilic myositis in childhood [11]. Definitive diagnosis requires protein and/or genetic analysis. Immunohistochemistry is helpful only in instances of total protein loss; mutations that cause partial loss of calpain-3 cannot be readily detected by this method. Immunoblot analysis is able to capture partial protein loss. However, immunoblot misses 20–30% of LGMD2A cases which have a mutation that impairs the function of the protein rather than its quantity [5]. A functional assay that detects loss of the normal autocatalytic activity of the protein can identify some but not all of the functional mutations. Genetic testing in the form of LGMD panel is becoming the principle method for confirming the diagnosis.

To date, there is no specific treatment for any of the LGMD subtypes. Once diagnosis is made, treatment for the condition is generally supportive. Physical therapy and orthotic intervention is important to maintain safe ambulation and independence for as long as possible. Passive range of motion promotes mobility and flexibility. Gentle and low impact aerobic exercise improves cardiovascular performance and reduces fatigue. Surgical correction of foot deformities, scoliosis, and contractures might be useful [12]. Given the risk of respiratory involvement, regular assessment of forced vital capacity and overnight pulse oximetry are very important [12, 13]. Non-invasive ventilation and cough assist devices may be needed in select individuals [14]. Finally, genetic counseling is important in family planning.

Pearls

Clinical Pearls

1. LGMD2A characteristically causes selective weakness and atrophy of the hamstrings, gluteal muscles, and hip adductors. Scapular weakness and joint contractures are other common features.
2. Muscles of the heart and face are spared in LGMD2A.
3. MRI of the thigh detects fatty infiltration in the adductors and hamstrings and can be used as a screening tool.
4. Mutation testing for LGMD2A can be done by next generation sequencing of the 24 coding exons of the *CAPN3* gene.

Pathology Pearls

1. The degree of pathology varies greatly and does not necessarily correlate with clinical severity.
2. A chronic active myopathy that lacks regenerating fibers, and eosinophilic myositis in children are relatively specific features of LGMD2A.
3. Although lobulated myopathy has often been associated with LGMD2A, it is neither sensitive nor specific. Lobulated myopathy can be seen in a variety of hereditary and non-hereditary conditions [15].
4. In muscle with chronic active myopathy, MHC class I immunostain is helpful in differentiating muscular dystrophies (usually negative) from inflammatory myopathies (usually positive). However, notable exceptions exist both ways. For example, dysferlinopathy (LGMD2B) and facioscapulohumeral dystrophy (FSHD) may have prominent inflammation and myofiber MHC1 upregulation. Conversely, inflammatory myopathies undergoing long-term steroid treatment may have negative MHC1 myofiber expression.

References

1. Groen EJ, Charlton R, Barresi R, Anderson LV, Eagle M, Hudson J, et al. Analysis of the UK diagnostic strategy for limb girdle muscular dystrophy 2A. Brain. 2007;130.(Pt 12:3237–49.
2. Fichna JP, Macias A, Piechota M, Korostynski M, Potulska-Chromik A, Redowicz MJ, et al. Whole-exome sequencing identifies novel pathogenic mutations and putative phenotype-influencing variants in Polish limb-girdle muscular dystrophy patients. Hum Genomics. 2018;12(1):34.
3. Liewluck T, Milone M. Untangling the complexity of limb-girdle muscular dystrophies. Muscle Nerve. 2018;58(2):167–77.
4. Mah JK, Korngut L, Fiest KM, Dykeman J, Day LJ, Pringsheim T, et al. A systematic review and meta-analysis on the epidemiology of the muscular dystrophies. Can J Neurol Sci. 2016;43(1):163–77.
5. Fanin M, Angelini C. Protein and genetic diagnosis of limb girdle muscular dystrophy type 2A: the yield and the pitfalls. Muscle Nerve. 2015;52(2):163–73.
6. Richard I, Hogrel JY, Stockholm D, Payan CA, Fougerousse F, Calpainopathy Study G, et al. Natural history of LGMD2A for delineating outcome measures in clinical trials. Ann Clin Transl Neurol. 2016;3(4):248–65.
7. Kramerova I, Kudryashova E, Venkatraman G, Spencer MJ. Calpain 3 participates in sarcomere remodeling by acting upstream of the ubiquitin-proteasome pathway. Hum Mol Genet. 2005;14(15):2125–34.
8. Nigro V, Savarese M. Genetic basis of limb-girdle muscular dystrophies: the 2014 update. Acta Myol. 2014;33(1):1–12.
9. Duno M, Sveen ML, Schwartz M, Vissing J. cDNA analyses of CAPN3 enhance mutation detection and reveal a low prevalence of LGMD2A patients in Denmark. Eur J Hum Genet. 2008;16(8):935–40.
10. Feng X, Luo S, Li J, Yue D, Xi J, Zhu W, et al. Fatty infiltration evaluation and selective pattern characterization of lower limbs in limb-girdle muscular dystrophy type 2A by muscle magnetic resonance imaging. Muscle Nerve. 2018;58:536–41.

11. Krahn M, Lopez de Munain A, Streichenberger N, Bernard R, Pecheux C, Testard H, et al. CAPN3 mutations in patients with idiopathic eosinophilic myositis. Ann Neurol. 2006;59(6):905–11.
12. Angelini C, Giaretta L, Marozzo R. An update on diagnostic options and considerations in limb-girdle dystrophies. Expert Rev Neurother. 2018;18(9):693–703.
13. Murphy AP, Straub V. The classification, natural history and treatment of the limb girdle muscular dystrophies. J Neuromuscul Dis. 2015;2(s2):S7–19.
14. Simonds AK. Recent advances in respiratory care for neuromuscular disease. Chest. 2006;130(6):1879–86.
15. Figarella-Branger D, El-Dassouki M, Saenz A, Cobo AM, Malzac P, Tong S, et al. Myopathy with lobulated muscle fibers: evidence for heterogeneous etiology and clinical presentation. Neuromuscul Disord. 2002;12(1):4–12.

Chapter 12
A 52-Year-Old Man with Proximal Limb Weakness and Hand Stiffness

Lan Zhou and Susan C. Shin

History

A 52-year-old man presented to our neuromuscular clinic for obtaining a second opinion on his myopathy. He first noted mild difficulty rising out of a chair from a seated position, climbing stairs, and doing pushups 5 years prior to the presentation. The weakness slowly progressed with significant involvement of both upper and lower extremities. He noted intermittent cramping and stiffness in the hands and toes. He reported mild difficulty swallowing sometimes, but denied slurred speech, droopy eyelids, double vision, shortness of breath, or palpitations. He had a past medical history of Asperger syndrome, asthma, pancreatitis, cataracts at age 30s, and non-insulin dependent diabetes mellitus diagnosed 5 years prior. He had bilateral cataract removal. His medications included metformin, albuterol, and aspirin. He was adopted and did not know his biological family members. He did not have children. He did not drink alcohol or smoke cigarettes.

Physical Examination

General examination was notable to frontal balding and residua from the bilateral cataract surgery. His cardiac examination was normal. His mental status was unremarkable. Cranial nerve functions were intact with normal extraocular movements

L. Zhou (✉)
Departments of Neurology and Pathology, Boston University Medical Center, Boston, MA, USA
e-mail: lanzhou@bu.edu

S. C. Shin
Department of Neurology, Icahn School of Medicine at Mount Sinai, New York, NY, USA
e-mail: susan.shin@mssm.edu

L. Zhou et al. (eds.), *A Case-Based Guide to Neuromuscular Pathology*,
https://doi.org/10.1007/978-3-030-25682-1_12

and no eyelid ptosis or dysarthria. Motor examination showed normal tone and bulk. Mild percussion myotonia was noted in the thenar muscles, greater on the right. Weakness was detected in the neck flexors (MRC 4/5) and bilateral deltoid (4/5), biceps (4/5), hip flexors (4/5), and knee extensors (4/5). He was unable to rise from a chair without using his hands to push. Deep tendon reflexes were 2+ throughout. Sensory examination was normal to all modalities. Toes were downgoing bilaterally. His gait was normal.

Investigations

The patient's serum creatine kinase (CK) level was normal. He had nerve conduction studies (NCS) and electromyography (EMG) twice by outside neurologists, one reportedly being normal and the other reportedly showing myotonic discharges in the proximal limb muscles. He underwent a right quadriceps muscle biopsy.

Muscle Biopsy Findings

The right quadriceps muscle biopsy (Fig. 12.1) showed increased fiber size variation with some scattered atrophic and hypertrophic muscle fibers, a few pyknotic nuclear clumps, a marked increase in internal nuclei, several round atrophic fibers with ringbinden (ring fibers), a single necrotic fiber, and type 2

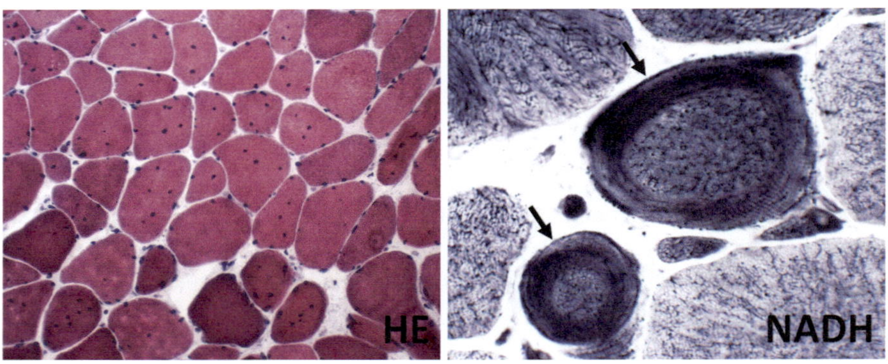

Fig. 12.1 Quadriceps muscle biopsy from the present patient. HE stain shows increased fiber size variation with a few atrophic and hypertrophic fibers, and numerous internal nuclei. Many fibers contain multiple internal nuclei. NADH stain shows two round fibers with ringbinden (ring fibers) (arrows)

fiber predominance. Many fibers contained multiple internal nuclei. There was no inflammation. These findings suggested myotonic dystrophy, especially myotonic dystrophy type 2 (DM2) in this clinical setting. There were very few angulated atrophic fibers which were esterase-positive, but no target fibers, fiber type grouping, or group atrophy. The findings suggested very mild denervation atrophy.

Additional Investigation After Muscle Biopsy Diagnosis

Based on the patient's clinical presentation, clinical and EMG myotonia, and muscle biopsy findings, the DM2 gene test was ordered. It showed a repeat expansion mutation of DM2 with the expanded repeat size of 13,170 base pairs (normal: <176 base pairs), diagnostic for DM2. CBC, comprehensive metabolic panel, HbA1C, thyroid function test, ANA, and Vitamin D level were all normal.

Final Diagnosis

Myotonic dystrophy type 2

Patient Follow-up

The diagnosis, management, and prognosis of DM2 were discussed with the patient. He received physical therapy for the proximal limb weakness with benefit. His clinical myotonia was mild, and he did not want to take a medication for it. He underwent cardiology evaluation with no significant abnormalities found. His glycemic control was optimal. He was followed annually by neurology, cardiology, endocrinology, and ophthalmology.

Discussion

Myotonic dystrophy is the most common form of muscular dystrophies seen in adults. It is a unique muscular dystrophy characterized by multisystem involvement, clinical and EMG myotonia, RNA toxicity being the disease-causing mechanism, and lack of dystrophic changes on muscle biopsy.

Myotonic dystrophy is an autosomal dominant disease. It has two types: myotonic dystrophy type 1 (DM1) and DM2. While both types manifest muscle atrophy, weakness, myotonia, early-onset cataract (before age 50 years), diabetes mellitus, gastrointestinal dysfunction, hypogonadism, and cardiac abnormalities including arrhythmia, conduction defects, and cardiomyopathy, there are several differences between the two types [1, 2]. DM1 has an early symptom onset with the presence of a congenital form, while the onset of DM2 is late, most often in the fourth and fifth decades of life with no congenital form [1]. DM1 mainly affects distal limb muscles such as finger flexors, wrist flexors, and ankle dorsiflexors, while DM2 predominantly involves proximal and axial muscles including neck flexors, arm abductors, hip flexors, and hip extensors. Frontal balding is common in both types, but facial weakness is mainly seen in DM1. Cardiac dysfunction and central nervous system involvement are less common in DM2 than in DM1 [3–6].

DM2 is also known as proximal myotonic myopathy (PROMM) [7–11]. It is less common than DM1. The prevalence of DM2 is uncertain, and it likely varies by population. DM2 is probably underdiagnosed as the disease manifestation is variable and can be very mild and non-specific [12]. Some patients may only have muscle pain, fatigue, or mild weakness. Clinical myotonia is usually mild and can be absent. Percussion of forearm extensors and thenar muscles is the most sensitive clinical test for myotonia. When clinical myotonia is prominent in a patient with DM2, a superimposed chloride or sodium channel gene mutation should be considered [13, 14]. CK is usually mildly elevated or normal. Needle EMG in resting muscles may show myotonia which can be evoked by percussion; the myotonic discharges tend to be waning in DM2 as opposed to waxing-waning in DM1 [15]. EMG myotonia can be minimal or absent in DM2.

Muscle biopsy is not necessary in myotonic dystrophy as gene testing is commercially available for making the definitive diagnosis. However, due to the heterogeneity of the clinical presentation in DM2, muscle biopsy may still be useful in patients with mild and non-specific symptoms and findings. Muscle biopsy in myotonic dystrophy usually does not show dystrophic changes which consist of prominent myofiber degeneration, regeneration, and necrosis, and endomysial inflammation and fibrosis [16–18]. It typically shows markedly increased internal nuclei and increased fiber size variation with angulated or rounded atrophic fibers and some hypertrophic fibers [16–18]. In DM1, it may also show sarcoplasmic mass and prominent type 1 fiber hypotrophy [19, 20]. In DM2, it usually shows prominent pyknotic nuclei clumps and type 2 fiber atrophy and/or hypertrophy but not type 1 fiber hypotrophy [16–18]. Ring fibers is an infrequent finding [16, 18], and it is caused by disorientation of peripheral myofibrils running at right angles to the main body of the fibre [21]. It is best viewed by NADH stain or electron microscopy (EM). Muscle biopsies in individual DM2 cases may not show all the pathological features; while some show ring fibers (Fig. 12.1), the others do not (Fig. 12.2). In general, the pathological changes are more prominent in type 2 fibers in DM2 but more involving type 1 fibers in DM1

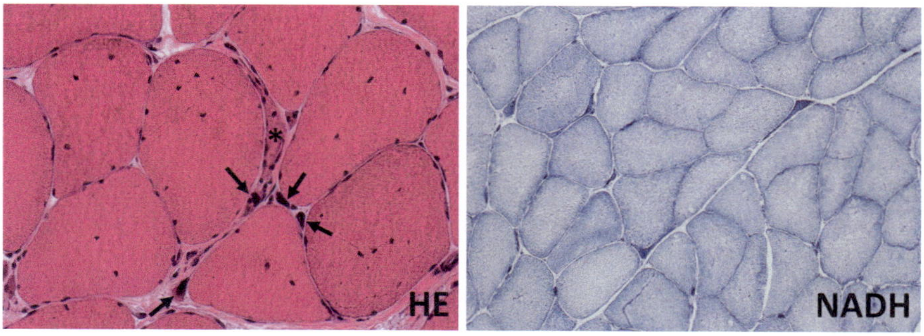

Fig. 12.2 Triceps muscle biopsy from another patient with DM2. HE stain shows markedly increased internal nuclei, many pyknotic nuclear clumps (arrows), a rare angulated atrophic fiber (*), and some hypertrophic fibers. NADH stain shows type 2 fiber predominance, occasional angulated atrophic fibers, and absent ring fibers

[17]. The pathological changes in DM2 do not correlate with individual clinical symptoms [16].

The pathogenic mechanism underlying myotonic dystrophy involves RNA toxicities. DM1 is caused by expanded CTG repeats in the 3′ untranslated region of the myotonic dystrophy protein kinase gene (*DMPK*) on chromosome 19q13 [22, 23]. DM2 is caused by expanded CCTG repeats in intron 1 of the zinger finger protein 9 gene (*ZNF9*) on chromosome 3q [24, 25]. These expanded repeats in the noncoding regions are transcribed into RNAs which exert a toxic gain-of-function to deregulate several RNA binding proteins including muscleblind-like proteins, resulting in aberrant RNA slicing, polyadenylation, or expression of hundreds of genes. The expanded RNA repeats may also affect cell signaling and are sometimes translated into neurotoxic peptides [26]. The multilevel toxicities and the large number of genes affected by the expanded RNA repeats account for the complex phenotype of myotonic dystrophy. The phenotype of DM2 is milder than that of DM1, which is most likely contributed by modifiers [27]. Currently, there is active therapy development to target and reduce the RNA toxicities by antisense oligonucleotides and others [26].

There is no cure for myotonic dystrophy at this point. Genetic counseling should be provided to every patient. Given the multisystem involvement, the symptomatic management of DM2 requires multiple clinical specialties, including neurology, cardiology, endocrinology, ophthalmology, gastroenterology, and rehabilitation. Myotonia, pain, and hypersomnolence are managed by neurologist. Grip myotonia is usually mild, and mexiletine may be used if bothersome [28]. A thorough cardiac evaluation is needed to identify and control the risks for major cardiac arrhythmia and cardiomyopathy [3]. Diabetes mellitus is more frequently seen in DM2 than in DM1, and it should be monitor and treated by endocrinologist. Periodic slit-lamp exam should be performed by ophthalmologist to detect cataract and treat accordingly. Rehabilitation is important for DM2 patients to manage their proximal limb weakness.

Pearls

Clinical Pearls

1. Myotonic dystrophy is the most common muscular dystrophy seen in adults.
2. DM2 is a multisystem disease which usually manifests adult-onset and slowly progressive muscle pain, fatigue, and stiffness, as well as mild proximal limb weakness. Diabetes mellitus, early-onset cataract, gallbladder dysfunction, and cardiac abnormalities are the commonly associated conditions.
3. Examination in patients with DM2 often shows frontal balding and mild proximal limb weakness. Facial weakness, a common feature in DM1, is usually not seen or mild in DM2.
4. EMG often shows myotonia in limb muscles, but clinical myotonia is usually mild or even absent in DM2. CK is usually mildly elevated but can be normal.
5. Muscle biopsy can be spared as the definitive diagnosis is made by the DM2 gene test. In patients with mild and nonspecific symptoms and findings, a muscle biopsy may still be useful to raise the suspicion and direct the gene test.
6. Due to the multisystem involvement, patients with DM2 should be managed by multiple clinical specialties, including neurology, cardiology, ophthalmology, endocrinology, gastroenterology, and rehabilitation.
7. The pathogenic mechanism underlying myotonic dystrophy involves RNA toxicities. There is active therapy development to target and reduce the RNA toxicities.

Pathology Pearls

1. Muscle biopsy in DM2 usually does not show dystrophic changes which consist of prominent myofiber degeneration, necrosis, and regeneration, and endomysial inflammation and fibrosis.
2. Muscle biopsy in DM2 usually shows a combination of markedly increased internal nuclei, pyknotic nuclear clumps, ring fibers, a few angulated atrophic fibers, and some hypertrophic fibers. These changes are more prominent in type 2 fibers. These features may not be all present in an individual muscle biopsy from a patient with DM2.
3. Type 1 fiber hypotrophy, a relatively common finding in DM1, is not a feature of DM2.

References

1. Day JW, Ricker K, Jacobsen JF, Rasmussen LJ, Dick KA, Kress W, et al. Myotonic dystrophy type 2: molecular, diagnostic and clinical spectrum. Neurology. 2003;60(4):657–64.
2. Meola G, Cardani R. Myotonic dystrophy type 2 and modifier genes: an update on clinical and pathomolecular aspects. Neurol Sci. 2017;38(4):535–46.
3. Sansone VA, Brigonzi E, Schoser B, Villani S, Gaeta M, De Ambroggi G, et al. The frequency and severity of cardiac involvement in myotonic dystrophy type 2 (DM2): long-term outcomes. Int J Cardiol. 2013;168(2):1147–53.
4. Wenninger S, Montagnese F, Schoser B. Core clinical phenotypes in myotonic dystrophies. Front Neurol. 2018;9:303.
5. Meola G, Sansone V, Perani D, Scarone S, Cappa S, Dragoni C, et al. Executive dysfunction and avoidant personality trait in myotonic dystrophy type 1 (DM-1) and in proximal myotonic myopathy (PROMM/DM-2). Neuromuscul Disord. 2003;13(10):813–21.
6. Romeo V, Pegoraro E, Ferrati C, Squarzanti F, Soraru G, Palmieri A, et al. Brain involvement in myotonic dystrophies: neuroimaging and neuropsychological comparative study in DM1 and DM2. J Neurol. 2010;257(8):1246–55.
7. Meola G, Sansone V. A newly-described myotonic disorder (proximal myotonic myopathy--PROMM): personal experience and review of the literature. Ital J Neurol Sci. 1996;17(5):347–53.
8. Meola G, Sansone V, Radice S, Skradski S, Ptacek L. A family with an unusual myotonic and myopathic phenotype and no CTG expansion (proximal myotonic myopathy syndrome): a challenge for future molecular studies. Neuromuscul Disord. 1996;6(3):143–50.
9. Ricker K, Koch MC, Lehmann-Horn F, Pongratz D, Otto M, Heine R, et al. Proximal myotonic myopathy: a new dominant disorder with myotonia, muscle weakness, and cataracts. Neurology. 1994;44(8):1448–52.
10. Thornton CA, Griggs RC, Moxley RT 3rd. Myotonic dystrophy with no trinucleotide repeat expansion. Ann Neurol. 1994;35(3):269–72.
11. Udd B, Krahe R, Wallgren-Pettersson C, Falck B, Kalimo H. Proximal myotonic dystrophy--a family with autosomal dominant muscular dystrophy, cataracts, hearing loss and hypogonadism: heterogeneity of proximal myotonic syndromes? Neuromuscul Disord. 1997;7(4):217–28.
12. Meola G, Biasini F, Valaperta R, Costa E, Cardani R. Biomolecular diagnosis of myotonic dystrophy type 2: a challenging approach. J Neurol. 2017;264(8):1705–14.
13. Bugiardini E, Rivolta I, Binda A, Soriano Caminero A, Cirillo F, Cinti A, et al. SCN4A mutation as modifying factor of myotonic dystrophy type 2 phenotype. Neuromuscul Disord. 2015;25(4):301–7.
14. Cardani R, Giagnacovo M, Botta A, Rinaldi F, Morgante A, Udd B, et al. Co-segregation of DM2 with a recessive CLCN1 mutation in juvenile onset of myotonic dystrophy type 2. J Neurol. 2012;259(10):2090–9.
15. Logigian EL, Ciafaloni E, Quinn LC, Dilek N, Pandya S, Moxley RT 3rd, et al. Severity, type, and distribution of myotonic discharges are different in type 1 and type 2 myotonic dystrophy. Muscle Nerve. 2007;35(4):479–85.
16. Schoser BG, Schneider-Gold C, Kress W, Goebel HH, Reilich P, Koch MC, et al. Muscle pathology in 57 patients with myotonic dystrophy type 2. Muscle Nerve. 2004;29(2):275–81.
17. Pisani V, Panico MB, Terracciano C, Bonifazi E, Meola G, Novelli G, et al. Preferential central nucleation of type 2 myofibers is an invariable feature of myotonic dystrophy type 2. Muscle Nerve. 2008;38(5):1405–11.
18. Vihola A, Bassez G, Meola G, Zhang S, Haapasalo H, Paetau A, et al. Histopathological differences of myotonic dystrophy type 1 (DM1) and PROMM/DM2. Neurology. 2003;60(11):1854–7.
19. Tohgi H, Kawamorita A, Utsugisawa K, Yamagata M, Sano M. Muscle histopathology in myotonic dystrophy in relation to age and muscular weakness. Muscle Nerve. 1994;17(9):1037–43.

20. Harper PS, van Engelen BG, Eymard B, Rogers M, Wilcox D. 99th ENMC international workshop: myotonic dystrophy: present management, future therapy. 9–11 November 2001, Naarden, The Netherlands. Neuromuscul Disord. 2002;12(6):596–9.
21. Dubowitz VS, Sewry CA, Oldfors A. In: Dubowitz VS, Sewry CA, Oldfors A, editors. Histological and Histochemical Changes. 4th ed. Oxford: Saunders Elsevier; 2013.
22. Brook JD, McCurrach ME, Harley HG, Buckler AJ, Church D, Aburatani H, et al. Molecular basis of myotonic dystrophy: expansion of a trinucleotide (CTG) repeat at the 3′ end of a transcript encoding a protein kinase family member. Cell. 1992;68(4):799–808.
23. Fu YH, Pizzuti A, Fenwick RG Jr, King J, Rajnarayan S, Dunne PW, et al. An unstable triplet repeat in a gene related to myotonic muscular dystrophy. Science. 1992;255(5049):1256–8.
24. Liquori CL, Ricker K, Moseley ML, Jacobsen JF, Kress W, Naylor SL, et al. Myotonic dystrophy type 2 caused by a CCTG expansion in intron 1 of ZNF9. Science. 2001;293(5531):864–7.
25. Ranum LP, Rasmussen PF, Benzow KA, Koob MD, Day JW. Genetic mapping of a second myotonic dystrophy locus. Nat Genet. 1998;19(2):196–8.
26. Thornton CA, Wang E, Carrell EM. Myotonic dystrophy: approach to therapy. Curr Opin Genet Dev. 2017;44:135–40.
27. Sellier C, Cerro-Herreros E, Blatter M, Freyermuth F, Gaucherot A, Ruffenach F, et al. rbFOX1/MBNL1 competition for CCUG RNA repeats binding contributes to myotonic dystrophy type 1/type 2 differences. Nat Commun. 2018;9(1):2009.
28. Logigian EL, Martens WB, RTt M, McDermott MP, Dilek N, Wiegner AW, et al. Mexiletine is an effective antimyotonia treatment in myotonic dystrophy type 1. Neurology. 2010;74(18):1441–8.

Chapter 13
A 51-Year-Old Woman with Long-Standing Exercise Intolerance

Lan Zhou

History

A 51-year-old Hispanic woman started to run 2–3 miles a day and 5 days a week when she was in high school. At the end of high school, the running became difficult as she would develop intense leg muscle pain, cramps, and fatigue which required frequent rest. She also noticed dark-color urine several times triggered by running at age 20s and 30s. She stopped running regularly at late 30s. She usually developed annoying muscle pain, cramps, and fatigue in the legs shortly after running. She had to slow down or stop for a few minutes to get the symptoms relieved. She also developed mild difficulty climbing stairs and uncomfortable heaviness feeling in her arms when carrying grocery bags at age 40s. She saw a local neurologist who found persistently elevated serum creatine kinase (CK) level in a range of 300s to 5,000s U/L. In one occasion, CK went up to 21,000 U/L when she had tea-color urine after jogging for 2 miles. She underwent a left quadriceps muscle biopsy with no definitive diagnosis. She was suspected to have an inflammatory myopathy. She had been treated with Prednisone, methotrexate, and Cytoxan for 2–1/2 years with no improvement. Her muscle pain and cramps as well as the degree of CK elevation correlated with her physical activity but not the treatment. She discontinued all the immunosuppressive agents 3 years prior to the presentation with no change of her symptoms of exercise intolerance. Her leg weakness, however, had been slowly progressed. She came to our clinic for a second opinion. Her birth history and developmental history were unremarkable. Her past medical history was significant for hypothyroidism, for which she took levothyroxine. Her family history was negative for a muscle disease. There was no consanguinity in her parents. She did not drink alcohol, smoke cigarettes, or abuse illicit drugs.

L. Zhou (✉)
Departments of Neurology and Pathology, Boston University Medical Center, Boston, MA, USA
e-mail: lanzhou@bu.edu

L. Zhou et al. (eds.), *A Case-Based Guide to Neuromuscular Pathology*,
https://doi.org/10.1007/978-3-030-25682-1_13

Physical Examination

General examination was unremarkable. Neurologic examination showed intact cranial nerve functions with no facial, ocular, or bulbar weakness. Motor examination revealed normal muscle tone and bulk, and mild weakness in the hip flexors (MRC 4/5). She could get up from a chair without using her hands to push but with difficulty. Sensation and coordination were normal. Deep tendon reflexes were 2+ throughout. Toes were downgoing bilaterally. Her gait was normal, including heel, toe, and tandem walking.

Investigations

Serum CK level was mildly elevated at 830 U/L. CBC, comprehensive metabolic panel, TSH, and free T4 were all normal. Plasma lactate and pyruvate levels as well as acylcarnitine profile were also unremarkable. Nerve conduction study (NCS) was normal. Electromyography (EMG) showed a non-irritable myopathy with myopathic motor unit potentials seen in the proximal limb muscles and paraspinal muscles. Her prior muscle biopsy slides were reviewed, which showed very tiny specimen with remarkable freezing artefact, precluding adequate interpretation. There was no obvious inflammation. A right quadriceps muscle biopsy was performed.

Muscle Biopsy Findings

The right quadriceps muscle biopsy (Fig. 13.1) showed a vacuolar myopathy with many fibers containing subsarcolemmal vacuoles or blebs. These vacuoles were not red rimmed or autophagic with no acid phosphatase reactivity.

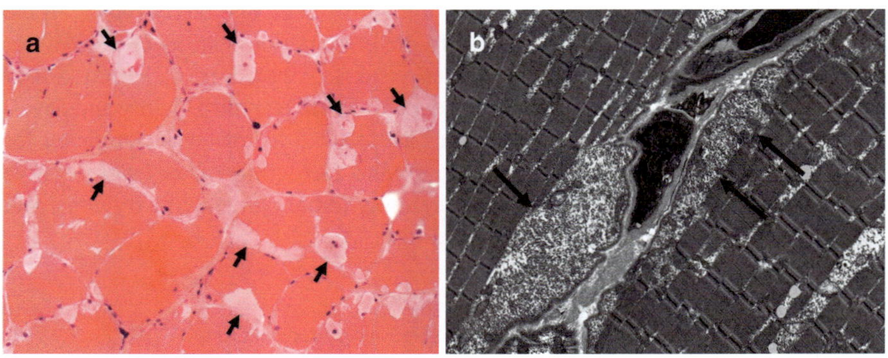

Fig. 13.1 Glycogen storage myopathy. (**a**), H&E stain shows many fibers containing subsarcolemmal vacuoles or blebs (arrows). (**b**), EM shows striking subsarcolemmal glycogen accumulations (arrows)

Electron microscopy (EM) showed striking subsarcolemmal accumulations of glycogen granules, corresponding to the blebs seen under light microscopy. There were very few scattered polygonal atrophic fibers but no myofiber necrosis, degeneration, or regeneration. The findings are typical for a glycogen storage myopathy.

Additional Investigation After the Muscle Biopsy Diagnosis

A part of the patient's muscle biopsy tissue was sent for myoglobinuria panel (biochemical analysis of enzyme activities involved in muscle energy metabolism, the deficiencies in which could cause recurrent rhabdomyolysis). It showed a reproducible and profound deficiency in myophosphorylase activity.

Final Diagnosis

Glycogen Storage Disease Type V (McArdle Disease)

Patient Follow-up

The test results were discussed with the patient. Due to the long distance, she preferred to be managed by her local physicians. She was recommended to obtain the *PYGM* gene test and genetic counseling. She was instructed to receive physical therapy, modify her exercise and diet, and take nutritional supplements.

Discussion

McArdle disease, also known as glycogen storage disease type V, is an autosomal recessive metabolic myopathy caused by mutations in the *PYGM* gene which encodes the muscle isoenzyme of glycogen phosphorylase (myophosphorylase) [1]. Myophosphorylase is one of the key enzymes involved in converting glycogen to glucose 1-phosphate (glycogenolysis) which enters the glycolytic pathways to produce the energy molecule ATP to support muscle activity. Deficiency in myophosphorylase causes abnormal glycogen accumulation and impaired energy metabolism in skeletal muscle.

Among the metabolic myopathies that are caused by the defects in carbohydrate metabolism, McArdle disease is the most common with an estimated prevalence of 1:100,000 in Dallas-Fort Worth of Texas [2] and 1:167,000 in Spain [3]. The usual symptom onset is in the first or second decade of life but it can vary. The clinical presentation of McArdle disease is heterogeneous. The majority of patients present with exercise intolerance, and they start to notice muscle symptoms when they become athletic at school ages. The common symptoms include myalgia, cramps, and fatigue in exercising muscles, which are usually developed a few minutes after isometric (e.g., carrying weights) or sustained aerobic exercise (e.g., jogging). The symptoms may improve after a brief rest or reducing the exercise intensity (second wind phenomenon). Recurrent rhabdomyolysis occurs in approximately 50% of the patients. These episodes may cause acute renal failure. Fixed proximal limb weakness can be detected in 11% of the patients, mostly in those above 40 years of age [3, 4].

The diagnosis of McArdle disease is often delayed due to the rarity and under-recognition of the disease. It can be misdiagnosed with inflammatory myopathy as seen in our case because of the persistent CK elevation and fixed proximal limb weakness. Misdiagnosis causes diagnostic delay in McArdle disease [5]. Making a correct diagnosis of McArdle disease at an early stage of the disease is important because patients can be managed appropriately to avoid unnecessary exposure to the side effects of immunosuppressive therapies.

Diagnostic evaluation of McArdle disease mainly includes serum CK, NCS/EMG, muscle biopsy, and gene test. Forearm non-ischemic test and cycle and walking test to detect the heart rate response to the second wind phenomenon may also be used to screen for McArdle disease [6, 7]. As exercise intolerance with an early age at onset is a common feature of metabolic myopathies which also include mitochondrial myopathies and lipid storage myopathies, one may also check serum lactate, pyruvate, carnitines, acylcarnitine profile, and urine organic acids during the initial evaluation. Resting serum CK is usually persistently elevated in McArdle disease. The CK elevation is mild or moderate at baseline and severe during the episodes of rhabdomyolysis. EMG may show myopathic changes but can be normal. Muscle biopsy is useful in evaluating a patient with a suspected metabolic myopathy. It can differentiate a glycogen storage myopathy from a lipid storage myopathy or a mitochondrial myopathy, as these individual metabolic myopathies have distinct pathological features. It can also rule out other chronic myopathies which can cause exercise intolerance and muscle weakness such as muscular dystrophy. The phosphorylase stain allows histochemical analysis of the myophosphorylase activity in muscle fibers to detect myophosphorylase deficiency. Myophosphorylase activity can also be measured by biochemical analysis using biopsied muscle tissue, and the diagnosis of McArdle disease can be established when the myophosphorylase enzyme activity is deficient. The *PYGM* gene test identifies specific mutations causing myophosphorylase deficiency. So far, 147 pathological mutations of the *PYGM* gene have been identified [8]. There is no genotype-phenotype correlation [9–14]. Some neurologists prefer genetic testing first; if negative, proceed with a muscle biopsy.

Muscle pathology of McArdle disease features the presence of subsarcolemmal vacuoles or blebs. These vacuoles are filled with glycogen granules, which may be striking on PAS stain (Fig. 13.2). Unlike lysosomal glycogen storage disease (e.g., Pompe disease), these vacuoles are not autophagic with no reactivity to acid phos-

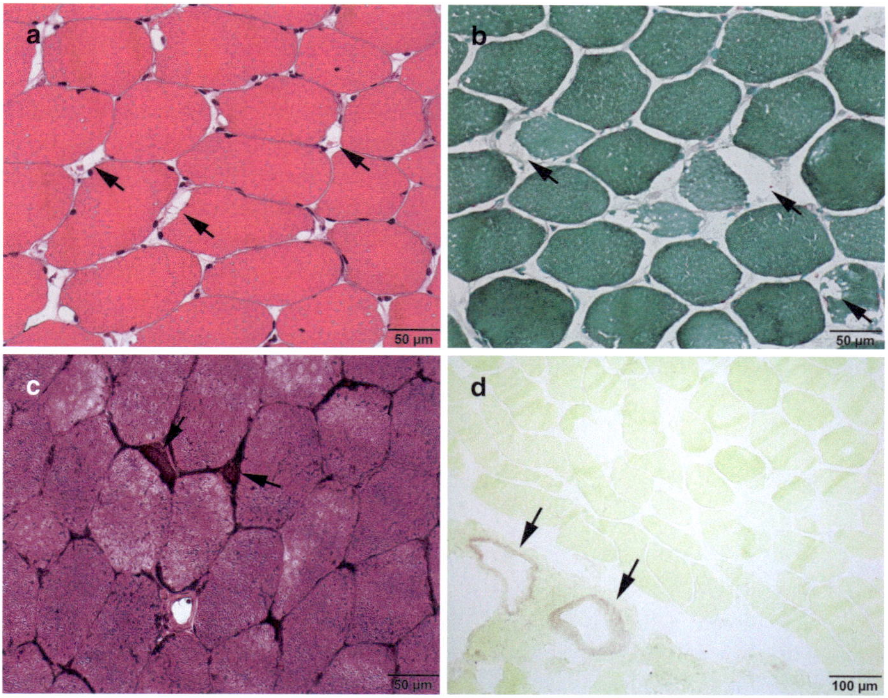

Fig. 13.2 Muscle biopsy from another patient, a 14-year-old female, with a history of rhabdomyolysis and muscle pain. (**a**), H&E shows subtle subsarcolemmal vacuoles in an otherwise unremarkable muscle (arrows). These vacuoles are negative for acid phosphatase stain (**b**, arrows), but contain PAS-positive granules (**c**, arrows) that are diastase digestible. Phosphorylase reactivity is completely absent in myofibers but retained in the wall of blood vessels (**d**, arrows). (This figure is provided by Dr. Chunyu Cai)

phatase (see Fig. 13.2). EM allows ultrastructural visualization of glycogen granules accumulated in the subsarcolemmal areas corresponding to the blebs seen under light microscopy (see Fig. 13.1) [15]. Phosphorylase reactivity is completely absent in muscle fibers but often retain in the wall of blood vessels (see Fig. 13.2) as blood vessel smooth muscle contains a different phosphorylase isoenzyme. The finding is specific to McArdle disease as long as the biopsied muscle tissue contains endogenous glycogen. A positive control should be used to avoid false-negative results of the phosphorylase stain. Muscle fiber type proportion or size is not altered [16].

Management of patients with McArdle disease consists of aerobic training, exercise and dietary modifications, and nutritional supplementation. The goal is to reduce exercise intolerance and to avoid rhabdomyolysis. Aerobic training is beneficial as it can improve fitness by improving cardiorespiratory capacity and increasing delivery of blood-born fuels without adverse events in patients with McArdle disease [17–20]. Intense isometric exercise (e.g., weight lifting) or maximal aerobic exercise (e.g., running, strenuous swimming, or cycling) should be avoided. As

McArdle disease is caused by the defect in the breakdown of glycogen to generate glucose for glycolysis, rich carbohydrate diet (65% carbohydrates) and taking carbohydrates (glucose, fructose, or sucrose) right before exercise have been shown beneficial to reduce exercise intolerance [21–23]. Combining aerobic exercise training and carbohydrates ingestion before exercise has been advocated [24, 25]. Low-dose creatine monohydrate also appears beneficial [26–28]. Large-scale, double-blinded, and placebo-controlled studies are needed to confirm the efficacy of nutritional and pharmacological treatments. Such studies may be difficult to do because the disease is rare. Genetic counseling should be provided to every patient. These patients should also be instructed to recognize myoglobinuria (pigmenturia). They should go to a local emergency department when pigmenturia occurs to obtain acute treatment (intravenous hydration, etc.) to avoid acute renal failure.

Pearls

Clinical Pearls

1. The clinical hallmark feature of McArdle disease is exercise intolerance with recurrent rhabdomyolysis triggered by strenuous exercise. The main differential diagnosis is the other metabolic myopathies such as lipid storage myopathies, mitochondrial myopathies, and other glycogen storage myopathies.
2. Patients with McArdle disease may manifest fixed proximal limb weakness especially after age 40 years, persistent CK elevation, and myopathic changes on EMG.
3. Recognition and early diagnosis of McArdle disease is important for initiating appropriate management and avoiding wrong diagnosis and treatment.
4. Diagnostic evaluation of McArdle disease mainly includes serum CK, NCS/EMG, muscle biopsy, and gene test.
5. Muscle biopsy is useful as it can differentiate McArdle disease from other glycogen storage myopathies, lipid storage myopathies, and mitochondrial myopathies to direct subsequent genetic testing. Myophosphorylase activity can be assessed by histochemical and biochemical analyses using muscle biopsy tissue. The diagnosis of McArdle disease can be established if myophosphorylase activity is absent.
6. The *PYGM* gene test identifies specific mutations in patients with McArdle disease. There is no genotype-phenotype correlation.
7. The current management of patients with McArdle disease consists of aerobic exercise training, dietary modifications, nutritional supplementation, and acute treatment of rhabdomyolysis when it occurs. Genetic counselling should be provided to every patient.

Pathology Pearls

1. Muscle pathology of McArdle disease features the presence of subsarcolemmal vacuoles or blebs filled with excessive glycogen granules. These vacuoles are not autophagic with no reactivity to acid phosphatase. These vacuoles contain excessive PAS-positive granules that are diastase digestible.
2. EM study is essential, which allows ultrastructural confirmation of subsarcolemmal accumulation of glycogen granules.
3. Phosphorylase stain shows complete absence of reactivity in muscle fibers, but the reactivity often retains in the wall of intramuscular blood vessels. The finding is specific to McArdle disease as long as the biopsied muscle tissue contains endogenous glycogen. A positive control should be used to avoid false-negative results.

References

1. Schmid R, Mahler R. Chronic progressive myopathy with myoglobinuria: demonstration of a glycogenolytic defect in the muscle. J Clin Invest. 1959;38:2044–58.
2. Haller RG. Treatment of McArdle disease. Arch Neurol. 2000;57(7):923–4.
3. Lucia A, Ruiz JR, Santalla A, Nogales-Gadea G, Rubio JC, Garcia-Consuegra I, et al. Genotypic and phenotypic features of McArdle disease: insights from the Spanish national registry. J Neurol Neurosurg Psychiatry. 2012;83(3):322–8.
4. Nadaj-Pakleza AA, Vincitorio CM, Laforet P, Eymard B, Dion E, Teijeira S, et al. Permanent muscle weakness in McArdle disease. Muscle Nerve. 2009;40(3):350–7.
5. Scalco RS, Morrow JM, Booth S, Chatfield S, Godfrey R, Quinlivan R. Misdiagnosis is an important factor for diagnostic delay in McArdle disease. Neuromuscul Disord. 2017;27(9):852–5.
6. Vissing J, Haller RG. A diagnostic cycle test for McArdle's disease. Ann Neurol. 2003;54(4):539–42.
7. Buckley JP, Quinlivan RM, Sim J, Eston RG, Short DS. Heart rate and perceived muscle pain responses to a functional walking test in McArdle disease. J Sports Sci. 2014;32(16):1561–9.
8. Nogales-Gadea G, Brull A, Santalla A, Andreu AL, Arenas J, Martin MA, et al. McArdle disease: update of reported mutations and polymorphisms in the PYGM gene. Hum Mutat. 2015;36(7):669–78.
9. Aquaron R, Berge-Lefranc JL, Pellissier JF, Montfort MF, Mayan M, Figarella-Branger D, et al. Molecular characterization of myophosphorylase deficiency (McArdle disease) in 34 patients from Southern France: identification of 10 new mutations. Absence of genotype-phenotype correlation. Neuromuscul Disord. 2007;17(3):235–41.
10. Bruno C, Cassandrini D, Martinuzzi A, Toscano A, Moggio M, Morandi L, et al. McArdle disease: the mutation spectrum of PYGM in a large Italian cohort. Hum Mutat. 2006;27(7):718.
11. Deschauer M, Morgenroth A, Joshi PR, Glaser D, Chinnery PF, Aasly J, et al. Analysis of spectrum and frequencies of mutations in McArdle disease. Identification of 13 novel mutations. J Neurol. 2007;254(6):797–802.
12. Martin MA, Rubio JC, Buchbinder J, Fernandez-Hojas R, del Hoyo P, Teijeira S, et al. Molecular heterogeneity of myophosphorylase deficiency (McArdle's disease): a genotype-phenotype correlation study. Ann Neurol. 2001;50(5):574–81.

13. Vieitez I, Teijeira S, Fernandez JM, San Millan B, Miranda S, Ortolano S, et al. Molecular and clinical study of McArdle's disease in a cohort of 123 European patients. Identification of 20 novel mutations. Neuromuscul Disord. 2011;21(12):817–23.
14. Santalla A, Nogales-Gadea G, Encinar AB, Vieitez I, Gonzalez-Quintana A, Serrano-Lorenzo P, et al. Genotypic and phenotypic features of all Spanish patients with McArdle disease: a 2016 update. BMC Genomics. 2017;18(Suppl 8):819.
15. Dubowitz V, Sewry CA, Oldfors A. Metablic myopathies I: glycogenoses and lysosomal myopathies. In: Muscle biopsy: a practical approach. 4th ed. Oxford: Saunders Elsevier; 2013. p. 423–45.
16. Henning F, Cunninghame CA, Martin MA, Rubio JC, Arenas J, Lucia A, et al. Muscle fiber type proportion and size is not altered in mcardle disease. Muscle Nerve. 2017;55(6):916–8.
17. Haller RG, Wyrick P, Taivassalo T, Vissing J. Aerobic conditioning: an effective therapy in McArdle's disease. Ann Neurol. 2006;59(6):922–8.
18. Mate-Munoz JL, Moran M, Perez M, Chamorro-Vina C, Gomez-Gallego F, Santiago C, et al. Favorable responses to acute and chronic exercise in McArdle patients. Clin J Sport Med. 2007;17(4):297–303.
19. Quinlivan R, Vissing J, Hilton-Jones D, Buckley J. Physical training for McArdle disease. Cochrane Database Syst Rev. 2011;12:CD007931.
20. Ollivier K, Hogrel JY, Gomez-Merino D, Romero NB, Laforet P, Eymard B, et al. Exercise tolerance and daily life in McArdle's disease. Muscle Nerve. 2005;31(5):637–41.
21. Andersen ST, Vissing J. Carbohydrate- and protein-rich diets in McArdle disease: effects on exercise capacity. J Neurol Neurosurg Psychiatry. 2008;79(12):1359–63.
22. Perez M, Mate-Munoz JL, Foster C, Rubio JC, Andreu AL, Martin MA, et al. Exercise capacity in a child with McArdle disease. J Child Neurol. 2007;22(7):880–2.
23. Vissing J, Haller RG. The effect of oral sucrose on exercise tolerance in patients with McArdle's disease. N Engl J Med. 2003;349(26):2503–9.
24. Amato AA. Sweet success—a treatment for McArdle's disease. N Engl J Med. 2003;349(26):2481–2.
25. Nogales-Gadea G, Santalla A, Ballester-Lopez A, Arenas J, Martin MA, Godfrey R, et al. Exercise and preexercise nutrition as treatment for McArdle disease. Med Sci Sports Exerc. 2016;48(4):673–9.
26. Quinlivan R, Beynon RJ, Martinuzzi A. Pharmacological and nutritional treatment for McArdle disease (Glycogen Storage Disease type V). Cochrane Database Syst Rev. 2008;2:CD003458.
27. Vorgerd M, Grehl T, Jager M, Muller K, Freitag G, Patzold T, et al. Creatine therapy in myophosphorylase deficiency (McArdle disease): a placebo-controlled crossover trial. Arch Neurol. 2000;57(7):956–63.
28. Vorgerd M, Zange J, Kley R, Grehl T, Husing A, Jager M, et al. Effect of high-dose creatine therapy on symptoms of exercise intolerance in McArdle disease: double-blind, placebo-controlled crossover study. Arch Neurol. 2002;59(1):97–101.

Chapter 14
A 37-Year-Old Woman with Leg Weakness and CK Elevation

Elisabeth Golden and Lan Zhou

History

A 37-year-old woman presented for evaluation of leg weakness. The symptom started about 6 months prior to the office visit and were gradually worsened. She had to rest during household chores. She had great difficulty with stairs, needed to use the hand rail, and felt as if there were weights on her legs. She would sometimes have to push with her arms to get out of chairs. Her arms would get tired when she would fix her hair. She had some minor anterior thigh discomfort but no stiffness, spasms, or cramps. She had mild non-radiating low back pain but no neck pain. She denied ocular or bulbar symptoms. She had very mild shortness of breath with exertion but no orthopnea. She denied constitutional symptoms, skin rashes, or joint swelling. She denied any history of pigmenturia. There was no history of myotoxic drug exposure. Her past medical history included gastro-esophageal reflux disease treated with proton pump inhibitor, vitamin B12 deficiency undergoing supplementation, and a remote episode of polyarthralgia with unclear diagnosis. Family history was negative for neuromuscular diseases, adverse reactions to anesthesia, or autoimmune diseases. She was a non-smoker, and she did not drink alcohol or use illicit drugs.

E. Golden (✉)
Department of Neurology and Neurotherapeutics,
University of Texas Southwestern Medical Center, Dallas, TX, USA
e-mail: Elisabeth.Golden@UTSouthwestern.edu

L. Zhou
Departments of Neurology and Pathology, Boston University Medical Center,
Boston, MA, USA
e-mail: lanzhou@bu.edu

L. Zhou et al. (eds.), *A Case-Based Guide to Neuromuscular Pathology*,
https://doi.org/10.1007/978-3-030-25682-1_14

Physical Examination

Her general examination was normal. Neurological examination showed normal mental status and cranial nerve functions. Muscle bulk was notable for bilateral calf hypertrophy. Tone was normal. There was mild weakness detected in the bilateral shoulder abductors, elbow flexors, hip flexors, and hip extensors (MRC 4+/5), as well as subtle weakness in the thigh abductors (5−/5). Sensory examination was normal. Deep tendon reflexes were slightly brisk and symmetric. Hoffmann sign was absent. Toes were downgoing bilaterally. Her gait and coordination were normal.

Investigations

Blood tests showed elevated creatine kinase (CK) at 1,139 U/L, mildly elevated sedimentation rate at 31 mm/hour (normal: 0–20) and C-reactive protein 6.9 mg/L (normal: < 5), minimally elevated AST 37 U/L (10–30) and ALT 41 U/L (6–29) but normal alkaline phosphatase. Renal function, thyroid function, and lactate level were all normal. Hepatitis B and C, HIV, and HTLV serology was negative. Antinuclear antigen (ANA), extractable nuclear antigen antibody (ENA) panel, rheumatoid factor, and myositis antibody panel were all negative. Acetylcholine receptor and muscle-specific kinase antibodies were negative. Very long chain fatty acid profile was normal. Dried blood spot analysis for acid alpha glucosidase activity was normal. Magnetic resonance imaging (MRI) of the brain and spine was unremarkable. Motor and sensory nerve conduction studies (NCS) were normal. Needle electromyography (EMG) study demonstrated an irritable myopathy, with findings most pronounced in the thoracic paraspinal muscles. A right biceps muscle biopsy was performed.

Muscle Biopsy Findings

This right biceps muscle biopsy (Fig. 14.1) showed a vacuolar myopathy with many fibers containing multiple small sarcoplasmic vacuoles. These fibers were mainly type 1 fibers, which appeared generally smaller than type 2 fibers. The sarcoplasmic vacuoles were not rimmed or autophagic; they contained excessive neutral lipids but not glycogens as demonstrated by Oil Red O and PAS stains. Some fibers with vacuolar changes also displayed incomplete ragged red appearance. There were no COX-deficient fibers. Electron microscopy (EM) confirmed the presence of abundant accumulations of lipid droplets associated with pleomorphic mitochondria between the myofibrils and less frequently under the sarcolemma. No abnormal cristae pattern or crystalline inclusions were seen. These findings are characteristic of a lipid storage myopathy.

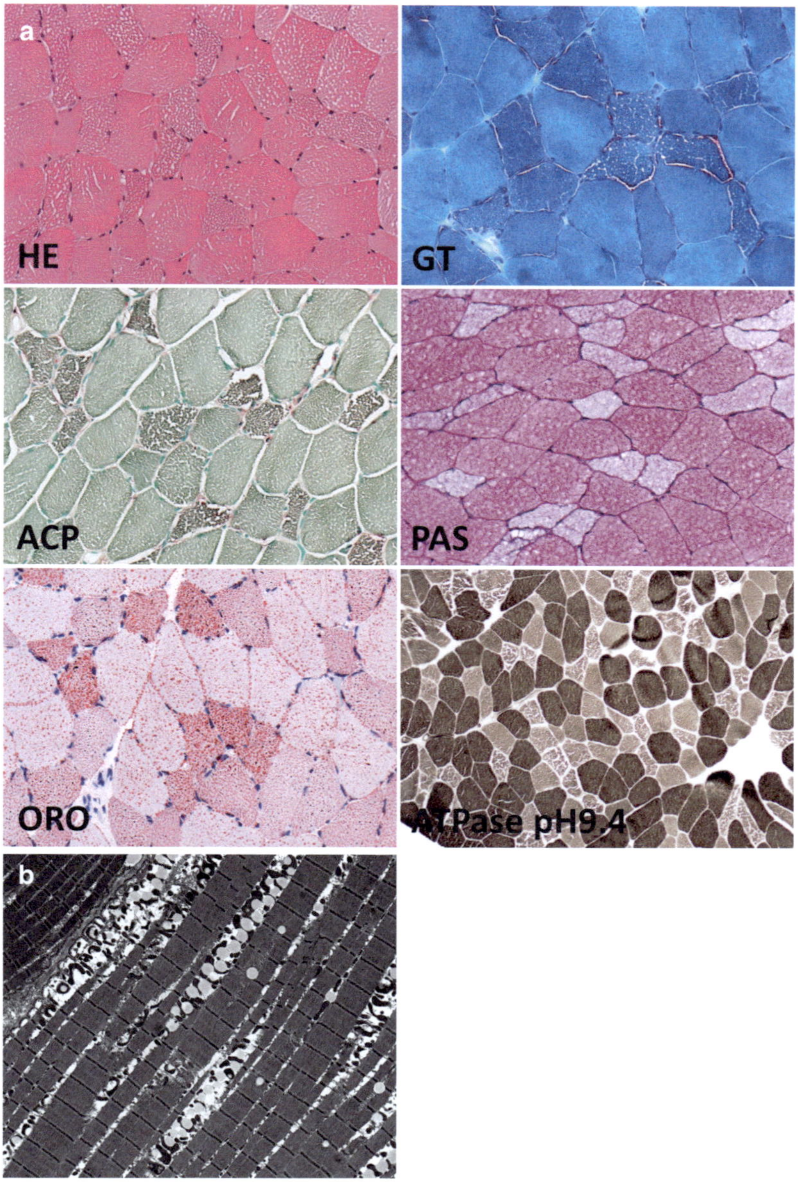

Fig. 14.1 Lipid storage myopathy. (**a**), HE stain shows many fibers containing multiple small sarcoplasmic vacuoles. Gomori trichrome stain (GT) shows these vacuoles are not red rimmed; a few of these fibers also display incomplete ragged red appearance. Acid phosphatase stain (ACP) shows no increase in acid phosphatase activity. PAS stain shows no abnormal glycogen accumulation. Oil Red O (ORO) stain shows some type 1 fibers containing intense larger red droplets, indicating excessive lipid accumulation. ATPase pH 9.4 stain shows the vacuolar changes are mostly seen in type 1 fibers (pale), and the type 1 fibers are generally smaller than the type 2 fibers (dark). (**b**), EM shows abundant sarcoplasmic accumulations of lipid droplets (round empty spaces with no membranes) associated with pleomorphic mitochondria between the myofibrils and under the sarcolemma

Additional Investigations After the Muscle Biopsy Diagnosis

After the muscle biopsy diagnosis of a lipid storage myopathy was obtained, the patient had additional laboratory tests. Urine organic acids were normal. Acylcarnitine profile showed low levels of essentially all species. Plasma total and free carnitine levels were very low; the esterified carnitine level was also decreased but to a lesser degree. The total carnitine level was 5 μmol/L (normal: 25–28), free carnitine level was 3 μmol/L (normal: 19–48), and the esterified carnitine level was 2 μmol/L (normal: 4–13). The esterified carnitine/free carnitine ratio was elevated at 0.63 (normal: 0.13–0.42).

Final Diagnosis

Lipid storage myopathy with carnitine deficiency

Patient Follow-up

The patient declined genetic testing for more specific characterization of her lipid storage myopathy. She was recommended to take empiric supplementation with L-carnitine and riboflavin. She was also referred for cardiology evaluation.

Discussion

Lipid storage myopathies (LSM), a type of metabolic myopathies, are genetic disorders caused by defects in the intracellular triacylglycerol catabolism and characterized by excessive lipid accumulation mainly in the muscle fibers. Body triacylglycerol is mostly derived from dietary fat with a small portion synthesized in adipocytes and liver. It is stored in subcutaneous and visceral adipose tissue with minimal amount in muscle, in the form of lipid droplets, to provide energy for muscle activity. Triacylglycerol catabolism takes several key steps. Triacylglycerol is first hydrolysed to fatty acids by lipases. Fatty acids are then transported in circulation and taken up by target cells. Within target cells, non-esterified fatty acids couple with coenzyme A (CoA) to form short-chain (< C8), medium-chain (C8–12), long-chain (C12–24), and very long-chain (> C24) acyl-CoAs by fatty acyl-CoA synthetases. While short- and medium-chain acyl-CoAs can passively diffuse across mitochondrial membranes, long- and very long-chain acyl-CoAs need the carnitine shuttle system. They bind free carnitine catalyzed by the carnitine palmitoyltransferase I (CPT I) to form acylcarnitines, which then translocate into mitochondrial matrix, where acylcarnitines dissociate back to acyl-CoAs and free carnitine catalyzed by the carnitine palmitoyltransferase II (CPT II). Acyl-CoAs then undergo beta-oxidation catalyzed by acyl-CoA dehydrogenases to generate acetyl-CoA molecules, which subsequently undergo tricarboxylic acid (TCA) cycle and oxidative phosphorylation to generate the energy molecule adenosine triphosphate (ATP) [1].

LSM are genetically and phenotypically heterogeneous. The onset can be early or late, and the disease presentation can be acute or chronic. Clinical presentations of infant-onset are similar across different types and are severe with multisystem involvement. Patients usually present with hypotonia, hypoketotic hypoglycemic encephalopathy, hepatomegaly, and cardiomyopathy. The late-onset presentations can be acute (recurrent rhabdomyolysis) or chronic (fixed slowly progressive muscle weakness), and the disease is relatively mild [2–5].

Recurrent rhabdomyolysis has been associated with defects in mitochondrial fatty acid transport or beta-oxidation, such as deficiencies in CPT II, very-long-chain acyl-CoA dehydrogenase (VLCAD), trifunctional protein, and lipin-1. CPT II deficiency mainly causes recurrent rhabdomyolysis in adults, which is frequently triggered by strenuous exercise and/or fasting [6, 7]. Lipin-1 deficiency is one of the most common causes of severe recurrent rhabdomyolysis in children [8, 9]. Muscle biopsy in these patients usually does not show significant abnormal lipid accumulation. In patients with CPT II deficiency, neurological examination, CK, EMG, and muscle biopsy are usually normal between the rhabdomyolysis attacks. During or shortly after the attacks, muscle biopsy may show a necrotizing myopathy with the presence of necrotic and regenerating muscle fibers. Besides acute management of rhabdomyolysis, these patients should avoid triggers such as fasting, prolonged exercise (> 30 minutes), infection, fever, cold, emotional stress, and high-fat diet. They may change diet to high-carbonhydrate and low-fat diet, take extra carbohydrate before and during exercise, and take frequent meals. They may also take carnitine. Bezafibrate did not improve fatty acid oxidation in patients with CPT II or VLCAD deficiency [10].

There are four types of LSM: neutral lipid storage disease with myopathy (NLSD-M), neutral lipid storage disease with ichthyosis (NLSD-I), primary carnitine deficiency (PCD), and multiple acyl-CoA deficiency (MADD).

NLSD-M is an autosome recessive disease caused by mutations in the patatin-like phospholipase domain containing 2 (*PNPLA2*) gene which encodes adipose triglyceride lipase (ATGL) [11]. NLSD-M may manifest gradually progressive muscle weakness (either distal- or proximal-predominant), exercise intolerance, myalgia, and cardiomyopathy with a disease onset in childhood or early adulthood [12, 13]. NLSD-I is caused by mutations in the comparative gene identification-58 (*CGI-58*) gene which encodes alpha/beta-hydrolase domain-containing protein 5 (ABHD5), a co-activator of ATGL [14]. It tends to cause less muscle weakness but prominent skin involvement with non-bullous congenital ichthyosiform erythroderma as well as cognitive, ophthalmologic, and hearing deficits, hepatomegaly, and intestinal involvement [15–17]. The disease onset of NLSD-I is earlier than that of NLSD-M. CK is typically elevated in NLSD-M but may be normal in NLSD-I. Lipid accumulation is seen in muscle as well as many other tissues. Lipid accumulation seen in leukocytes on routine peripheral blood smear is called "Jordan's anomaly" [4, 18]. There is no specific treatment for NLSD. Topical application of urea-containing emollients may be used for skin ichthyosis. Dietary changes with high-carbonhydrate and low-fat diet supplemented with medium-chain triacylglycerols are beneficial.

PCD is caused by mutations in the solute carrier family 22 member 5 (*SLC22A5*) gene which encodes organic cation/carnitine transporter 2 (OCTN2) responsible for the cellular uptake of carnitine [19, 20]. The *SLC22A5* mutations impair the carnitine transport into cells and carnitine reuptake by kidneys, thus causing carnitine wasting. As carnitine is required for long-chain and very long-chain fatty acid transport from cytoplasm into mitochondria, carnitine deficiency causes impaired utilization of fatty acids for energy production. PCD has a wide clinical spectrum. Infant- or childhood-onset may manifest progressive limb weakness, cardiomyopathy, hepatomegaly, and recurrent episodes of hepatic encephalopathy, while adult-onset may only show subtle fatigability, mild progressive limb weakness, or no symptoms at all (though cardiac involvement may still be present) [6, 21]. Previously asymptomatic women may decompensate during pregnancy [22]. CK may or may not be elevated, and total carnitine and acylcarnitine levels are extremely low. Urine organic acids are normal. Lipid accumulation is seen in muscle and liver. Treatment with lifelong L-carnitine supplementation, 100–400 mg/kg/day in four daily doses, titrated to normalize plasma carnitine levels, can improve skeletal and cardiac muscle function and yield a favorable prognosis [23–26]. Pivalic acid containing antibiotics should be avoided. Patients should also have regular screening for cardiac involvement with echocardiogram and electrocardiogram [18, 22].

MADD, also known as glutaric acidemia type II, is an autosomal recessive disorder caused by dysfunction of flavoproteins, which normally function to transfer electrons from acyl-coA dehydrogenases to coenzyme Q10 in the electron transport chain [18]. The disease is caused predominantly by mutations in the electron transfer flavoprotein (*ETFA*, *ETFB*) or ETF dehydrogenase (*ETFDH*) genes. It can also be caused by mutations in the other genes associated with riboflavin transport such as *SLC52A1*, *SLC52A2*, and *SLC52A3,* or flavin adenine dinucleotide (FAD) transport or synthesis such as *SLC25A32* and *FLAD1*. Mutations in the *ETFA* and *ETFB* tend to cause the severe neonatal-onset form, while *ETFDH* mutations are linked to the mild adult-onset form [27]. Most late-onset cases present with a gradual onset of muscle weakness, exercise intolerance, and myalgia, although a third present with acute and episodic metabolic decompensation with lethargy, vomiting, hypoglycemia, acidosis, and liver dysfunction [28]. Cardiomyopathy can be seen in both neonatal- and late-onset forms. Lipid accumulation can be seen in muscle and liver. There may be secondary carnitine deficiency, but blood acylcarnitines of all species are usually increased. Serum CK may be normal or elevated, though note that labs may be normal if not drawn during an episode of metabolic decompensation. A subset of MADD patients respond to riboflavin very well, and all the riboflavin-responsive cases appear associated with *ETFDH* mutations [27–30]. Riboflavin should be initiated at 100–400 mg daily. Carnitine and coenzyme Q10 supplementation may also be considered, particularly if there is evidence of secondary deficiency [4]. The mechanism of riboflavin-responsiveness is still not entirely clear, but supplementation likely increases mitochondrial FAD concentration, which could increase FAD binding and/or increase the chaperone effect of FAD to improve flavoprotein folding [27]. Patients should also avoid fasting [18].

Diagnostic evaluation of LSM should include blood and urine biochemical analyses, muscle biopsy, and genetic testing. Biochemical analyses to measure blood and urine carnitines, plasma acylcarnitine species, and urine organic acids are helpful to distinguish different types of LSM, but the definitive diagnosis relies on the gene tests. In PCD, plasma total and free carnitine levels as well as acylcarnitine species are usually severely reduced. Urine excretion of carnitine is increased. Urine organic acids are normal. In MADD, free carnitine may be normal or low (secondary deficiency), all acylcarnitine species are elevated, and urine C5 to C10 dicarboxylic acids are elevated [4, 18]. It may also show secondary CoQ10 deficiency. In CPT II deficiency, plasma C16 and C18 acylcarnitines are increased, but the free carnitine level is normal. Our patient showed markedly reduced blood free and total carnitines as well as low acylcarnitines but normal urine organic acids. She was well-nourished, had no significant hepatic or renal dysfunction, and was not on any medications which could cause carnitine deficiency. Therefore, she was most likely to have lipid storage myopathy from primary carnitine deficiency. Unfortunately, she refused the gene test to confirm the diagnosis and the genetic cause.

Muscle biopsy plays an essential role in diagnosing LSM as seen in our case, as the clinical presentation with mild, progressive, and proximal limb muscle weakness is quite non-specific, and can be seen with inflammatory myopathies, late-onset Pompe disease, and limb-girdle muscular dystrophies. We initially suspected an inflammatory myopathy given her weakness pattern, moderate CK elevation, and irritable myopathic changes on EMG. Bilateral calf hypertrophy also raised a suspicion for a limb-girdle muscle dystrophy. But her muscle biopsy showed no inflammation or dystrophic changes; it showed prominent sarcoplasmic lipid accumulation in type 1 fibers, characteristic for a LSM.

Muscle biopsy in LSM such as PCD typically shows a vacuolar myopathy with many small vacuoles present in the sarcoplasm of predominantly type 1 fibers. These vacuoles are not red rimmed in the Gomori trichrome stain. They are not of lysosomal origin with increased acid phosphatase activity (autophagic) as seen in Pompe disease. They are not filled with excessive PAS-positive glycogen as seen in glycogen storage disease. These vacuoles are filled with excessive neutral lipids that can be readily revealed by Oil Red O or Sudan black stain. Oil Red O stain shows intense and larger red lipid droplets in the affected type 1 fibers. EM often shows prominent accumulation of lipid droplets between the myofibrils and under the sarcolemma. The lipid droplets are often adjacent to mitochondria. Mitochondrial abnormalities such as increased proliferation, subsarcolemmal accumulation, and pleomorphism are often present [31].

It is important to obtain a specific diagnosis of LSM, as some of the LSM are treatable. PCD can be successfully treated with a high-dose of L-carnitine supplementation (100–400 mg/kg/day). Early carnitine therapy not only improves muscle strength, but also prevents cardiomyopathy and other irreversible organ damage [23–26]. A subset of MADD patients respond very well to riboflavin, and all riboflavin-responsive cases are associated with *ETFDH* mutations [27]. Riboflavin should be initiated at 100–400 mg daily. There is still no specific effective treatment for NLSD-M or NLSD-I. Besides the specific supplementations, it is critical for patients with LSM to avoid various triggers of rhabdomyolysis and to modify lifestyle and diet.

Pearls

Clinical Pearls

1. Lipid storage myopathies, especially those with late-onset, can present with mild, progressive, proximal limb weakness, mimicking inflammatory myopathy, muscular dystrophy, and late-onset Pompe disease, among others.
2. Although recurrent rhabdomyolysis is a feature of many patients with metabolic myopathies, lack of a history of rhabdomyolysis does not exclude a metabolic myopathy.
3. Muscle biopsy plays an essential role in diagnosing LSM.
4. Once the diagnosis of LSM is made by a muscle biopsy, biochemical analyses of blood and urine carnitine levels, acylcarnitine profile, and urine organic acids can help differentiate different types of LSM to direct gene test.
5. As PCD and some MADD patients respond very well to L-carnitine and riboflavin, respectively, it is important to make a specific genetic diagnosis for a patient with LSM.
6. It is critical for patients with LSM to avoid various triggers of rhabdomyolysis and to modify lifestyle and diet.

Pathology Pearls

1. Muscle biopsy in LSM such as PCD typically shows a vacuolar myopathy with many small sarcoplasmic vacuoles mainly in type 1 fibers. These vacuoles are not rimmed; they do not show increased acid phosphatase activity or contain PAS-positive glycogen accumulation. These vacuoles contain excessive neutral lipids which can be revealed by Oil Red O or Sudan black stain. Oil Red O stain shows intense larger red droplets in type 1 fibers.
2. EM is very useful in evaluating LSM, which typically shows prominent accumulation of lipid droplets between myofibrils and under sarcolemma. The lipid droplets are often adjacent to mitochondria. Mitochondrial structural changes such as increased proliferation, subsarcolemmal accumulation, and pleomorphism can be seen in PCD. But crystalline inclusions are absent in contrast to primary mitochondria diseases.
3. Muscle biopsy in LSM does not show dystrophic changes.

References

1. Vasiljevski ER, Summers MA, Little DG, Schindeler A. Lipid storage myopathies: current treatments and future directions. Prog Lipid Res. 2018;72:1–17.
2. Angelini C. Disorders of lipid metabolism. Handb Clin Neurol. 2007;86:183–91.
3. Laforet P, Vianey-Saban C. Disorders of muscle lipid metabolism: diagnostic and therapeutic challenges. Neuromuscul Disord. 2010;20(11):693–700.
4. Liang WC, Nishino I. Lipid storage myopathy. Curr Neurol Neurosci Rep. 2011;11(1):97–103.
5. Pennisi EM, Garibaldi M, Antonini G. Lipid Myopathies. J Clin Med. 2018;7(12):472.
6. Di Mauro S, Trevisan C, Hays A. Disorders of lipid metabolism in muscle. Muscle Nerve. 1980;3(5):369–88.
7. DiMauro S, DiMauro PM. Muscle carnitine palmityltransferase deficiency and myoglobinuria. Science. 1973;182(4115):929–31.
8. Michot C, Hubert L, Brivet M, De Meirleir L, Valayannopoulos V, Muller-Felber W, et al. LPIN1 gene mutations: a major cause of severe rhabdomyolysis in early childhood. Hum Mutat. 2010;31(7):E1564–73.
9. Zeharia A, Shaag A, Houtkooper RH, Hindi T, de Lonlay P, Erez G, et al. Mutations in LPIN1 cause recurrent acute myoglobinuria in childhood. Am J Hum Genet. 2008;83(4):489–94.
10. Orngreen MC, Madsen KL, Preisler N, Andersen G, Vissing J, Laforet P. Bezafibrate in skeletal muscle fatty acid oxidation disorders: a randomized clinical trial. Neurology. 2014;82(7):607–13.
11. Fischer J, Lefevre C, Morava E, Mussini JM, Laforet P, Negre-Salvayre A, et al. The gene encoding adipose triglyceride lipase (PNPLA2) is mutated in neutral lipid storage disease with myopathy. Nat Genet. 2007;39(1):28–30.
12. Ohkuma A, Nonaka I, Malicdan MCV, Noguchi S, Ohji S, Nomura K, et al. Distal lipid storage myopathy due to PNPLA2 mutation. Neuromuscul Disord. 2008;18(8):671–4.
13. Reilich P, Horvath R, Krause S, Schramm N, Turnbull DM, Trenell M, et al. The phenotypic spectrum of neutral lipid storage myopathy due to mutations in the PNPLA2 gene. J Neurol. 2011;258(11):1987–97.

14. Lefevre C, Jobard F, Caux F, Bouadjar B, Karaduman A, Heilig R, et al. Mutations in CGI-58, the gene encoding a new protein of the esterase/lipase/thioesterase subfamily, in Chanarin-Dorfman syndrome. Am J Hum Genet. 2001;69(5):1002–12.
15. Dorfman ML, Hershko C, Eisenberg S, Sagher F. Ichthyosiform dermatosis with systemic lipidosis. Arch Dermatol. 1974;110(2):261–6.
16. Igal RA, Rhoads JM, Coleman RA. Neutral lipid storage disease with fatty liver and cholestasis. J Pediatr Gastroenterol Nutr. 1997;25(5):541–7.
17. Bruno C, Bertini E, Di Rocco M, Cassandrini D, Ruffa G, De Toni T, et al. Clinical and genetic characterization of Chanarin-Dorfman syndrome. Biochem Biophys Res Commun. 2008;369(4):1125–8.
18. Sharp LJ, Haller RG. Metabolic and mitochondrial myopathies. Neurol Clin. 2014;32(3):777–99. ix
19. Filippo CA, Ardon O, Longo N. Glycosylation of the OCTN2 carnitine transporter: study of natural mutations identified in patients with primary carnitine deficiency. Biochim Biophys Acta. 2011;1812(3):312–20.
20. Nezu JI, Tamai I, Oku A, Ohashi R, Yabuuchi H, Hashimoto N, et al. Primary systemic carnitine deficiency is caused by mutations in a gene encoding sodium ion-dependent carnitine transporter. Nat Genet. 1999;21(1):91–4.
21. Engel AG, Angelini C. Carnitine deficiency of human skeletal muscle with associated lipid storage myopathy: a new syndrome. Science. 1973;179(4076):899–902.
22. Magoulas PL, El-Hattab AW. Systemic primary carnitine deficiency: an overview of clinical manifestations, diagnosis, and management. Orphanet J Rare Dis. 2012;7:68.
23. Agnetti A, Bitton L, Tchana B, Raymond A, Carano N. Primary carnitine deficiency dilated cardiomyopathy: 28 years follow-up. Int J Cardiol. 2013;162(2):e34–5.
24. Cederbaum SD, Auestad N, Bernar J. Four-year treatment of systemic carnitine deficiency. N Engl J Med. 1984;310(21):1395–6.
25. Chapoy PR, Angelini C, Brown WJ, Stiff JE, Shug AL, Cederbaum SD. Systemic carnitine deficiency—a treatable inherited lipid-storage disease presenting as Reye's syndrome. N Engl J Med. 1980;303(24):1389–94.
26. Kishimoto S, Suda K, Yoshimoto H, Teramachi Y, Nishino H, Koteda Y, et al. Thirty-year follow-up of carnitine supplementation in two siblings with hypertrophic cardiomyopathy caused by primary systemic carnitine deficiency. Int J Cardiol. 2012;159(1):e14–5.
27. Olsen RK, Olpin SE, Andresen BS, Miedzybrodzka ZH, Pourfarzam M, Merinero B, et al. ETFDH mutations as a major cause of riboflavin-responsive multiple acyl-CoA dehydrogenation deficiency. Brain. 2007;130(Pt 8):2045–54.
28. Grunert SC. Clinical and genetical heterogeneity of late-onset multiple acyl-coenzyme A dehydrogenase deficiency. Orphanet J Rare Dis. 2014;9:117.
29. Liang WC, Ohkuma A, Hayashi YK, Lopez LC, Hirano M, Nonaka I, et al. ETFDH mutations, CoQ10 levels, and respiratory chain activities in patients with riboflavin-responsive multiple acyl-CoA dehydrogenase deficiency. Neuromuscul Disord. 2009;19(3):212–6.
30. Ohkuma A, Noguchi S, Sugie H, Malicdan MC, Fukuda T, Shimazu K, et al. Clinical and genetic analysis of lipid storage myopathies. Muscle Nerve. 2009;39(3):333–42.
31. Dubowitz V, Sewry C, Oldfors A. Metabolic Myopathies II: lipid-related disprders and mitochondrial myopathies. 4th ed. London: Elsevier; 2013.

Chapter 15
A 25-Year-Old Woman with Droopy Eyelids and Double Vision

Lan Zhou and Chunyu Cai

History

A 25-year-old woman started to notice bilateral droopy eyelids and binocular double vision 5 years prior to the presentation. The symptoms were non-fatigable and had gradually worsened. The patient denied any limb weakness or trouble chewing, swallowing, or breathing. She had previously seen several neurologists, and the workup of myasthenia gravis was unrevealing, which included acetylcholine receptor (AChR) antibody, muscle specific kinase (MuSK) antibody, and repetitive nerve stimulation test (RNS). She was suspected to have a mitochondrial disease. She denied palpitation, dizziness or hearing problems. She had a past medical history of non-insulin dependent diabetes mellitus and asthma. Her medications included glyburide, saxagliptin, and Vitamin D. Family history was significant for an "enlarged heart" in her maternal grandmother and maternal aunt. She did not drink alcohol or smoke cigarettes. She was a sales assistant.

Physical Examination

General examination was notable for the patient's short stature (4′ 10″). There was no evidence of cataracts in either eye. Cardiac examination was unremarkable. Cranial nerve examination revealed bilateral, non-fatigable, partial eyelid ptosis,

L. Zhou (✉)
Departments of Neurology and Pathology, Boston University Medical Center, Boston, MA, USA
e-mail: lanzhou@bu.edu

C. Cai
Department of Pathology, University of Texas Southwestern Medical Center, Dallas, TX, USA
e-mail: chunyu.cai@UTSouthwestern.edu

L. Zhou et al. (eds.), *A Case-Based Guide to Neuromuscular Pathology*,
https://doi.org/10.1007/978-3-030-25682-1_15

and slow extraocular muscle movements. The patient had difficulty with upper gaze, the right eye could not fully adduct or abduct, and the left eye could not fully adduct. Hearing was symmetrical and intact to finger rubs. Motor examination revealed normal tone and bulk, and mild weakness in the arm abductors, finger extensors, and hip flexors (MRC 4/5). Deep tendon reflexes were reduced (1+) at the biceps, triceps, and brachioradialis, and normal (2+) at the knees and ankles. Toes were downgoing bilaterally. Sensation, coordination, and gait were normal.

Investigations

Serum creatine phosphokinase (CPK) level was normal at 57 U/L (25–175 U/L). CBC and comprehensive metabolic panel were normal. Serum lactate, pyruvate, TSH, and free T4 levels were all normal. The blood mitochondrial DNA point mutations and deletions screen testing did not show any point mutations or deletions. Brain MRI without contrast showed mild cerebral and cerebellar atrophy for her age. Nerve conduction study (NCS), electromyography (EMG), and RNS were normal. A left deltoid muscle biopsy was performed.

Muscle Biopsy Findings

The left deltoid muscle biopsy (Fig. 15.1) showed the presence of many ragged red fibers and COX-deficient fibers. There were a few scattered atrophic fibers but no necrotic, degenerating, or regenerating fibers. Electron microscopy (EM) revealed multiple subsarcolemmal and intrasarcoplasmic mitochondrial aggregations. Many of these mitochondria contained paracrystalline inclusions. Some mitochondria were swollen. Myofilaments appeared normal. The findings are characteristic of a primary mitochondrial disease.

Additional Investigation After the Muscle Biopsy Diagnosis

A part of the patient's muscle biopsy tissue was sent for the next-generation sequencing for mitochondrial DNA point mutations and deletions. It showed a large heteroplasmic mtDNA deletion (3.37 kb). Low level multiple deletions were also observed. The sequence of 15 genes, mutations in which could potentially result in mtDNA deletions, was negative.

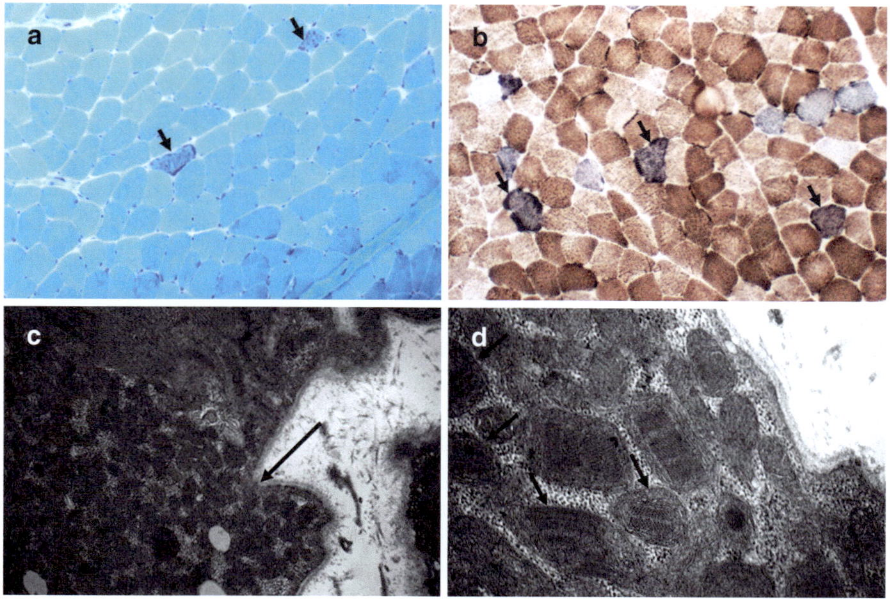

Fig. 15.1 Mitochondrial myopathy. (**a**), Gomori trichrome (GT) stain shows two ragged red fibers (arrows). (**b**), COX/SDH stain shows many COX-deficient fibers (blue), some of which show ragged blue appearance (arrows). (**c**, **d**), EM shows a large subsarcolemmal accumulation of pleomorphic mitochondria (**c**, arrow); many of these mitochondria contain paracrystalline inclusions (**d**, arrows)

Final Diagnosis

Mitochondrial Myopathy, Kearns-Sayre syndrome (KSS)

Patient Follow-up

The patient received genetic counseling. She underwent cardiac evaluation. Her EKG revealed conduction blocks, for which she had a pacemaker implanted. Her cardiac function was normal. Her ophthalmological evaluation was unremarkable except for bilateral eyelid ptosis. She underwent a blepharoplasty surgery for her eyelid ptosis. Her hearing evaluation was normal. Her diabetes was controlled well by her endocrinologist. She also took mitochondrial cocktail (CoQ10, creatine, alpha-lipoic acid, and vitamins) and underwent physical therapy. Her weakness did not deteriorate during the 2-year follow-up. She was able to function better and keep her job.

Discussion

Mitochondrial diseases are a heterogeneous group of genetic disorders caused by defects in the mitochondrial oxidative phosphorylation (OXPHOS) function. The mitochondrial OXPHOS process produces the energy molecule ATP to support cellular activities. Mitochondrial diseases often affect the tissues with a high metabolic demand such as brain, heart, skeletal muscle, and nerve. When skeletal muscle is predominantly affected, the disease is also called mitochondrial myopathy [1, 2].

The OXPHOS system (respiratory chain) contains fiver enzyme complexes (complex I–V). The components involved in the OXPHOS are encoded by nuclear or mitochondrial genes. The majority of these genes are nuclear DNA (nDNA), the defects in which cause diseases with Mendelian inheritance. The mitochondrial genome is small, which contains 16,569 base pairs. The mitochondrial DNA (mtDNA) encodes 13 proteins, 22 transfer RNAs, and two ribosomal RNAs. The defects in the mitochondrial genes cause diseases with maternal transmission as mtDNA is maternally inherited. Unlike nuclear gene, each mitochondrial gene has multiple copies within a cell. Individual cells may have variable proportions of mutant to wild-type mtDNA copies, and this phenomenon is called heteroplasmy. Dysfunction of individual cells and tissues occurs when the heteroplasmy reaches a threshold level. The mutant heteroplasmy is usually low in blood but high in muscle and brain. The mtDNA abnormalities can be primary or secondary to the nuclear gene mutations. Such mutations affect the mtDNA maintenance, resulting in multiple large-scale mtDNA deletions and/or mtDNA depletion with reduced mtDNA copy number.

Mitochondrial diseases are clinically heterogeneous. Patients may present with short statue, eyelid ptosis, chronic progressive external ophthalmoplegia (CPEO), fixed proximal limb weakness, exercise intolerance, recurrent rhabdomyolysis, cardiac conduction block, hearing loss, retinopathy, anemia, migraine headaches, seizure, stroke, ataxia, peripheral neuropathy, diabetes mellitus, and intestinal pseudo-obstruction, among others. CPEO is a common presentation of adult-onset mitochondrial diseases. It can be associated with either primary mtDNA mutations or mtDNA abnormalities secondary to nDNA mutations. Mitochondrial diseases can cause several neurological syndromes, including metabolic encephalopathy, lactic acidosis, stroke-like episodes (MELAS), myoclonic epilepsy with ragged red fibers (MERRF), Kearns Sayre syndrome (KSS), mitochondrial neurogastrointestinal encephalopathy (MNGIE), neuropathy, ataxia, retinitis pigmentosa syndrome (NARP), Leber hereditary optic neuropathy (LHON), Leigh syndrome, Pearson syndrome, and others [1]. KSS has a symptom onset in childhood or early adulthood (before age 20 years) with the presence of CPEO and at least one of the following clinical presentations, including cardiac conduction defects, cardiomyopathy, short statue, retinopathy, hearing loss, ataxia, cognitive defect, and tremor [3]. The disease is usually sporadic caused by a single large-scale mtDNA deletion. The heteroplasmy, but not the deletion size, inversely correlates with the age at onset [3]. Our patient showed typical features of KSS, and her mtDNA testing revealed a large heteroplasmic deletion.

Diagnostic evaluation of mitochondrial diseases includes biochemical testing of blood, cerebrospinal fluid (CSF), and urine, muscle biopsy, and DNA testing. Serum CK and NCS/EMG may also be used to evaluate a mitochondrial disease with myopathy and/or neuropathy, although they are frequently normal in mitochondrial myopathy as seen in our case. It has been recommended that the initial evaluation should include the measurements of lactate and pyruvate in plasma and CSF, amino acids in plasma, urine, and CSF, acylcarnitine profile in plasma, and organic acids in urine. The sensitivity and specificity of lactate and pyruvate elevation in primary mitochondrial diseases are not high enough. However, these biochemical tests may help differentiate mitochondrial diseases from other inborn errors of metabolism [4]. The diagnosis of mitochondrial diseases becomes relatively easy nowadays owing to the development of the new genetic testing methodologies including next-generation sequencing (NGS) and whole-exome sequencing. NGS has become the first-line testing for mitochondrial and nuclear genome analysis [4]. Muscle biopsy still plays an essential role in investigating mtDNA deletion and duplication syndromes such as KSS, CPEO, and Pearson syndrome. The muscle biopsy tissue can be used for enzyme histochemistry, EM study, mitochondrial biochemical and functional analysis, and mtDNA analysis. Since mtDNA mutations tend to be restrict to one or a few tissues, and the mutant heteroplasmy is low in blood but high in muscle, muscle biopsy tissue is ideal for mtDNA analysis to improve the diagnostic sensitivity. In general, mitochondrial DNA deletions are rarely present in blood but usually present in skeletal muscle. As seen in our case, the mtDNA testing was negative in blood but positive in the biopsied muscle tissue.

There are several hallmark pathological features of mitochondrial myopathy, including ragged red fibers (RRF), COX-deficient fibers, and paracrystalline (parking lot) inclusions [5, 6]. The RRF are seen in the Gomori trichrome (GT) stain which highlights mitochondria [7]. It is caused by marked proliferation and subsarcolemmal aggregation of mitochondria, likely due to a compensatory production of mitochondria in response to the reduced ATP synthesis. The RRF usually appear as "ragged blue fibers" on the SDH enzyme histochemical stain, and "COX-deficient fibers" on COX enzyme histochemical stain. The SDH enzyme (complex II) is unique in that all its subunits are encoded by nuclear DNA, thus not affected by mtDNA mutations. The COX enzyme (complex IV), on the other hand, is encoded by both mtDNA and nuclear DNA. As a result, mutations or deletions of mtDNA often lead to a selective loss of COX reactivity and retention of SDH reactivity on enzyme histochemical stains. These "COX-deficient fibers" are best seen with sequential staining of COX and SDH in the same section, where COX-deficient fibers stand out as blue fibers in a background of brown fibers. Less commonly, RRF can be COX positive, such as in most patients with MELAS syndrome [8]. It has been shown that RRF are present in 80% and COX-deficient fibers in 76.7% of patients with KSS [3]. Paracrystalline inclusions, one of the most characteristic findings of mitochondrial diseases, although not specific, are seen by EM study. They represent crystal formation of mitochondrial creatine kinase [9]. They give a parking lot appearance. EM may also show mitochondrial subsarcolemmal accumulation, size and shape pleomorphism, concentric layering of cristae membranes, and other abnormal cristae patterns (Figs. 15.1 and 15.2). SDH strongly positive blood vessels are indicative of MELAS [5].

The muscle biopsy features of mitochondrial abnormalities are not present in all primary mitochondrial diseases or specific to primary mitochondrial diseases. They are often rare or absent in pediatric patients with primary mitochondrial diseases [5] (Fig. 15.2). Muscle biopsy is normal in some mitochondrial diseases such as Leigh syndrome and NARP [6, 10]. On the other hand, RRF and COX-deficient fibers can be seen with normal aging, as aging is associated with accumulation of mitochondrial abnormalities [11]. There is no widely accepted threshold how many RRF or COX deficient fibers should be considered substantially increased. We follow the recommendation that the presence of >2% RRF, >2% COX-deficient fibers below age 50 years, or >5% COX-deficient fibers above age 50 years is considered major criteria for mitochondrial abnormality; any RRF in patients under 30 years of age, 1–2% RRF in patients between 30 and 50 years, and >2% fibers with subsarcolemmal mitochondria accumulation in children under 16 years would be considered minor criteria [12]. Several notable exceptions exist. First, RRF and COX-deficient fibers may be seen in a large numbers in patients with human immunodeficiency virus (HIV) infection with or without Zidovudine (AZT) therapy [13], sporadic inclusion body myositis, and some cases of polymyositis [14]. Second, external ocular muscles and axial muscles such as paraspinal and scalene muscles often show a high number of COX-deficient fibers without a primary mitochondrial disorder associated. The consensus report from the mitochondrial medicine society recommended using vastus lateralis as the preferred site for muscle biopsy in the evaluation of mitochondrial diseases [4]. Third, myofibers with drying artifact or mild cautery artifact may have selective loss of COX activity but relatively preserved SDH reactivity. The same is true for atrophic perifascicular fibers in dermatomyositis patients [15]. This abnormality is particularly evident on COX/SDH double stain. In general, any zonal loss of COX reactivity should not be considered evidence of a primary mitochondria disorder.

Management of patients with mitochondrial myopathy requires a multidisciplinary team as these patients often have multisystem involvement. Genetic counseling should be provided. A thorough cardiac evaluation is crucial even in asymptomatic patients. In our patient with no cardiac symptoms, her cardiac evaluation revealed significant cardiac conduction blocks, and the pacemaker was implanted to prevent syncope and sudden death. These patients should also be screened and/or treated for central nervous system abnormalities, retinopathy,

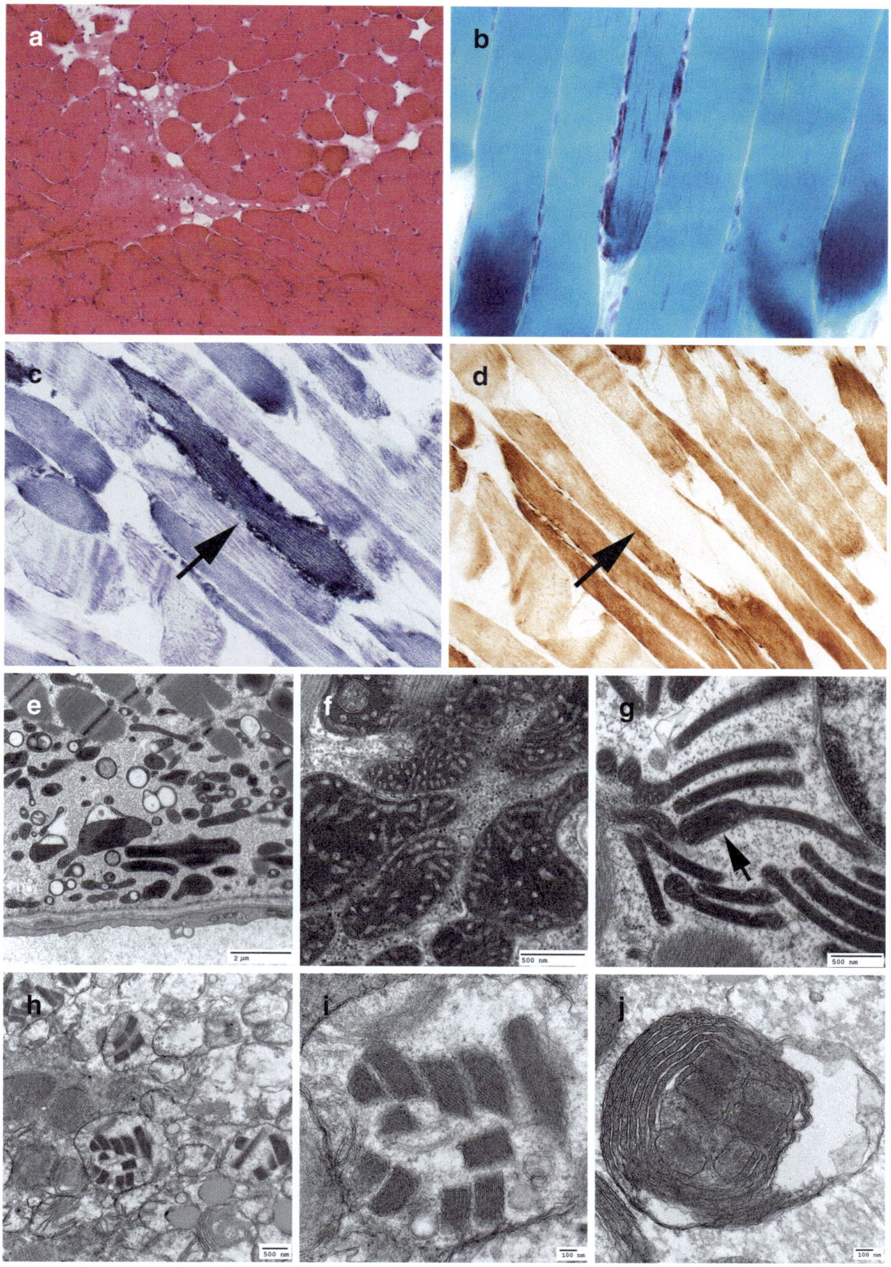

Fig. 15.2 (**a**–**g**), Images from a child with TWINKLE (mitochondrial DNA helicase) deficiency. (**a**), H&E shows relatively normal myofiber morphology. (**b**), Gomori trichrome stain shows rare ragged red fibers. These fibers are dark on SDH (**c,** arrow, "ragged blue fiber") and pale on COX (**d**, arrow, COX deficient fiber). Electron microscopy shows marked variation in mitochondria size, shape, and cristae pattern (**e**), such as a lattice-like cristae pattern (**f**) or cristae compaction (**g**). Images (**h**–**j**) are from a separate pediatric patient with MNGIE syndrome, and demonstrate frequent "parking lot" like crystalloid mitochondria inclusions, which are likely due to cristae compaction

hearing loss, and diabetes mellitus. Blepharoplasty is helpful when ptosis is severe enough to affect the vision or cosmetic appearance. It has been shown that endurance exercise is safe and beneficial, as it can increase muscle mitochondrial enzyme activity and improve quality of life [16–20]. Supplementation with CoQ10, creatine, alpha-lipoic acid, and vitamins also appears beneficial [21–23] and should be offered [4], although there are very few randomized, double-blinded, and placebo-controlled studies to prove the efficacy.

Pearls

Clinical Pearls

1. Mitochondrial diseases can be caused by mutations in nuclear or mitochondrial genes with Mendelian inheritance or maternal transmission, respectively.
2. Mitochondrial diseases characteristically involve multiple systems. They tend to affect muscle, heart, brain, and nerve.
3. Early-onset, progressive, bilateral eyelid ptosis and ophthalmoplegia should raise a suspicion for a mitochondrial myopathy. The main differential considerations include other hereditary myopathies that affect ocular muscles and myasthenia gravis.
4. KSS is caused by a single large-scale mtDNA deletion. Besides bilateral eyelid ptosis and ophthalmoplegia, patients with KSS may also manifest fixed proximal limb weakness, cardiac conduction block, cardiomyopathy, hearing loss, retinopathy, and diabetes mellitus, among others. These conditions should be screened in every patient and treated if present.
5. Diagnostic evaluation of mitochondrial myopathy includes biochemical testing, EMG, muscle biopsy, and DNA testing. Serum CK and EMG are often normal. Plasma lactate and pyruvate elevation is neither very sensitive nor specific. NGS has become the first-line testing for mitochondrial and nuclear genome analysis for diagnosing mitochondrial diseases. Muscle biopsy can be spared if the genetic testing is positive in blood.
6. Muscle biopsy is still frequently needed for diagnosing mtDNA deletion and duplication syndromes such as KSS, CPEO, and Pearson syndrome. The mutant mtDNA may be detected in muscle biopsy tissue but not in blood due to the mutant heteroplasmy being high in muscle and low in blood.
7. The current treatment of mitochondrial myopathy is mainly symptomatic to improve the quality of life. Endurance exercise is beneficial. Supplementation with CoQ10, alpha-lipoic acid, creatine, and vitamins should be offered.

Pathology Pearls

1. The hallmark pathological features of mitochondrial myopathy include ragged red fibers (RRF), COX-deficient fibers, paracrystalline (parking lot) inclusions, and other mitochondrial ultrastructural abnormalities.
2. Mitochondrial myopathy with primary mtDNA abnormalities such as KSS typically shows many RRF, COX-deficient fibers, and paracrystalline inclusions.
3. RRF and COX deficient fibers are often absent or rare in pediatric patients with primary mitochondrial diseases. Mild subsarcolemmal accumulation of mitochondria is a more common finding in this population.
4. Muscle biopsy is usually normal in some mitochondrial diseases such as Leigh syndrome and NARP.
5. A large number of RRF or COX-deficient fibers can be seen in IBM, polymyositis with COX-deficient fibers, and HIV-associated myopathy with or without AZT therapy. RRF and COX-deficient fibers can also be seen in association with aging and in normal extra-ocular and axial muscles.
6. Zonal loss of COX reactivity is usually not associated with a primary mitochondria defect, and typically seen in perifascicular atrophic fibers in dermatomyositis patients and artifacts.

References

1. Gorman GS, Chinnery PF, DiMauro S, Hirano M, Koga Y, McFarland R, et al. Mitochondrial diseases. Nat Rev Dis Primers. 2016;2:16080.
2. Ahmed ST, Craven L, Russell OM, Turnbull DM, Vincent AE. Diagnosis and treatment of mitochondrial myopathies. Neurotherapeutics. 2018;15(4):943–53.
3. Mancuso M, Orsucci D, Angelini C, Bertini E, Carelli V, Comi GP, et al. Redefining phenotypes associated with mitochondrial DNA single deletion. J Neurol. 2015;262(5):1301–9.
4. Parikh S, Goldstein A, Koenig MK, Scaglia F, Enns GM, Saneto R, et al. Diagnosis and management of mitochondrial disease: a consensus statement from the Mitochondrial Medicine Society. Genet Med. 2015;17(9):689–701.
5. Bourgeois JM, Tarnopolsky MA. Pathology of skeletal muscle in mitochondrial disorders. Mitochondrion. 2004;4(5–6):441–52.
6. Dubowitz V, Sewry C, Oldfors A. Metabolic myopathies II: lipid-related disorders and mitochondrial myopathies. In: Muscle biopsy: a practical approach. 4th ed. Saunders Elsevier; 2013. p. 446–84.
7. Engel WK, Cunningham GG. Rapid examination of muscle tissue. An improved trichrome method for Fresh-Frozen biopsy sections. Neurology. 1963;13:919–23.
8. Vogel H. Mitochondrial myopathies and the role of the pathologist in the molecular era. J Neuropathol Exp Neurol. 2001;60(3):217–27.
9. Eppenberger-Eberhardt M, Riesinger I, Messerli M, Schwarb P, Muller M, Eppenberger HM, et al. Adult rat cardiomyocytes cultured in creatine-deficient medium display large mitochondria with paracrystalline inclusions, enriched for creatine kinase. J Cell Biol. 1991;113(2):289–302.
10. Holt IJ, Harding AE, Petty RK, Morgan-Hughes JA. A new mitochondrial disease associated with mitochondrial DNA heteroplasmy. Am J Hum Genet. 1990;46:428–33.

11. Cao Z, Wanagat J, McKiernan SH, Aiken JM. Mitochondrial DNA deletion mutations are concomitant with ragged red regions of individual, aged muscle fibers: analysis by laser-capture microdissection. Nucleic Acids Res. 2001;29(21):4502–8.
12. Bernier FP, Boneh A, Dennett X, Chow CW, Cleary MA, Thorburn DR. Diagnostic criteria for respiratory chain disorders in adults and children. Neurology. 2002;59(9):1406–11.
13. Morgello S, Wolfe D, Godfrey E, Feinstein R, Tagliati M, Simpson DM. Mitochondrial abnormalities in human immunodeficiency virus-associated myopathy. Acta Neuropathol. 1995;90(4):366–74.
14. Rifai Z, Welle S, Kamp C, Thornton CA. Ragged red fibers in normal aging and inflammatory myopathy. Ann Neurol. 1995;37(1):24–9.
15. Woo M, Chung SJ, Nonaka I. Perifascicular atrophic fibers in childhood dermatomyositis with particular reference to mitochondrial changes. J Neurol Sci. 1988;88(1–3):133–43.
16. Cejudo P, Bautista J, Montemayor T, Villagomez R, Jimenez L, Ortega F, et al. Exercise training in mitochondrial myopathy: a randomized controlled trial. Muscle Nerve. 2005;32(3):342–50.
17. Jeppesen TD, Duno M, Schwartz M, Krag T, Rafiq J, Wibrand F, et al. Short- and long-term effects of endurance training in patients with mitochondrial myopathy. Eur J Neurol. 2009;16(12):1336–9.
18. Jeppesen TD, Schwartz M, Olsen DB, Wibrand F, Krag T, Duno M, et al. Aerobic training is safe and improves exercise capacity in patients with mitochondrial myopathy. Brain. 2006;129(Pt 12):3402–12.
19. Taivassalo T, Gardner JL, Taylor RW, Schaefer AM, Newman J, Barron MJ, et al. Endurance training and detraining in mitochondrial myopathies due to single large-scale mtDNA deletions. Brain. 2006;129(Pt 12):3391–401.
20. Taivassalo T, Shoubridge EA, Chen J, Kennaway NG, DiMauro S, Arnold DL, et al. Aerobic conditioning in patients with mitochondrial myopathies: physiological, biochemical, and genetic effects. Ann Neurol. 2001;50(2):133–41.
21. Glover EI, Martin J, Maher A, Thornhill RE, Moran GR, Tarnopolsky MA. A randomized trial of coenzyme Q10 in mitochondrial disorders. Muscle Nerve. 2010;42(5):739–48.
22. Rodriguez MC, MacDonald JR, Mahoney DJ, Parise G, Beal MF, Tarnopolsky MA. Beneficial effects of creatine, CoQ10, and lipoic acid in mitochondrial disorders. Muscle Nerve. 2007;35(2):235–42.
23. Tarnopolsky MA, Roy BD, MacDonald JR. A randomized, controlled trial of creatine monohydrate in patients with mitochondrial cytopathies. Muscle Nerve. 1997;20(12):1502–9.

Chapter 16
A 58-Year-Old Man with Hypercapnic Respiratory Failure

Lan Zhou, Patrick Kwon, and Susan C. Shin

History

A 58-year-old Caucasian man presented to the emergency room with worsening shortness of breath and bilateral lower extremity edema for 2 weeks. Eleven years ago, he suffered a myocardial infarction, which resulted in left ventricular apical akinesis and systolic congestive heart failure (CHF) (ejection fraction 28%). This required treatment with anticoagulation. When he was a young adult, he had mild supine breathing difficulty requiring two pillows to sleep and was never athletic. He did not, however, have any obvious disability. Over the past 2 years, he noticed mild progressive proximal upper and lower extremity weakness manifested by difficulty in walking upstairs, showering, and standing from a seated position. Additionally, he developed more prominent breathing difficulties and lower extremity edema requiring diuretics. He saw a neuromuscular specialist who suspected a limb girdle muscular dystrophy (LGMD), but the LGMD gene panel was negative. Over the past decade, his creatine kinase (CK) levels fluctuated between 300–900 U/L; however, over the past several months his CK had been normal. His medications included rosuvastatin, warfarin, digoxin, furosemide and enalapril. He used to smoke cigarettes but did not drink alcohol. He did not have a family history of a muscle disease.

L. Zhou (✉)
Departments of Neurology and Pathology, Boston University Medical Center, Boston, MA, USA
e-mail: lanzhou@bu.edu

P. Kwon
Department of Neurology, New York University Langone–Brooklyn, New York, NY, USA
e-mail: Patrick.Kwon@nyumc.org

S. C. Shin
Department of Neurology, Icahn School of Medicine at Mount Sinai, New York, NY, USA
e-mail: Susan.shin@mssm.edu

L. Zhou et al. (eds.), *A Case-Based Guide to Neuromuscular Pathology*,
https://doi.org/10.1007/978-3-030-25682-1_16

While in the emergency room, he was noted to be in hypercapnic respiratory failure ($PaCO_2 > 100$ mmHg, PaO_2 88 mmHg); therefore, he was intubated and admitted to the intensive care unit (ICU). Cardiac enzymes and EKG did not reveal a new acute myocardial infarction. He was treated for CHF exacerbation with the lower extremity edema resolved. However, his $PaCO_2$ remained markedly elevated, and he was unable to be weaned off the ventilator. Neurology consult was requested for possible respiratory muscle weakness.

Physical Examination

The patient was intubated. His mental status, cranial nerve functions, sensory examination, deep tendon reflexes, and coordination were all normal. Motor examination showed normal tone and bulk throughout. On manual muscle testing, weakness was detected in his neck flexors and extensors (MRC: 4/5), and bilateral deltoids (4/5), biceps (4+/5), triceps (5−/5), hip extensors (5−/5), knee extensors (5−/5), and knee flexors (5−/5). His distal limb muscles were strong.

Investigations

His complete blood count, comprehensive metabolic panel, serum CK, thyroid-stimulating hormone, vitamin B12, folate, acetylcholine receptor antibodies, MuSK-antibody, and Vitamin D level were all unremarkable. International normalized ratio (INR) was 2.2. Nerve conduction studies (NCS) were normal. Needle electromyography (EMG) of selected upper and lower limb muscles was also normal. Paraspinal and iliacus muscles were not examined by needle EMG due to the patient being on an anticoagulant. Fluoroscopic sniff test and diaphragmatic ultrasound showed paralysis of bilateral hemidiaphragms. A right deltoid muscle biopsy was performed.

Muscle Biopsy Findings

The right deltoid muscle biopsy (Fig. 16.1) showed a mild chronic active vacuolar myopathy with a few scattered atrophic and hypertrophic muscle fibers, rare necrotic and regenerating fibers, several fibers containing autophagic vacuoles with increased acid phosphatase activity, and some fibers containing acid phosphatase-positive globular inclusions in the sarcoplasm. Electron microscopy (EM) showed sarcoplasmic vacuoles containing lysosomal debris and globular inclusions with lipofuscin pigments, and small lakes of freely dispersed glycogen granules. The findings are highly suggestive of a lysosomal glycogen storage disease, acid maltase deficiency.

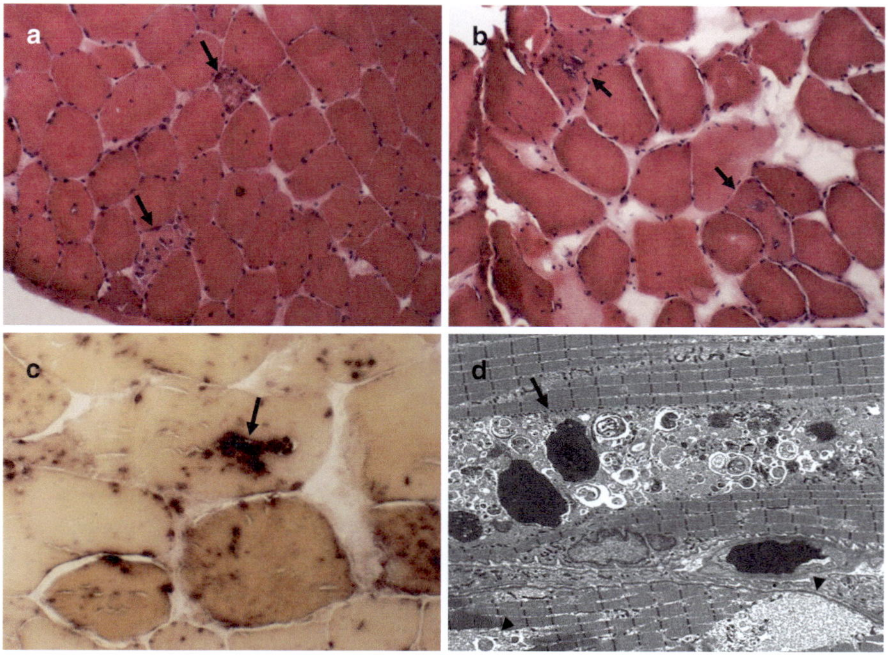

Fig. 16.1 HE stain shows increased internalized nuclei, a few necrotic fibers and myophagocytosis (**a**, arrows), and several fibers containing blue-rimmed sarcoplasmic vacuoles (**b**, arrows). Acid phosphatase stain shows a few fibers containing aid phosphatase-positive globular inclusions (**c**, arrow). EM (**d**) shows a sarcoplasmic vacuole (arrow) containing lysosomal debris and globular inclusions with lipofuscin pigments, and small lakes of freely dispersed glycogen granules (arrowheads). (The EM picture was provided by Dr. Dennis K. Burns)

Additional Investigation After Muscle Biopsy Diagnosis

Given the combination of limb-girdle weakness, prominent respiratory muscle weakness, and the muscle biopsy findings, the patient's blood sample was sent for dried blood spot assay, which showed a markedly reduced acid α-glucosidase activity at 2.8 pmol/punch/hour (normal: ≥10) with a normal neutral α-glucosidase activity at 110.35 pmol/punch/hour (normal: 23.8–132.6). The subsequent sequencing of the lysosomal acid alpha-glucosidase (GAA) gene revealed a c.-32-13 T > G sequence alteration on one allele and a deletion of exon 18 on the other; both were known pathogenic.

Final Diagnosis

Late-onset Pompe disease

Patient Follow-up

The patient required tracheostomy due to the inability to be weaned off the ventilator. He was started on enzyme replacement therapy (ERT), receiving alglucosidase alfa (20 mg/kg body weight) biweekly. After 12 months, his exercise tolerance, pulmonary function tests, and proximal limb weakness all improved. The patient required assist control ventilation at night but did not require any ventilator support during the day. The ERT was continued. His lowest forced vital capacity (FVC) during the hospitalization was 0.7 Liter (L) which improved to 2.03 L (53% predicted) 2 years after the hospitalization and enzyme replacement therapy.

Discussion

Pompe disease, also known as acid maltase deficiency or glycogenosis type II, is a rare autosomal recessive metabolic disorder caused by a partial or a complete deficiency in lysosomal acid α-1,4-glucosidase activity. The disease has multisystem involvement, including skeletal muscle. The inability to metabolize glycogen leads to intralysosomal and cytoplasmic build-ups of glycogen in skeletal muscle causing glycogen storage myopathy. The two forms of the disease are infantile-onset and late-onset [1, 2].

Late-onset Pompe disease (LOPD) has an estimated frequency of 1:57,000 according to one study [3]. It presents after 1 year of age, most commonly between the second and sixth decade with slowly progressive limb-girdle weakness and respiratory muscle weakness but usually without significant cardiac involvement, although Wolff-Parkinson-White syndrome has been reported [4–6]. It tends to more affect axial muscles and respiratory muscles with more than 70% of patients progressing into respiratory failure, which is the most common cause of death [7]. Although limb-girdle weakness is the most common presenting symptom, respiratory insufficiency can precede the onset of limb weakness [6]. Since the presentation is mild and non-specific at the early stage, the diagnosis can be delayed for years or missed entirely [6, 8], as seen in our case. In one retrospective study, 48% of patients carried wrong diagnoses initially [8].

Diagnosis of LOPD requires a high clinical suspicion based on the clinical presentation and test findings. Serum CK can be mildly elevated or normal in LOPD. NCS is usually normal. Needle EMG often shows myopathic motor unit potentials with increased membrane irritability and myotonia [1, 6], which can be restricted to the paraspinal muscles [9]. Limb muscle EMG can be normal in LOPD as seen in our case, and paraspinal muscles should be examined when LOPD is suspected [10]. Although patients may have EMG myotonia, they do not have clinical myotonia.

Muscle biopsy in Pompe disease typically shows a vacuolar myopathy with increased acid phosphatase activity and increased sarcoplasmic glycogen accumulation. EM often shows glycogen granules accumulated freely in sarcoplasm and/or in membrane bound lysosomes [11, 12]. While infantile-onset Pompe disease usually shows many large sarcoplasmic vacuoles, LOPD often shows a few fibers containing small vacuoles or no vacuoles at all [13–16], which makes the muscle biopsy diagnosis of LOPD quite challenging. It could be due to the lack of significant involvement of the limb muscles biopsied. Glycogen accumulation can be evaluated by PAS stain and EM, but glycogen can be washed out by the preparation in some cases. Therefore, negative muscle biopsy does not exclude the diagnosis of LOPD. It has been shown that even in muscle biopsies of LOPD with no vacuolar changes, sarcoplasmic acid phosphatase-positive globular inclusions can be seen [15]. These inclusions contain lipofuscin pigments [16, 17]. The sarcoplasmic inclusions have been reported and described in all forms of Pompe disease [15, 16, 18–20]. They are different from cytoplasmic bodies as they do not contain Z-band materials and they are acid phosphatase-positive. The acid phosphatase-positive globular inclusion is a useful diagnostic marker especially for LOPD [15].

Diagnosis of LOPD has become easier owing to the development of a fast and reliable screening test, dried blood spot assay [21]. It is the gold standard for diagnosing Pompe disease [22]. The test measures the acid α-glucosidase activity, which is reduced but not absent in LOPD. It is important to also measure the neutral α-glucosidase activity, which should be normal in LOPD, to ensure the quality of the specimen. The common practice now is to order dried blood spot first, which is relatively inexpensive. If it shows reduced acid α-glucosidase activity, then proceed with the GAA gene test. More than 200 mutations have been reported [1]. The GAA mutations discovered in our patient are common. Deletion of exon 18, which leads to a complete loss of the enzyme catalytic function, is commonly seen in the infantile form. The c. -32-13 T > G mutation is seen in over 50% of LOPD. This mutation changes a single nucleotide within the first intron of the GAA gene, which affects the splicing of the exon 2.

Early diagnosis of LOPD is essential because enzyme replacement therapy (ERT) is available to improve or stabilize LOPD [23–26]. Early diagnosis requires the awareness of this disease. It has been advocated that the dried blood spot assay should be ordered for every patient with unexplained limb-girdle weakness but prominent axial and respiratory muscle weakness, especially when EMG shows myotonia in paraspinal muscles [8]. Normal CK, normal limb muscle EMG, and lack of characteristic findings on limb muscle biopsy, however, do not exclude LOPD. Muscle biopsy can be spared as the dried blood spot assay is fast, reliable, inexpensive, and non-invasive. The subsequent GAA gene test is definitive.

Recombinant human acid alpha-glucosidase (rhGAA) was developed in 1990s. Alglucosidase alfa (Myozyme) was approved by the U.S. Food and Drug Administration (FDA) and the European Medicines Agency in 2006 for treating Pompe disease, and Lumizyme was approved in 2010 for treating LOPD in the USA. The randomized Late-Onset Treatment Study (LOTS) showed that biweekly infusion of alglucosidase alfa (20 mg/kg body weight) improved limb and respiratory functions [26]. The open-labeled exploratory muscle biopsy, imaging, and functional assessment (EMBASSY) showed that the muscle tissue glycogen was reduced and the limb and respiratory functions were improved in adult patients with LOPD after 6 months of the alglucosidase alfa treatment [25]. Although both studies only included ambulatory patients without invasive ventilation and no trials have been done in patients with severe LOPD as seen in our case, the consensus committee of the American Association of Neuromuscular & Electrodiagnostic Medicine (AANEM) recommends treating these patients with alglucosidase alfa for at least 1 year, and the ERT should be continued if no decline in symptoms or signs [27]. The side effects of alglucosidase alfa are mild to moderate, and the hypersensitivity should be monitored especially in patients who develop a high alpha-glucosidase antibody titer [27]. A new therapy, reveglucosidase alfa, has been developed to improve the lysosome uptake of the enzyme [28]. Future studies will test whether this new treatment is safe and more effective.

Pearls

Clinical Pearls

1. LOPD may predominantly affect respiratory muscles resulting in respiratory failure. Limb girdle weakness can be very mild. LOPD should be considered as a potential cause of hypercapnic respiratory failure even in a patient with coexisting cardiopulmonary disease.
2. Patients with LOPD often present with mild limb girdle weakness but prominent axial and respiratory muscle weakness.
3. Serum CK may be intermittently normal in LOPD.
4. Needle EMG can be normal in limb muscles in LOPD. Paraspinal muscles should be sampled as they may be the only muscles that show abnormalities, including myotonia.
5. Normal CK, normal limb muscle EMG, or lack of pathological features in limb muscle biopsy does not exclude LOPD.
6. Early diagnosis of LOPD is challenging, and it requires a high clinical suspicion. The gold standard diagnostic test is the dried blood spot followed by the GAA gene test. Muscle biopsy can be spared as the dried blood spot screening test is fast, reliable, and inexpensive. The GAA gene test provides a definitive genetic diagnosis.
7. Early diagnosis of LOPD is essential as the enzyme replacement therapy is useful to reduce glycogen accumulation in muscle cells and to improve limb and respiratory muscle functions.

Pathology Pearls

1. Muscle biopsy in LOPD often shows myopathic changes, small autophagic vacuoles, acid phosphatase-positive sarcoplasmic globular inclusions, and excessive glycogen accumulation.
2. EM in LOPD often shows glycogen granules accumulated freely in sarcoplasm and/or in membrane bound lysosomes. It may also show

vacuoles containing lysosomal debris, glycogen granules, and globular inclusions with lipofuscin pigments.
3. Vacuolar changes can be absent in LOPD muscle biopsy.
4. Acid phosphatase-positive sarcoplasmic globular inclusions is a useful diagnostic marker for LOPD.

References

1. American Association of N, Electrodiagnostic M. Diagnostic criteria for late-onset (childhood and adult) Pompe disease. Muscle Nerve. 2009;40(1):149–60.
2. van der Ploeg AT, Reuser AJ. Pompe's disease. Lancet. 2008;372(9646):1342–53.
3. Ausems MG, Verbiest J, Hermans MP, Kroos MA, Beemer FA, Wokke JH, et al. Frequency of glycogen storage disease type II in the Netherlands: implications for diagnosis and genetic counselling. Eur J Hum Genet. 1999;7(6):713–6.
4. Disease AWGoMoP, Kishnani PS, Steiner RD, Bali D, Berger K, Byrne BJ, et al. Pompe disease diagnosis and management guideline. Genet Med. 2006;8(5):267–88.
5. Kishnani PS, Howell RR. Pompe disease in infants and children. J Pediatr. 2004;144(5 Suppl):S35–43.
6. Muller-Felber W, Horvath R, Gempel K, Podskarbi T, Shin Y, Pongratz D, et al. Late onset Pompe disease: clinical and neurophysiological spectrum of 38 patients including long-term follow-up in 18 patients. Neuromuscul Disord. 2007;17(9–10):698–706.
7. Winkel LP, Hagemans ML, van Doorn PA, Loonen MC, Hop WJ, Reuser AJ, et al. The natural course of non-classic Pompe's disease; a review of 225 published cases. J Neurol. 2005;252(8):875–84.
8. Hobson-Webb LD, Kishnani PS. How common is misdiagnosis in late-onset Pompe disease? Muscle Nerve. 2012;45(2):301–2.
9. Barohn RJ, McVey AL, DiMauro S. Adult acid maltase deficiency. Muscle Nerve. 1993;16(6):672–6.
10. Hobson-Webb LD, Dearmey S, Kishnani PS. The clinical and electrodiagnostic characteristics of Pompe disease with post-enzyme replacement therapy findings. Clin Neurophysiol. 2011;122(11):2312–7.
11. Schlenska GK, Heene R, Spalke G, Seiler D. The symptomatology, morphology and biochemistry of glycogenosis type II (Pompe) in the adult. J Neurol. 1976;212(3):237–52.
12. Bembi B, Cerini E, Danesino C, Donati MA, Gasperini S, Morandi L, et al. Diagnosis of glycogenosis type II. Neurology. 2008;71(23 Suppl 2):S4–11.
13. Golsari A, Nasimzadah A, Thomalla G, Keller S, Gerloff C, Magnus T. Prevalence of adult Pompe disease in patients with proximal myopathic syndrome and undiagnosed muscle biopsy. Neuromuscul Disord. 2018;28(3):257–61.
14. Lorenzoni PJ, Kay CSK, Higashi NS, D'Almeida V, Werneck LC, Scola RH. Late-onset Pompe disease: what is the prevalence of limb-girdle muscular weakness presentation? Arq Neuropsiquiatr. 2018;76(4):247–51.
15. Tsuburaya RS, Monma K, Oya Y, Nakayama T, Fukuda T, Sugie H, et al. Acid phosphatase-positive globular inclusions is a good diagnostic marker for two patients with adult-onset Pompe disease lacking disease specific pathology. Neuromuscul Disord. 2012;22(5):389–93.
16. Schoser BG, Muller-Hocker J, Horvath R, Gempel K, Pongratz D, Lochmuller H, et al. Adult-onset glycogen storage disease type 2: clinico-pathological phenotype revisited. Neuropathol Appl Neurobiol. 2007;33(5):544–59.

17. Feeney EJ, Austin S, Chien YH, Mandel H, Schoser B, Prater S, et al. The value of muscle biopsies in Pompe disease: identifying lipofuscin inclusions in juvenile- and adult-onset patients. Acta Neuropathol Commun. 2014;2:2.
18. Jay V, Christodoulou J, Mercer-Connolly A, McInnes RR. "Reducing body"-like inclusions in skeletal muscle in childhood-onset acid maltase deficiency. Acta Neuropathol. 1992;85(1):111–5.
19. Raben N, Ralston E, Chien YH, Baum R, Schreiner C, Hwu WL, et al. Differences in the predominance of lysosomal and autophagic pathologies between infants and adults with Pompe disease: implications for therapy. Mol Genet Metab. 2010;101(4):324–31.
20. Sharma MC, Schultze C, von Moers A, Stoltenburg-Didinger G, Shin YS, Podskarbi T, et al. Delayed or late-onset type II glycogenosis with globular inclusions. Acta Neuropathol. 2005;110(2):151–7.
21. Umapathysivam K, Hopwood JJ, Meikle PJ. Determination of acid alpha-glucosidase activity in blood spots as a diagnostic test for Pompe disease. Clin Chem. 2001;47(8):1378–83.
22. Vissing J, Lukacs Z, Straub V. Diagnosis of Pompe disease: muscle biopsy vs blood-based assays. JAMA Neurol. 2013;70(7):923–7.
23. Park JS, Kim HG, Shin JH, Choi YC, Kim DS. Effect of enzyme replacement therapy in late onset Pompe disease: open pilot study of 48 weeks follow-up. Neurol Sci. 2015;36(4):599–605.
24. Toscano A, Schoser B. Enzyme replacement therapy in late-onset Pompe disease: a systematic literature review. J Neurol. 2013;260(4):951–9.
25. van der Ploeg A, Carlier PG, Carlier RY, Kissel JT, Schoser B, Wenninger S, et al. Prospective exploratory muscle biopsy, imaging, and functional assessment in patients with late-onset Pompe disease treated with alglucosidase alfa: the EMBASSY study. Mol Genet Metab. 2016;119(1–2):115–23.
26. van der Ploeg AT, Clemens PR, Corzo D, Escolar DM, Florence J, Groeneveld GJ, et al. A randomized study of alglucosidase alfa in late-onset Pompe's disease. N Engl J Med. 2010;362(15):1396–406.
27. Cupler EJ, Berger KI, Leshner RT, Wolfe GI, Han JJ, Barohn RJ, et al. Consensus treatment recommendations for late-onset Pompe disease. Muscle Nerve. 2012;45(3):319–33.
28. Byrne BJ, Geberhiwot T, Barshop BA, Barohn R, Hughes D, Bratkovic D, et al. A study on the safety and efficacy of reveglucosidase alfa in patients with late-onset Pompe disease. Orphanet J Rare Dis. 2017;12(1):144.

Chapter 17
A 65-Year-Old Man with Asymmetrical Leg Weakness and Foot Tingling

Lan Zhou and Chunyu Cai

History

A 65-year-old Caucasian man was referred for evaluation of neuropathy. Nine years prior to the presentation, he developed tingling in both feet. He then developed aching pain in the thighs. Two years prior to the presentation, he developed leg weakness with difficulty climbing stairs and picking up his feet, worse on the left. He noticed atrophy in the left calf muscles but no fasciculations. He also developed pain but not numbness or weakness in his hands. He admitted to chronic low back pain and hip pain, which was non-radiating. He denied bowel or bladder symptoms. He was evaluated by an outside neurologist and had nerve conduction study (NCS) and electromyography (EMG) done three times. They all reportedly showed chronic, predominantly axonal, sensorimotor polyneuropathy and right carpal tunnel syndrome. Lumbosacral spine MRI only showed a small disc protrusion at L5/S1 with no spinal canal or neural foraminal stenosis. He had been on a statin drug for 25 years for hyperlipidemia. He stopped it for 1 month at one time with no change of his symptoms. He had a past medical history of hypertension, hyperlipidemia, mitral valve prolapse, and right carpal tunnel syndrome. The only surgery that he had was the right carpal tunnel release. His medications included aspirin, carvedilol, lisinopril, zocor, and gabapentin. His family history was positive for hypertension

L. Zhou (✉)
Departments of Neurology and Pathology, Boston University Medical Center, Boston, MA, USA
e-mail: lanzhou@bu.edu

C. Cai
Department of Pathology, University of Texas Southwestern Medical Center, Dallas, TX, USA
e-mail: chunyu.cai@UTSouthwestern.edu

L. Zhou et al. (eds.), *A Case-Based Guide to Neuromuscular Pathology*,
https://doi.org/10.1007/978-3-030-25682-1_17

and hyperlipidemia but negative for muscle or nerve diseases. He was married with two children. He did not drink alcohol or smoke cigarettes. He was a retired real estate agent.

Physical Examination

General examination was unremarkable. There was no cataract, spine tenderness, spine scoliosis, or joint contracture. Neurologic examination showed normal mental status and cranial nerve functions. Motor examination revealed reduced muscle tone in the left leg with atrophy in the distal leg muscles. Weakness was detected in the bilateral hip flexors (MRC: 4+/5), left foot and toe dorsiflexors (MRC 4−/5), left foot and toe plantar flexors (3/5), left foot evertor (4−/5), and right toe dorsiflexors (4+/5). There was no muscle fasciculation or scapular winging. Pinprick sensation was reduced from the toes to ankles. Vibratory sensation was reduced at the toes. Joint position sense was intact. Deep tendon reflexes were 2+ at the biceps, triceps, brachioradialis, and knees, and absent at the ankles. Toes were downgoing bilaterally. He was able to walk but could not walk on his heels, toes, or in tandem.

Investigations

A repeat NCS showed reduced bilateral peroneal and tibial compound muscle action potential (CMAP) amplitudes, worse on the left, and normal distal motor latencies and conduction velocities. Left sural conduction response was absent, and right sural sensory nerve action potential (SNAP) amplitude was markedly reduced with normal peak latency and conduction velocity. Needle EMG of selected left lower limb muscles showed a few fibrillation potentials and positive sharp waves in the tibialis anterior and medial gastrocnemius muscles, early recruitment of small-amplitude and short-duration motor unit potentials in the tibialis anterior, medial gastrocnemius, and vastus lateralis muscles. Needle EMG of the right flexor digitorum profundus muscles also showed a few small-amplitude and short-duration motor unit potentials but normal recruitment and no abnormal spontaneous activities. Overall, the NCS/EMG showed an irritable myopathy mainly affecting distal leg muscles, and a distal sensory polyneuropathy. Serum creatine kinase (CK) level was elevated at 481 U/L. Aldolase level was also elevated at 8.5 U/L (normal <7.7). Complete blood count (CBC), comprehensive metabolic panel (CMP), ESR, TSH, free T4, HbA1C, vitamin B12, and serum immunofixation were all normal. ANA, ENA, ANCAs, myositis antibody panel, anti-cytosolic 5′-nucleotide 1A (cN1A; NT5C1A) autoantibody, and anti-3-hydroxy-3-methyglutaryl-coenzyme A reductase (HMGCR) autoantibody were all negative. A right vastus lateralis muscle biopsy was performed.

Muscle Biopsy Findings

The right vastus lateralis muscle biopsy (Fig. 17.1) showed a chronic active myopathy with marked fiber size variation, rare rimmed vacuoles and occasional scattered necrotic and regenerating fibers. The most distinctive feature was the presence of over a dozen of myofibers containing small sarcoplasmic spherical proteinaceous aggregates, which were eosinophilic on the H&E stain (Fig. 17.1a), dark blue on the Gomori

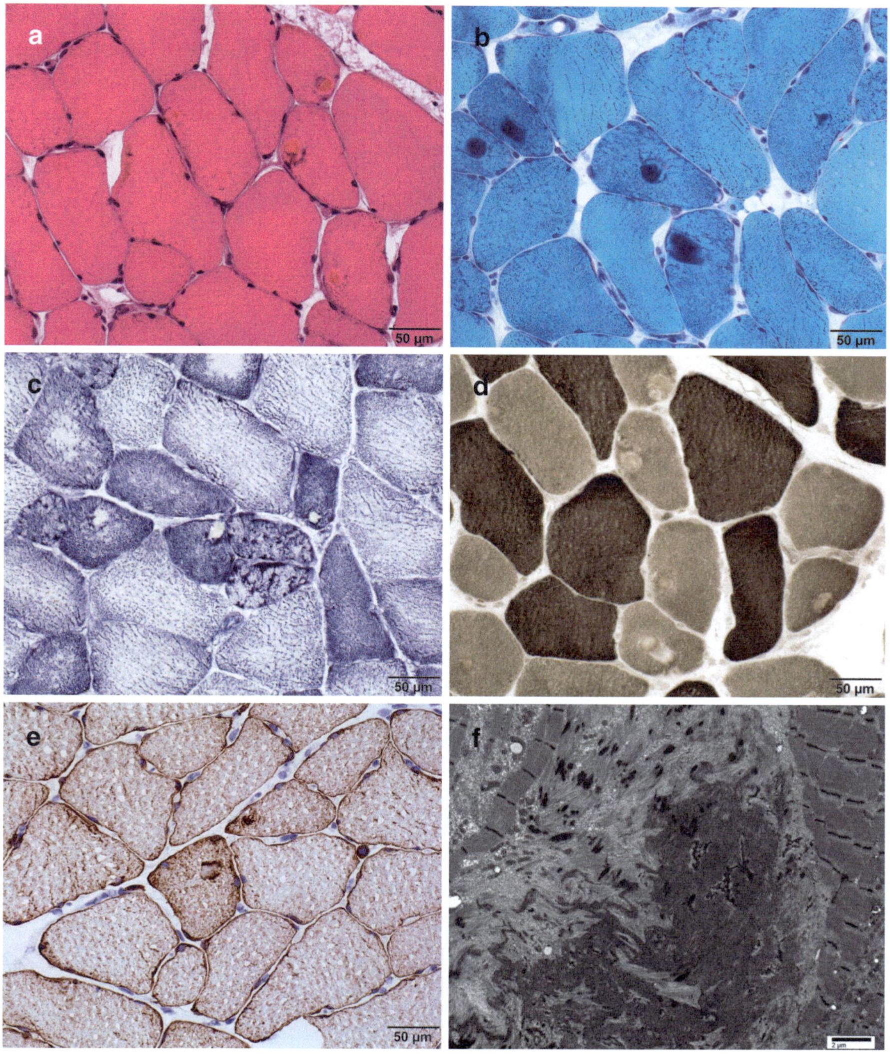

Fig. 17.1 Myofibrillar myopathy. (**a**) H&E stain. (**b**) Gomori trichrome stain. (**c**) NADH-TR stain. (**d**) ATPase stain at pH 9.4. (**e**) Desmin immunostain. (**f**) Granulofilamentous material on electron microscopy

trichrome stain (Fig. 17.1b), metachromatic on the crystal violet stain, and pale on the NADH-TR (Fig. 17.1c), SDH, COX and ATPase (Fig. 17.1d) stains, involving predominantly type 1 myofibers. The protein aggregates in most of the fibers were immunoreactive to desmin (Fig. 17.1e). A small focus of endomysial lymphocytic inflammation was present. There was no diffuse upregulation of class I major histocompatibility complex (MHC1), except for focal reactivity in the necrotic fibers and near the inflammatory cells. There was no excessive COX-deficient fibers. Very mild neurogenic changes including rare esterase positive denervated atrophic fibers and subtle fiber type grouping were also present. Electron microscopy (EM) showed a sarcoplasmic accumulation of granulofilamentous materials which appeared to be a mixture of Z-line material, electron dense material, and disrupted myofilaments (Fig. 17.1f). The findings are characteristic of myofibrillar myopathy. Focal areas of maldistribution of mitochondria were also noted with streaks separating myofibrils, rendering a lobulated appearance on light microscopy.

Final Diagnosis

Myofibrillar Myopathy

Patient Follow-up

The patient underwent genetic testing. The muscular dystrophy gene panel showed one copy of a possible pathogenic variant, c.5568T > A (p.C1856X), in the *SMCHD1* gene. The *DUX4* gene expression-permissive 4q35 haplotype was not tested, as his presentation was atypical for facioscapulohumeral muscular dystrophy. There was no mutation detected in the *desmin, myotilin, FHL1, or DNAJB6* gene. The other genes, mutations in which could also cause myofibrillar myopathy, including *αB-crystallin*, Z-line alternatively spliced PDZ motif-containing protein (*ZASP*), *filamin C*, and *bcl-2-associated athanogene 3 (Bag3)* genes were not included in this muscular dystrophy gene panel. Due to the patient's insurance status, these genes had not been tested. The patient underwent physical therapy, and his weakness slightly progressed over the next 1–1/2 years. But his gait improved after wearing ankle foot orthotic brace (AFO). He was referred to cardiology for cardiac evaluation which revealed a very mild dilated cardiomyopathy, and it was treated. His pulmonary function test was unremarkable.

Discussion

Myofibrillar myopathies are a group of heterogeneous genetic myopathies that share distinct muscle pathology features [1]. They are caused by mutations in the genes that encode proteins in Z line or associated with Z line, which play important roles in maintaining intermyofibrillar architecture. The genes that are primarily involved in myofibrillar myopathies include *desmin (DES)*, *αB-crystallin (CRYAB)*, *myotilin (MYOT)*, *ZASP (LDB3)*, *filamin C (FLNC)*, *Bag3 (BAG3)*, and *four-and-a-half-LIM domain 1 protein (FHL1)*. Many cases are sporadic. The inheritance in the majority of the cases with a positive family history is autosome dominant except for the FHL1-associated cases which are X-linked. Recessive mutations are very rare. A large number of cases with myofibrillar myopathies have no gene mutations found, which indicates that some causative genes have not been identified yet [2–5].

Age of symptom onset in myofibrillar myopathies is variable, ranging from childhood to late adulthood with adult onset being more common [4], especially in the cases with mutations in the *LDB3*, *MYOT*, and *FLNC* genes. Childhood cases are often severe and the progression is rapid. Myofibrillar myopathies can affect skeletal muscles and cardiac muscles. Limb weakness is often distal starting from lower limbs. It gradually progresses to involve upper limb muscles and proximal limb muscles. Some patients may show Achilles and finger contractures and atypical predominant scapuloperoneal weakness. Facial weakness is uncommon. Some older patients may report slurred speech and difficulty swallowing. Cardiac involvement is relatively common in the disease that is caused by mutations in the *DES*, *FLNC*, *FHL1*, or *BAG3* gene. Patients may have arrhythmia, conduction defects, and/or dilated or hypertrophic cardiomyopathy. Cardiac involvement is rare in the disease that is caused by mutations in the *MYOT* or *LDB3* gene. Respiratory weakness is mainly seen in early-onset severe cases and is also common in cases with *FLNC* mutations. Peripheral neuropathy is common especially in patients with *BAG3* mutations. Early-onset cataract is a feature associated with *CRYAB* mutations.

The common causes of distal limb numbness and asymmetrical distal lower limb weakness in an elderly patient like ours include polyradiculopathy, lumbosacral plexopathy, and polyneuropathy. Myofibrillar myopathy is often misdiagnosed with these conditions and a correct diagnosis is often delayed. EMG plays a pivotal role in raising a suspicion for a myopathy. EMG in myofibrillar myopathies usually shows myopathic changes more prominent in the affected distal lower limb muscles as seen in our case. It may also show a coexisting distal polyneuropathy [4]. CK in myofibrillar myopathies is either normal or mildly elevated. The combination of a distal predominant myopathy and a distal polyneuropathy should raise a suspicion for a myofibrillar myopathy. The differential diagnosis in this setting includes sporadic inclusion body myositis (sIBM) and other distal myopathies [6]. For the distal limb muscles, sIBM more affects finger flexors than foot dorsiflexors. The more severe foot and toe plantar flexor weakness seen in our patient is atypical for sIBM. Muscle MRI may show different patterns of muscle involvement in myofibrillar myopathies caused by different gene mutations.

Muscle biopsy plays a key role in making a diagnosis of a myofibrillar myopathy and differentiating it from other distal myopathies. Subsequent genetic testing can identify genetic causes in many patients but not all [3]. As the disease more affects distal limb muscles and the muscle involvement can be asymmetrical, choosing an affected muscle for biopsy based on the clinical weakness, EMG findings, and muscle MRI findings is important as it can increase the biopsy yield.

The defining feature of myofibrillar myopathy is the presence of sarcoplasmic protein aggregates in a background of chronic myopathy. These protein aggregates have been referred to as hyaline structures, spheroid bodies, or Mallory bodies. They are eosinophilic on H&E, dark blue on Gomori trichrome, but pale on mitochondria enzyme stains (NADH-TR, SDH, and COX) and ATPase stains (Fig. 17.1). Cytoplasmic bodies can also be seen in myofibrillar myopathy, but much less specific. Cytoplasmic bodies are usually smaller than hyaline structures, composed of a dark red core surrounded by a pale halo on Gomori trichrome (Fig. 17.2a). On EM, cytoplasmic bodies are composed of an electron dense core surrounded by a halo of radiating filaments that show continuity with myofibrils (Fig. 17.2b). Replicated triads can be prominent (Fig. 17.2b). NADH-TR stain may also reveal widespread myofibrillar disarray (Fig. 17.2c), sometimes referred to as nonhyaline structures [7]. Both hyaline and nonhyaline structures are immunoreactive to desmin (Fig. 17.2d). These aggregates are also reported to be immunoreactive to alpha B crystalline, myotilin and dystrophin [4]. On EM, both hyaline and nonhyaline structures are composed of disintegrated Z band material, electron dense material, and disorganized myofilaments, which are collectively referred to as granulofilamentous material (Fig. 17.2e). Vacuoles containing degenerating membranous organelles can also be seen in some cases of myofibrillar myopathy (Fig. 17.2f); those vacuoles typically lack tubulofilamentous inclusions seen in inclusion body myositis (IBM).

Morphological differential considerations of myofibrillar myopathy include target/targetoid fibers, central cores, multi-minicores, lobulated myofibers, and chronic myopathies from any cause with markedly abnormal myofibrillar architecture. Most of those lack well-formed hyaline structures. Target/targetoid fibers are seen in chronic active denervation atrophy, and they often coexist with angular atrophic fibers and fiber type grouping. Central cores and multi-minicores are most common in children. The muscle biopsy usually shows type 1 fiber predominance and lacks active myopathic changes such as necrotic, myophagocytic, or regenerating fibers. Lobulated fibers (Fig. 17.2g) have been commonly associated with calpain deficiency but can be seen in a variety of hereditary and nonhereditary conditions. On EM, the lobulated appearance is rendered by maldistribution of mitochondria from their normal Z-band location into streaks that separate myofibrils into bundles (Fig. 17.2h). The presence of specific diagnostic features of other chronic myopathies, such as lymphocytic invasion and diffuse myofiber MHC1 upregulation in IBM and polymyositis, and muscle dystrophic changes with detectable membrane protein defects by immunostaining panel in various muscular dystrophies, overrides the morphological diagnosis of myofibrillar myopathy.

There is no effective disease-modifying therapy for myofibrillar myopathies currently. Several disease animal models have been generated to study the disease-causing mechanisms and to develop targeted therapies to control sarcomere disruption and protein aggregation [2]. At this point, the management of patients with myofibrillar myopathies is mainly supportive to maximize functions and prevent falls. Since cardiac involvement is relatively common in patients with myofibrillar myopathies, these patients should be referred to cardiology for a thorough

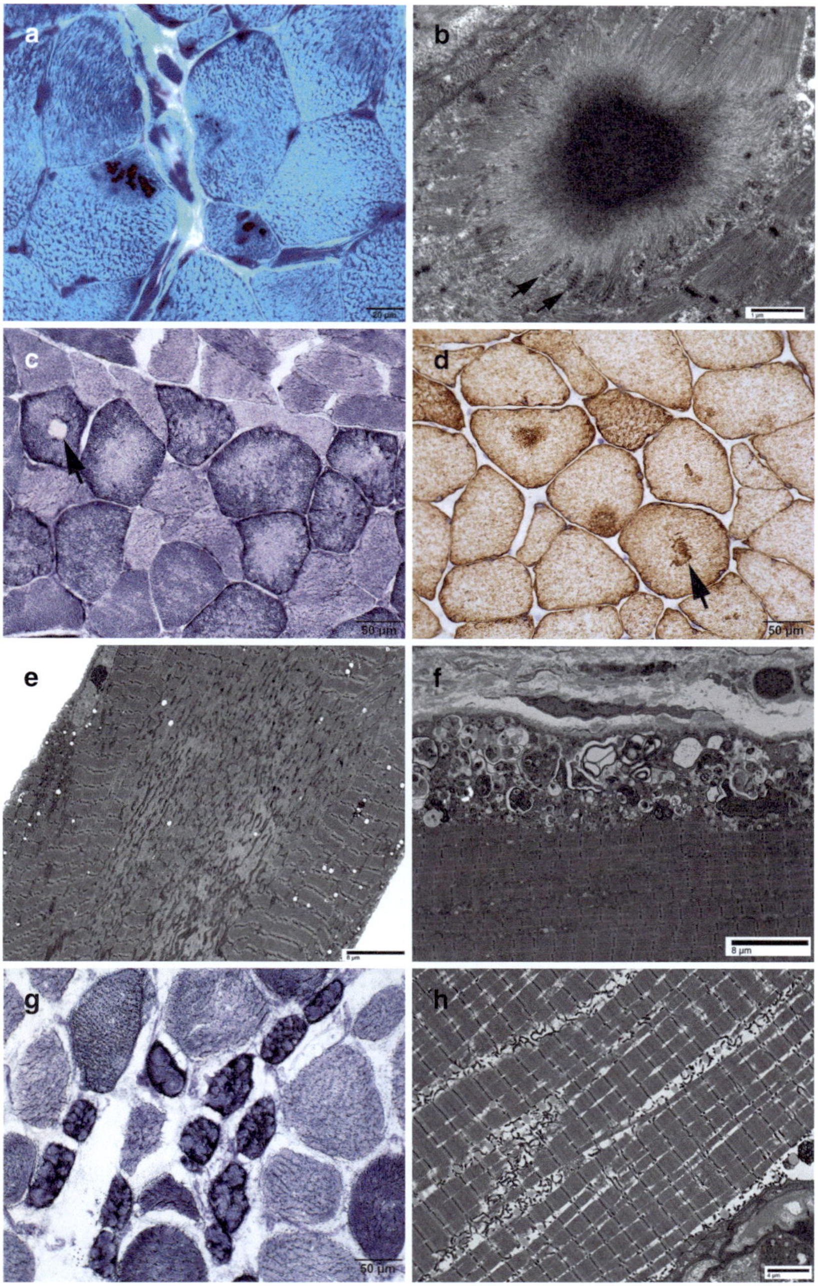

Fig. 17.2 (**a**, **b**) Cytoplasmic bodies from an 8-year-old girl with plectin (PLEC) associated muscular dystrophy. (**a**) Gomori trichrome and (**b**) EM (arrows: replicated triads). (**c–e**) Hyaline and Non-hyaline structures from a 72-year-old man with myofibrillar myopathy. (**c**) NADH-TR, (**d**) Desmin immunostaining, and (**e**) EM (arrows: hyaline structures). (**f**) A vacuole with degenerating membranous organelles in an 83-year-old man with myofibrillar myopathy. (**g–h**) Myopathy with lobulated fibers from a 67-year-old woman. (**g**) NADH-TR shows prominent lobulated changes in type 1 myofibers. (**h**) EM shows maldistribution of mitochondria that form subsarcolemmal and sarcoplasmic bands

cardiac evaluation and for the management of associated cardiac defects if present. These patients may also undergo swallow evaluation and pulmonary function test. Genetic counseling should be provided.

Pearls

Clinical Pearls

1. Myofibrillar myopathies are a group of heterogeneous genetic myopathies that are primarily caused by mutations in the genes encoding desmin, αB-crystallin, myotilin, ZASP, filamin C, Bag3, and FHL1. The disease is mainly autosomal dominant except for the FHL1-associated disease which is X-linked.
2. Patients with myofibrillar myopathies commonly show adult onset of symptoms. The onset is often late. The early-onset disease is usually more severe and rapidly progressive.
3. Myofibrillar myopathies predominantly affect distal limb muscles with initial weakness in the distal lower limb muscles. Cardiac involvement is common which may manifest arrhythmia, conduction defects, and/or dilated or hypertrophic cardiomyopathy. Peripheral neuropathy is common especially in patients with *BAG3* mutations.
4. The combination of a distal predominant myopathy and a distal polyneuropathy should raise a suspicion for a myofibrillar myopathy.
5. Muscle biopsy plays a key role in the diagnosis of a myofibrillar myopathy. Subsequent genetic testing can identify genetic causes in many patients but not all.
6. Currently there is no effective therapy for myofibrillar myopathies. The management is mainly supportive. Patients should be referred to cardiology for a thorough cardiac evaluation and for the management of associated cardiac defects if present.

Pathology Pearls

1. The characteristic feature of myofibrillar myopathy is the presence of sarcoplasmic hyaline structures in a background of chronic myopathy. Cytoplasmic bodies, non-hyaline structures, rimmed vacuoles, and uneven oxidative enzyme staining are common findings in myofibrillar myopathy but less specific.

2. The hyaline structures are dark on Gomori trichrome, pale on ATPase, NADH-TR, COX, and SDH stains, and immunoreactive to desmin.
3. On EM, the hyaline and non-hyaline structures are composed of disorganized filaments, Z-disk material, and electron dense material, which are collectively referred to as granulofilamentous material.

References

1. Dubowitz V, Sewry CA, Oldfors AO. Myopathies with vacuoles. In: Dubowitz V, Sewry CA, Oldfors AO, editors. Muscle biopsy: a practical approach. 4th ed. Sanders Elsevier; 2013. p. 406–22.
2. Batonnet-Pichon S, Behin A, Cabet E, Delort F, Vicart P, Lilienbaum A. Myofibrillar myopathies: new perspectives from animal models to potential therapeutic approaches. J Neuromuscul Dis. 2017;4(1):1–15.
3. Selcen D, Muntoni F, Burton BK, Pegoraro E, Sewry C, Bite AV, et al. Mutation in BAG3 causes severe dominant childhood muscular dystrophy. Ann Neurol. 2009;65(1):83–9.
4. Selcen D, Ohno K, Engel AG. Myofibrillar myopathy: clinical, morphological and genetic studies in 63 patients. Brain. 2004;127(Pt 2):439–51.
5. Schroder R, Schoser B. Myofibrillar myopathies: a clinical and myopathological guide. Brain Pathol. 2009;19(3):483–92.
6. Dimachkie MM, Barohn RJ. Distal myopathies. Neurol Clin. 2014;32(3):817–42, x
7. Nakano S, Engel AG, Waclawik AJ, Emslie-Smith AM, Busis NA. Myofibrillar myopathy with abnormal foci of desmin positivity. I. Light and electron microscopy analysis of 10 cases. J Neuropathol Exp Neurol. 1996;55(5):549–62.

Chapter 18
A 40-Year-Old Man with Muscle Pain and Fatigue

Lan Zhou

History

A 40-year-old Caucasian man presented with over 1 year of muscle pain and fatigue. He was diagnosed with hyperlipidemia 2 years prior to the presentation. It was unsatisfactorily controlled by dietary modification and exercise. He was started on Atorvastatin 20 mg once daily by his primary care physician. Two weeks later, he developed pain and fatigue mainly in his thigh muscles. Atorvastatin was switched to Rosuvastatin and then to Pravastatin. His muscle symptoms continued to progress, and they involved the upper arm muscles as well. He felt that his thigh muscles and upper arm muscles were heavy. He became tired easily, and could no longer run 1 mile per day. His serum creatine kinase (CK) level was tested several times, and it was persistently elevated in the range of 300s to 500s U/L. His baseline CK level before taking statin drugs was unknown. Eight months prior, statin drug was completely discontinued, but his muscle symptoms remained although less severe. He was evaluated by a local neurologist. Nerve conduction study (NCS) and needle electromyography (EMG) study were reportedly normal. He underwent a left quadriceps muscle biopsy with no definitive diagnosis. Dysferlin and myotonic dystrophy type 2 (DM2) gene tests were negative. He was referred to our clinic for further evaluation and a repeat muscle biopsy. His past medical history was significant for hyperlipidemia. He was not on any medications when presenting to our clinic. His family history was positive for hypertension and hyperlipidemia but not myopathy. He did not drink alcohol or smoke cigarettes. He was an engineer.

L. Zhou (✉)
Departments of Neurology and Pathology, Boston University Medical Center, Boston, MA, USA
e-mail: lanzhou@bu.edu

L. Zhou et al. (eds.), *A Case-Based Guide to Neuromuscular Pathology*,
https://doi.org/10.1007/978-3-030-25682-1_18

Physical Examination

His general examination was unremarkable. Neurological examination showed normal mental status and intact cranial nerve functions. Motor examination revealed normal muscle tone and bulk. Strength was minimally reduced in the bilateral iliopsoas muscles (MRC 5−/5) but normal in other limb muscles. Neck muscles were strong. He was able to get up from a chair without using his hands to push. There was no scapular winging or calf hypertrophy. Sensation and coordination were normal. Deep tendon reflexes were 2+ throughout. Toes were downgoing bilaterally. His gait was normal.

Investigations

Complete blood count (CBC) and comprehensive metabolic panel were normal. A repeat serum creatine kinase (CK) level was mildly elevated at 308 U/L. TSH, free T4, and vitamin D levels were normal. ANA, ENA, myositis antibody panel, and 3-hydroxy-3-methylglutaryl-coenzyme A reductase (HMGCR) antibody were all negative. A repeat NCS/EMG was normal. His left quadriceps muscle biopsy slides were reviewed.

Muscle Biopsy Findings

The left quadriceps muscle biopsy (Fig. 18.1) showed a few scattered polygonal atrophic fibers. There was no necrotic, degenerating, or regenerating fiber. The atrophic fibers were not esterase positive. There was no ragged red fiber or COX-deficient fiber. There was no inflammation. Myophosphorylase, phosphofructokinase,

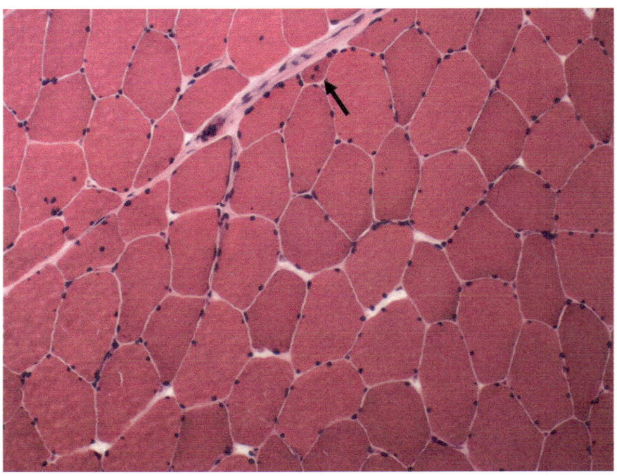

Fig. 18.1 Hematoxylin and eosin stain (HE) shows a rare atrophic fiber (arrow)

and myoadenylate deaminase stains showed positive sarcoplasmic reactivity with no evidence of deficiencies in these enzymes. Electron microscopy (EM) was reportedly unremarkable. The findings are non-diagnostic and insignificant.

Final Diagnosis

Mild Toxic Myopathy Induced by Statin Use

Patient Follow-up

The diagnosis of a mild toxic myopathy induced by statin use was discussed with the patient. He was reassured that his muscle symptoms would continue to improve with time. A repeat muscle biopsy was not needed. He was instructed to take coenzyme Q10 (CoQ10) and multivitamins. Six months later, he returned for follow-up. He reported near-complete resolution of his muscle symptoms. Examination showed no weakness. His CK level was minimally elevated at 283 U/L. His hyperlipidemia was relatively controlled by ezetimibe, low-fat diet, and daily exercise.

Discussion

Statin drugs, the HMGCR inhibitors, have been widely used for treating dyslipidemia and reducing the risk for cardiovascular and cerebrovascular diseases [1]. Muscle symptoms, including myalgia, fatigue, and weakness, represent a major side effect of this class of drugs, which can be seen in up to 20% of statin users [2]. Statin drugs can cause rhabdomyolysis, an immune-mediated necrotizing myopathy, and more commonly a mild toxic myopathy [3–8]. All statin drugs on the market can cause myopathy, which include lovastatin, simvastatin, pravastatin, atorvastatin, and fluvastatin [9]. The risk factors for statin-induced myopathies include age at or above 65 years, comorbidities such as diabetes mellitus, renal dysfunction, and cardiovascular disease, co-administration of certain drugs, and SLCO1B1 gene variants [10–12].

Rhabdomyolysis induced by statin is a very rare but serious type of myopathy [13, 14]. It is caused by the direct myotoxicity of statin. It can occur when initiating a statin drug or after increasing the dosage of a statin drug. These cases are mainly encountered in an emergency department or in an inpatient setting. Besides acute management of rhabdomyolysis, statin use should be discontinued immediately.

Immune-mediated necrotizing myopathy induced by statin is an autoimmune myopathy [15]. It is caused by the autoimmunity triggered by statin use [4–6]. The disease is characterized by progressive, symmetric, and proximal limb weakness, marked CK elevation, the presence of HMGCR autoantibody, muscle biopsy features of a necrotizing myopathy with diffuse or multifocal myofiber upregulation of class I major histocompatibility complex (MHC-1), and the need for immunosuppressive therapy [4–6]. The mean age of onset is 64.7 years in one series [4] and 55 years in the other [16]. The proximal limb weakness may develop weeks or years after statin exposure or even after statin withdrawal [4]. The initial serum CK while taking statin is markedly elevated, ranging from 3,000 to 17,280 U/L in one series of 25 patients [4]. Mean CK upon initial presentation is 6,853 U/L according to a systemic review of 100 published cases with immune-mediated necrotizing myopathy induced by statin [17]. This review also shows that HMGCR antibody is present in all cases tested [17]. HMGCR antibody is not present in asymptomatic statin users or statin users who develop self-limited mild toxic myopathy [18], which makes this autoantibody a useful marker for immune-mediated necrotizing myopathy induced by statin. HMGCR antibody can also be present in statin-naïve patients with autoimmune myopathy [19]. EMG in patients with immune-mediated necrotizing myopathy induced by statin often shows irritable myopathy with the presence of abnormal spontaneous activities in the forms of fibrillation potentials, positive sharp waves, and myotonic or pseudomyotonic discharges [4]. Muscle biopsy shows a necrotizing myopathy with minimal or absent lymphocytic infiltrates but with diffuse or multifocal myofiber upregulation of MHC-1 [6]. The disease course is characterized by the lack of improvement or worsening of muscle symptoms and CK elevation after statin withdrawal, the need for immunosuppressive therapy, and frequent relapse after tapering off immunosuppressive therapy [4, 6].

Mild toxic myopathy as seen in the present case is much more common than rhabdomyolysis and immune-mediated necrotizing myopathy induced by statin. It is caused by the direct myotoxicity of statin. The disease usually manifests muscle pain, fatigue, and/or mild weakness which predominantly affects proximal limb muscles. By using the development of muscle symptoms after statin use with no other causes of muscle symptoms identified as the definition for statin myopathy, and by excluding patients with rhabdomyolysis or immune-mediated necrotizing myopathy induced by statin use, we identified a cohort of 69 patients with mild toxic myopathy induced by statin (mild statin myopathy) to characterize their clinical features and outcomes after statin withdrawal [8]. Myalgia was the most common muscle symptom, as over 90% of the patients in our cohort reported myalgia. This is consistent with the finding by another study [20]. Although 68.1% of our patients also reported muscle weakness, only 26.1% had mild proximal limb weakness detectable by exam. CK was normal in nearly 25% of our patients, mildly elevated at or below 1,000 U/L in 52.2%, and above 1,000 U/L in 23.2%, with the highest CK level being 2,607 U/L. Despite that all of our patients had muscle symptoms and over 75% had CK elevation, only 25% of the patients who underwent EMG showed myopathic changes on EMG [8]. NCS/EMG is useful to rule out other neuromuscular disorders, but it is relatively insensitive to detect mild statin myopathy.

The diagnosis of mild statin myopathy can be made based on clinical grounds. Muscle biopsy is not needed as there is no muscle pathology signature for this condition. Among 16 patients in our cohort who underwent muscle biopsies, 3 showed rare degenerating and regenerating fibers, 2 showed occasional regenerating fibers, 3 showed rare COX-deficient fibers, and 1 showed mild type 2 fiber atrophy. EM only showed a mild increase in mitochondrial number in rare fibers in 3 cases, and it was completely normal in the others [8]. These findings are very mild and non-specific. Therefore, muscle biopsy is not helpful in diagnosing mild statin myopathy. The muscle biopsy in our patient also showed mild non-specific changes, but his clinical presentation was consistent with a mild statin myopathy. The purpose of a muscle biopsy is mainly to rule out immune-mediated necrotizing myopathy induced by statin and other underlying myopathies unmasked by statin use. The muscle pathology features of immune-mediated necrotizing myopathy are illustrated in the chapter of immune-mediated necrotizing myopathy.

Mild statin myopathy can be differentiated from immune-mediated necrotizing myopathy induced by statin based on the clinical features. Unlike immune-mediated necrotizing myopathy, mild statin myopathy is characterized by mild or no muscle weakness, normal or mildly elevated CK, absent HMGCR autoantibody, improvement of muscle symptoms and CK elevation after statin withdrawal, and no need for immunosuppressive therapy. However, we still frequently receive requests for performing muscle biopsies for patients with mild statin myopathy. The most common reason for referring physicians to request muscle biopsies is to rule out immune-mediated myopathy induced by statin use or other myopathies unmasked by statin use, as patients' CK elevation or muscle symptoms do not resolve as fast as expected after statin withdrawal. To avoid unnecessary muscle biopsies in this clinic setting and to obtain data to guide the biopsy threshold, we studied the outcomes of mild statin myopathy after statin withdrawal [8].

For the duration of follow-up (Mean ± SD: 29.6 ± 33.1 months) in our cohort of 69 patients, muscle symptoms completely recovered in 50/69 (72.5%), improved in 9/69 (13.0%), and did not change in 10/69 (14.5%). None of our patients reported worsening of muscle symptoms. Among the 10 patients who reported no change of their muscle symptoms, only 1 showed mild, persistent, detectable proximal weakness, and CK trended down in all. Among 50/69 (72.5%) patients who had their muscle symptoms completely resolved, the recovery was achieved within 1 month in 12 (24.0%), 3 months in 31 (62.0%), 6 months in 45 (90.0%), 1 year in 48 (96.0%), 3 years in 49 (98.0%), and 5 years in all (100%). 13/69 (18.8%) patients had muscle symptoms lingering beyond 14 months. Therefore, the symptom recovery in mild statin myopathy can be prolonged. One may hold muscle biopsy especially in those who have mild improving muscle symptoms even the improvement is relatively slow. The outcomes of mild statin myopathy after statin withdrawal do not correlate with the duration of statin exposure, duration of follow-up, initial CK elevation or myopathic changes on EMG [8]. There are no features that would allow us to accurately determine who may have a prolonged recovery course. The confounding factors of muscle symptoms should be screened, such as thyroid dysfunction, connective tissue diseases, and administration of non-statin myotoxic drugs.

Although 85.5% of our patients had muscle symptoms completely resolved (72.5%) or improved (13.0%) for the duration of follow up, the CK level remained elevated, although trended down, in 41/52 (78.8%). Baseline CK levels (before statin exposure) were retrievable in 34/69 (49.3%) patients, and they were all normal. The findings suggest that the normalization of CK often lags behind the improvement or resolution of muscle symptoms after statin withdrawal. Mild persistent CK elevation alone should not be an indication for muscle biopsy.

Management of patients with mild statin myopathy may include statin withdrawal and CoQ10 supplementation. Statin drugs should be immediately discontinued when the diagnosis of rhabdomyolysis or immune-mediated necrotizing myopathy is made. The decision of discontinuing statin in mild toxic myopathy should be made by weighing the benefits and risks. In some cases, the muscle symptoms are very mild, but the benefit of statin use to reduce the risk of cardiovascular and cerebrovascular diseases is significant. Such patients may be managed by close monitoring. If their muscle symptoms become significantly worse with time, the decision of statin withdrawal should be reconsidered. In this setting, treating neurologists should make a decision by discussing the benefits and risks of statin withdrawal not only with patients but also with physicians who treat patients with statin. It has been shown that CoQ10 can reduce muscle symptoms but not serum CK [21], and it may be offered to patients with mild statin myopathy.

Pearls

Clinical Pearls

1. Statin drugs can cause rhabdomyolysis, immune-mediated necrotizing myopathy, and mild toxic myopathy. The mild toxic myopathy is the most common.
2. Myalgia is the most common symptom of mild statin myopathy. The other common muscle symptoms include muscle fatigue and weakness.
3. Although the majority of patients with mild statin myopathy report muscle weakness, a few have muscle weakness detectable by exam.
4. Over 18% of patients with mild statin myopathy can have muscle symptoms lasting for more than 1 year after statin withdrawal. It is difficult to predict who will have a prolonged recovery course.
5. CK normalization often lags behind muscle symptom improvement or resolution. Mild persistent CK elevation alone should not be an indication for muscle biopsy.
6. EMG is often normal in mild statin myopathy.
7. Mild statin myopathy can be diagnosed and differentiated from immune-mediated necrotizing myopathy based on the clinical features.
8. Muscle biopsy is not needed for diagnosing mild statin myopathy.
9. Management of mild statin myopathy consists of statin withdrawal if the benefit outweighs the risk, and CoQ10 supplementation.

Pathology Pearls

1. Muscle biopsy findings in mild toxic myopathy induced by statin use are mild and non-specific. They may include a few atrophic fibers, degenerating fibers, and regenerating fibers with no myofiber upregulation of MHC1.
2. The purpose of a muscle biopsy is to rule out immune-mediated necrotizing myopathy induced by statin use and other myopathies unmasked by statin use. Muscle pathologic features of immune-mediated necrotizing myopathy are illustrated in the chapter of immune-mediated necrotizing myopathy.

References

1. Gu Q, Paulose-Ram R, Burt VL, Kit BK. Prescription cholesterol-lowering medication use in adults aged 40 and over: United States, 2003–2012. NCHS Data Brief. 2014(177):1–8.
2. Fernandez G, Spatz ES, Jablecki C, Phillips PS. Statin myopathy: a common dilemma not reflected in clinical trials. Cleve Clin J Med. 2011;78(6):393–403.
3. Christopher-Stine L, Casciola-Rosen LA, Hong G, Chung T, Corse AM, Mammen AL. A novel autoantibody recognizing 200-kd and 100-kd proteins is associated with an immune-mediated necrotizing myopathy. Arthritis Rheum. 2010;62(9):2757–66.
4. Grable-Esposito P, Katzberg HD, Greenberg SA, Srinivasan J, Katz J, Amato AA. Immune-mediated necrotizing myopathy associated with statins. Muscle Nerve. 2010;41(2):185–90.
5. Mammen AL, Chung T, Christopher-Stine L, Rosen P, Rosen A, Doering KR, et al. Autoantibodies against 3-hydroxy-3-methylglutaryl-coenzyme A reductase in patients with statin-associated autoimmune myopathy. Arthritis Rheum. 2011;63(3):713–21.
6. Needham M, Fabian V, Knezevic W, Panegyres P, Zilko P, Mastaglia FL. Progressive myopathy with up-regulation of MHC-1 associated with statin therapy. Neuromuscul Disord. 2007;17(2):194–200.
7. Thompson PD, Clarkson P, Karas RH. Statin-associated myopathy. JAMA. 2003;289(13):1681–90.
8. Armour R, Zhou L. Outcomes of statin myopathy after statin withdrawal. J Clin Neuromuscul Dis. 2013;14(3):103–9.
9. Rosenson RS, Baker SK, Jacobson TA, Kopecky SL, Parker BA, The National Lipid Association's Muscle Safety Expert P. An assessment by the Statin Muscle Safety Task Force: 2014 update. J Clin Lipidol. 2014;8(3 Suppl):S58–71.
10. Nguyen KA, Li L, Lu D, Yazdanparast A, Wang L, Kreutz RP, et al. A comprehensive review and meta-analysis of risk factors for statin-induced myopathy. Eur J Clin Pharmacol. 2018;74(9):1099–109.
11. Needham M, Mastaglia FL. Statin myotoxicity: a review of genetic susceptibility factors. Neuromuscul Disord. 2014;24(1):4–15.
12. Group SC, Link E, Parish S, Armitage J, Bowman L, Heath S, et al. SLCO1B1 variants and statin-induced myopathy--a genomewide study. N Engl J Med. 2008;359(8):789–99.
13. Davidson MH, Clark JA, Glass LM, Kanumalla A. Statin safety: an appraisal from the adverse event reporting system. Am J Cardiol. 2006;97(8A):32C–43C.
14. Law M, Rudnicka AR. Statin safety: a systematic review. Am J Cardiol. 2006;97(8A):52C–60C.
15. Mammen AL. Statin-associated autoimmune myopathy. N Engl J Med. 2016;374(7):664–9.
16. Pasnoor M, Barohn RJ, Dimachkie MM. Toxic myopathies. Curr Opin Neurol. 2018;31(5):575–82.
17. Nazir S, Lohani S, Tachamo N, Poudel D, Donato A. Statin-associated autoimmune myopathy: a systematic review of 100 cases. J Clin Rheumatol. 2017;23(3):149–54.

18. Mammen AL, Pak K, Williams EK, Brisson D, Coresh J, Selvin E, et al. Rarity of anti-3-hydroxy-3-methylglutaryl-coenzyme A reductase antibodies in statin users, including those with self-limited musculoskeletal side effects. Arthritis Care Res (Hoboken). 2012;64(2):269–72.
19. Mohassel P, Mammen AL. Anti-HMGCR myopathy. J Neuromuscul Dis. 2018;5(1):11–20.
20. Hansen KE, Hildebrand JP, Ferguson EE, Stein JH. Outcomes in 45 patients with statin-associated myopathy. Arch Intern Med. 2005;165(22):2671–6.
21. Qu H, Guo M, Chai H, Wang WT, Gao ZY, Shi DZ. Effects of coenzyme Q10 on statin-induced myopathy: an updated meta-analysis of randomized controlled trials. J Am Heart Assoc. 2018;7(19):e009835.

Chapter 19
A 42-Year-Old Woman with Progressive Limb Weakness and Breathing Difficulty

Lan Zhou and Dennis K. Burns

History

A 42-year-old Caucasian woman presented to our neuromuscular clinic for evaluation of progressive limb weakness and exertional shortness of breath. She was diagnosed with systemic lupus erythematosus (SLE) 2 years prior to the presentation and treated with Prednisone (20–40 mg once daily). Six months prior, hydroxychloroquine (Plaquenil) 200 mg twice daily was added. Three months prior, she started to notice difficulty holding arms up when blow drying her hairs. She also noticed difficulty climbing stairs. She developed easy fatigability associated with mild shortness of breath after walking a few blocks. She denied eyelid ptosis, double vision, or difficulty chewing or swallowing. She reported that her limb weakness had gradually worsened. She saw her rheumatologist who suspected steroid myopathy, and prednisone was tapered off 1 month prior with no improvement of her weakness. She was referred to our clinic for further evaluation. Her past medical history was significant for SLE and hypertension. Medications included Plaquenil, losartan, and calcium supplement. Family history was significant for lupus. She did not drink alcohol or smoke cigarettes. She was an office manager.

L. Zhou (✉)
Departments of Neurology and Pathology, Boston University Medical Center, Boston, MA, USA
e-mail: lanzhou@bu.edu

D. K. Burns
Department of Pathology, Neuropathology Section, University of Texas Southwestern Medical Center, Dallas, TX, USA
e-mail: dennis.burns@UTSouthwestern.edu

L. Zhou et al. (eds.), *A Case-Based Guide to Neuromuscular Pathology*,
https://doi.org/10.1007/978-3-030-25682-1_19

Physical Examination

Her general examination was unremarkable. There was no skin rash or ankle edema. Neurological examination showed normal mental status and intact cranial nerve functions. Motor examination revealed normal muscle tone and bulk. Mild weakness was detected in the bilateral deltoid (MRC 4/5), biceps (4+/5), iliopsoas (4/5), and quadriceps (4+/5) muscles. She could not get up from a chair without using her hands to push. Sensation and coordination were normal. Deep tendon reflexes were diffusely reduced (1+). Toes were downgoing bilaterally. Her gait was normal.

Investigations

Complete blood count (CBC) showed mild anemia. Comprehensive metabolic panel showed normal renal and hepatic functions. Serum creatine kinase (CK) level was mildly elevated at 290 U/L. TSH and free T4 were normal. Acetylcholine receptor antibody (AChR-Ab) and muscle specific kinase antibody (MuSK-Ab) were negative. Chest CT was normal. Echocardiogram was also normal with an ejection fraction of 65%. Nerve conduction study (NCS) and repetitive nerve stimulation (RNS) were unrevealing. Needle electromyography (EMG) showed an irritable myopathy with some fibrillation potentials and positive sharp waves in the proximal limb muscles and early recruitment of small-amplitude and short-duration motor unit potentials. A left deltoid muscle biopsy was performed.

Muscle Biopsy Findings

The left deltoid muscle biopsy (Fig. 19.1a) showed a vacuolar myopathy with conspicuous sarcoplasmic vacuoles in many severely atrophic fibers. These vacuoles were red rimmed in Gomori trichrome stain, and had strong acid phosphatase reactivity, consistent with a lysosomal origin. There was no accumulation of periodic acid Schiff (PAS)-positive granules in the vacuoles. There were occasional degenerating and regenerating fibers but no necrotic fibers or inflammation. Electron microscopy (EM) revealed numerous myeloid profiles and prominent collections of curvilinear bodies (Fig. 19.1b).

Final Diagnosis

Hydroxychloroquine Myopathy

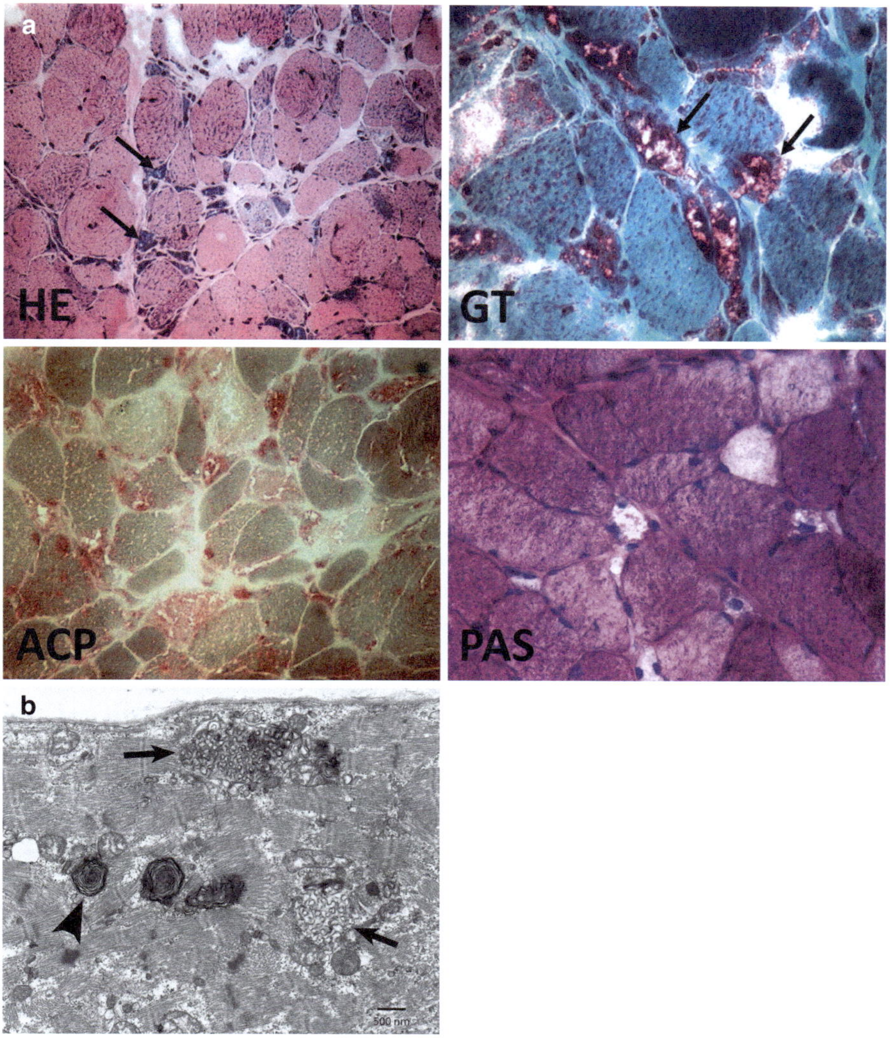

Fig. 19.1 Hydroxychloroquine myopathy. (**a**), Hematoxylin and eosin stain (HE) shows many scattered severely atrophic fibers, which are basophilic and contain sarcoplasmic vacuoles (arrows). Gomori trichrome stain (GT) shows the sarcoplasmic vacuoles are red rimmed (arrows). Acid phosphatase stain (ACP) shows strong reactivity in the vacuoles (arrows). PAS stain shows no abnormal accumulation of PAS-positive granules. (**b**), EM reveals osmiophilic lamellar myeloid profiles (arrow heads), accompanied by collections of well-developed curvilinear bodies (arrows). The findings in this clinical setting are consistent with a toxic myopathy induced by hydroxychloroquine

Patient Follow-up

Hydroxychloroquine was discontinued. The patient underwent physical therapy. She reported marked improvement of her weakness and endurance 2 months later when she returned for follow-up. She could walk a mile without feeling fatigue or shortness of breath. Examination showed minimal weakness in the bilateral deltoid and iliopsoas muscles (5−/5). Weakness in the biceps and quadriceps muscles resolved. She was able to get up from a chair without her hands to push.

Discussion

Hydroxychloroquine and its predecessor chloroquine were first introduced as antimalarial drugs. They were subsequently found to also have anti-inflammatory properties and have been widely used for treating connective tissue diseases, including SLE, rheumatoid arthritis, and Sjogren's syndrome, among others [1–4]. They are 4-aminoquinolones and amphiphilic cationic drugs with a high affinity for the lipid-rich membranes of lysosomes. Once the drugs enter lysosomes, they tend to accumulate, where they neutralize lysosomal contents and raise intra-lysosomal pH. This in turn inhibits lysosomal enzyme activities and affects lysosomal protein, phospholipid, and glycogen degradation [5]. The toxicity mainly affects muscle, nerve, myocardium and retina. Hydroxychloroquine is less toxic than chloroquine [6–9].

Hydroxychloroquine myopathy is considered to be rare, but it is probably underrecognized and underreported. The risk factors include Caucasian race, renal dysfunction, and concomitant use of other myotoxic drugs. The occurrence of hydroxychloroquine myopathy does not appear to be dose-dependent [10, 11]. The disease may predominantly affect proximal limb muscles or in severe cases may affect both proximal and distal limb muscles as well as respiratory muscles with resultant respiratory failure [12–14]. Therefore, it is important to make an early diagnosis to avoid mortality and morbidity.

As hydroxychloroquine is often used along with corticosteroids to treat connective tissue diseases, a myopathy that develops in this clinical setting may represent hydroxychloroquine myopathy, steroid myopathy, and/or an inflammatory myopathy associated with connective tissue diseases. Serum CK and EMG findings can sometimes be helpful in differentiating these conditions. Serum CK is usually normal in steroid myopathy while it is usually elevated in inflammatory myopathies. CK can be normal or mildly elevated in hydroxychloroquine myopathy. EMG often shows an irritable myopathy in hydroxychloroquine myopathy and inflammatory myopathy but a non-irritable myopathy or no myopathic findings in steroid myopathy. Diffuse myotonic discharges, if present, can help indicate hydroxychloroquine myotoxicity [12]. A muscle biopsy is necessary for a definitive diagnosis.

Muscle biopsies in hydroxychloroquine myopathy, steroid myopathy, and inflammatory myopathy have very different and distinctive features. The muscle biopsy in hydroxychloroquine myopathy is characterized by the presence of a vacuolar myopathy with autophagic rimmed vacuoles and, at an ultrastructural level, the accumulation of myeloid profiles and curvilinear bodies due to the enzymatic degradation of lysosomal membranes. The muscle fibers with vacuolar changes are often severely atrophic and basophilic [12, 13]. These vacuoles are red rimmed in

GT stain as they contain membranous debris. Unlike lysosomal glycogen storage diseases such as late-onset Pompe disease, sarcoplasmic vacuoles in hydroxychloroquine myopathy do not contain excessive glycogen accumulation. EM study shows distinctive curvilinear bodies, a characteristic finding only seen in chloroquine/hydroxychloroquine and other amphiphilic cationic myopathies and some variants of neuronal ceroid lipofuscinosis [11, 15]. Steroid myopathy is characterized by type 2b myofiber atrophy, a non-specific finding which can also be seen in disuse, cachexia, alcohol abuse, connective tissue diseases, and a number of endocrinopathies. Inflammatory myopathy is characterized by primary endomysial and/or perimysial inflammation, morphological evidence of myofiber injury and either diffuse of selective perifascicular MHC1 upregulation. Although inclusion body myositis (IBM) also shows red rimmed vacuoles, these vacuoles contain tubulofilamentous inclusions but not curvilinear bodies. In addition, biopsies from patients with IBM often have many cytochrome c oxidase (COX)-deficient fibers. Clinically, IBM tends to affect men above 50 years of age with predominant involvement of finger flexors and knee extensors. Therefore, the clinical presentation and muscle biopsy findings in our patient are consistent with hydroxychloroquine myopathy.

The management of hydroxychloroquine myopathy is simple, and the disease can be reversible by discontinuing hydroxychloroquine. Patients may show significant improvement over several months if diagnosed and managed early as seen in our case [10, 13]. However, the disease can also be severe and life-threatening due to the respiratory muscle involvement [12, 14]. It is thus important to make an early diagnosis by a muscle biopsy.

Pearls

Clinical Pearls

1. Hydroxychloroquine myopathy is rare but probably underrecognized and underreported. The risk factors include Caucasian race, renal dysfunction, and concomitant use of other myotoxic drugs.
2. Patients with hydroxychloroquine myopathy often present with proximal limb weakness which can progress into diffuse weakness with respiratory failure.
3. Serum CK is mildly elevated or normal in hydroxychloroquine myopathy. EMG shows an irritable myopathy and sometimes diffuse myotonic discharges.
4. As hydroxychloroquine is often used along with steroids to treat connective tissue diseases, a myopathy that develops in this clinical setting may represent hydroxychloroquine myopathy, steroid myopathy, and/or an inflammatory myopathy associated with connective tissue diseases. A muscle biopsy is needed to differentiate these diagnoses.

5. The management of hydroxychloroquine myopathy is to discontinue hydroxychloroquine. Hydroxychloroquine myopathy is reversible if diagnosed and managed early.

Pathology Pearls

1. Muscle biopsy in hydroxychloroquine myopathy is characterized by a vacuolar myopathy with the presence of autophagic rimmed vacuoles, myeloid profiles and curvilinear bodies due to the enzymatic degradation of lysosomal membranes. There is no inflammation.
2. Hydroxychloroquine myopathy can be differentiated from steroid myopathy as steroid myopathy shows type 2 fiber atrophy, a non-specific finding which can also be seen with disuse, cachexia, alcohol abuse, connective tissue diseases, and a number of endocrinopathies.

References

1. Ruiz-Irastorza G, Ramos-Casals M, Brito-Zeron P, Khamashta MA. Clinical efficacy and side effects of antimalarials in systemic lupus erythematosus: a systematic review. Ann Rheum Dis. 2010;69(1):20–8.
2. Saag KG, Teng GG, Patkar NM, Anuntiyo J, Finney C, Curtis JR, et al. American College of Rheumatology 2008 recommendations for the use of nonbiologic and biologic disease-modifying antirheumatic drugs in rheumatoid arthritis. Arthritis Rheum. 2008;59(6):762–84.
3. Tang C, Godfrey T, Stawell R, Nikpour M. Hydroxychloroquine in lupus: emerging evidence supporting multiple beneficial effects. Intern Med J. 2012;42(9):968–78.
4. Fox RI. Mechanism of action of hydroxychloroquine as an antirheumatic drug. Semin Arthritis Rheum. 1993;23(2 Suppl 1):82–91.
5. Stauber WT, Hedge AM, Trout JJ, Schottelius BA. Inhibition of lysosomal function in red and white skeletal muscles by chloroquine. Exp Neurol. 1981;71(2):295–306.
6. McChesney EW. Animal toxicity and pharmacokinetics of hydroxychloroquine sulfate. Am J Med. 1983;75(1A):11–8.
7. Finbloom DS, Silver K, Newsome DA, Gunkel R. Comparison of hydroxychloroquine and chloroquine use and the development of retinal toxicity. J Rheumatol. 1985;12(4):692–4.
8. Scherbel AL, Schuchter SL, Harrison JW. Comparison of effects of two antimalarial agents, hydroxychloroquine sulfate and chloroquine phosphate, in patients with rheumatoid arthitis. Cleve Clin Q. 1957;24(2):98–104.
9. Sundelin SP, Terman A. Different effects of chloroquine and hydroxychloroquine on lysosomal function in cultured retinal pigment epithelial cells. APMIS. 2002;110(6):481–9.
10. Stein M, Bell MJ, Ang LC. Hydroxychloroquine neuromyotoxicity. J Rheumatol. 2000;27(12):2927–31.
11. Khoo T, Otto S, Smith C, Koszyca B, Lester S, Blumbergs P, et al. Curvilinear bodies are associated with adverse effects on muscle function but not with hydroxychloroquine dosing. Clin Rheumatol. 2017;36(3):689–93.

12. Abdel-Hamid H, Oddis CV, Lacomis D. Severe hydroxychloroquine myopathy. Muscle Nerve. 2008;38(3):1206–10.
13. Bolanos-Meade J, Zhou L, Hoke A, Corse A, Vogelsang G, Wagner KR. Hydroxychloroquine causes severe vacuolar myopathy in a patient with chronic graft-versus-host disease. Am J Hematol. 2005;78(4):306–9.
14. Siddiqui AK, Huberfeld SI, Weidenheim KM, Einberg KR, Efferen LS. Hydroxychloroquine-induced toxic myopathy causing respiratory failure. Chest. 2007;131(2):588–90.
15. Neville HE, Maunder-Sewry CA, McDougall J, Sewell JR, Dubowitz V. Chloroquine-induced cytosomes with curvilinear profiles in muscle. Muscle Nerve. 1979;2(5):376–81.

Chapter 20
A 49-Year-Old Man with Limb Weakness and Painful Skin Lesions

Kara Stavros, Rajeev Motiwala, Lan Zhou, and Susan C. Shin

History

A 49-year-old man presented with a 2-week history of severe weakness, myalgias, and malaise. He also reported skin rashes over his trunk and limbs for several weeks. He denied double vision, difficulty in chewing, swallowing, or breathing, or increased distal limb numbness. He had a past medical history of end-stage renal disease on peritoneal dialysis for 10 years. He also had a history of hypertension and diabetes mellitus. The family history was positive for hypertension and diabetes mellitus. He did not smoke cigarettes or drink alcohol.

Physical Examination

The patient appeared cachectic with diffuse muscle wasting. Widespread ecchymosis and large areas of skin hardening with black discoloration were seen most concentrated on pressure sensitive areas such as the back, shoulders, upper thighs and

K. Stavros (✉)
Department of Neurology, Warren Alpert Medical School of Brown University, Rhode Island Hospital, Providence, RI, USA
e-mail: kara_stavros1@brown.edu

R. Motiwala
Department of Neurology, New York University, New York, NY, USA

L. Zhou
Departments of Neurology and Pathology, Boston University Medical Center, Boston, MA, USA

S. C. Shin
Department of Neurology, Icahn School of Medicine at Mount Sinai, New York, NY, USA

L. Zhou et al. (eds.), *A Case-Based Guide to Neuromuscular Pathology*,
https://doi.org/10.1007/978-3-030-25682-1_20

gluteal regions. Proximal muscles, especially beneath the regions of skin changes, were exquisitely tender to palpation. Neurological examination showed normal mental status and cranial nerve functions. Weakness was detected in the bilateral deltoid (4−/5), biceps (4/5), triceps (4/5), hip flexors (3/5), and knee extensors (4−/5). Sensory examination revealed reduced pinprick sensation in a stocking-glove distribution, impaired vibratory sensation at the toes, and intact joint position sense. Deep tendon reflexes were absent throughout.

Investigations

His initial serum creatine kinase level was markedly elevated at 10,000 IU/L (24–204 IU/L). Myositis antibody panel was negative. TSH and free T4 were normal. PTH level was markedly elevated at 2,345 pg/ml (16–97 pg/ml). Calcium level was 9.7 mg/dL (8.5–10.5 mg/dl), and ionized calcium was 0.98 mmol/L (1.14–1.29 mmol/L). Nerve conduction studies revealed a length-dependent axonal sensorimotor polyneuropathy. Needle electromyography revealed an irritable myopathy affecting the proximal muscles in the upper and lower extremities. Two lesional skin biopsies by dermatology were non-diagnostic and showed only diffuse tissue necrosis. A right quadriceps muscle biopsy was performed.

Muscle Biopsy Findings

The right quadriceps muscle biopsy revealed mild type 2 fiber atrophy and calcification of the walls of several perimysial blood vessels (Fig. 20.1). Myofiber necrosis, inflammation, or perifascicular atrophy was not present.

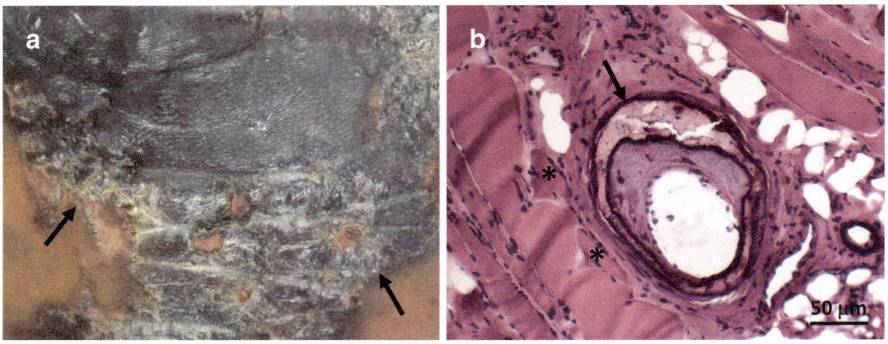

Fig. 20.1 Calciphylaxis. (**a**), A picture of the patient's back shows a large area of skin eschar (arrows). (**b**), Muscle biopsy with HE stain shows calcification of media tunica and thickening of intima of a perimysial arteriole (arrow), and some atrophic fibers (∗)

Final Diagnosis

Systemic calciphylaxis affecting skin and muscle

Patient Follow-up

The patient underwent multiple skin wound debridements and parathyroidectomy. Despite these treatment measures, the patient died from sepsis 4 months after the initial presentation.

Discussion

Calciphylaxis is a rare disorder that predominantly affects patients on dialysis for chronic renal failure [1, 2]. It is characterized by systemic vascular calcification. The disorder carries a high morbidity and mortality especially in patients with ulcerative skin lesions. Clinical manifestations most commonly affect the skin, however vascular calcifications can affect any organ in the body including skeletal muscle, brain, lung, mesentery, and eyes [1, 3–5].

Muscle involvement in calciphylaxis can present with a painful proximal myopathy that progresses over several months. Medial calcification and intimal proliferation of arterioles cause luminal narrowing which leads to muscle ischemia and resultant pain [6]. Although mural calcification predominantly involves small arterioles, it can also affect small venules and capillaries [6, 7]. A few case reports described patients with calciphylaxis who developed prominent muscle involvement manifesting with weakness, myalgias, and rhabdomyolysis [6–11]. In one case the myopathy symptoms preceded the development of skin lesions and were the first presenting symptoms of calciphylaxis [8]. Although a myopathy with skin abnormalities raises a concern for dermatomyositis [9], the ischemic necrotic skin lesions seen in calciphylaxis (Fig. 20.1a) are very different from skin rashes seen with dermatomyositis.

Laboratory studies may show higher levels of PTH, calcium, and phosphorous but are not reliable indicators of calciphylaxis. Definitive diagnosis of calciphylaxis requires a skin biopsy, which shows arteriolar medial calcification, intimal fibrosis and thrombotic occlusion [12]. However, as in this case, advanced tissue necrosis can cause the sample to be non-diagnostic. Muscle biopsy can be useful in such cases especially when myopathy is suspected to be a part of the clinical picture. Muscle biopsy shows calcification of the walls of perimysial arterioles, venules, and endomysial capillaries [6, 7].

Management includes wound debridement, pain control, dialysis, nutritional management, and parathyroidectomy in patients with refractory hyperparathyroidism. However, despite these measures, morbidity and mortality remain high.

Pearls

Clinical Pearls

1. Calciphylaxis should be considered as a cause of painful myopathy in dialysis patients who present with characteristic skin lesions.
2. Muscle biopsy may be useful to confirm the diagnosis if skin biopsy is non-diagnostic.
3. Calciphylaxis tends to affect skin, and the ischemic necrotic skin lesion is distinctive with hardening and black discoloration that most frequently seen in areas with abundant body fat.
4. The prognosis of calciphylaxis is usually poor.

Pathology Pearls

1. Biopsy of an affected muscle in a patient with systemic calciphylaxis may show mural calcification, intimal proliferation, and luminal narrowing or occlusion of small perimysial arterioles, venules, and endomysial capillaries.

References

1. Nigwekar SU, Kroshinsky D, Nazarian RM, Goverman J, Malhotra R, Jackson VA, et al. Calciphylaxis: risk factors, diagnosis, and treatment. Am J Kidney Dis. 2015;66(1):133–46.
2. Nigwekar SU, Thadhani R, Brandenburg VM. Calciphylaxis. N Engl J Med. 2018;379(4):399–400.
3. Adrogue HJ, Frazier MR, Zeluff B, Suki WN. Systemic calciphylaxis revisited. Am J Nephrol. 1981;1(3–4):177–83.
4. Fine A, Zacharias J. Calciphylaxis is usually non-ulcerating: risk factors, outcome and therapy. Kidney Int. 2002;61(6):2210–7.
5. Weenig RH, Sewell LD, Davis MD, McCarthy JT, Pittelkow MR. Calciphylaxis: natural history, risk factor analysis, and outcome. J Am Acad Dermatol. 2007;56(4):569–79.
6. Aouizerate J, Valleyrie-Allanore L, Limal N, Ayache SS, Gherardi RK, Audard V, et al. Ischemic myopathy revealing systemic calciphylaxis. Muscle Nerve. 2017;56(3):529–33.
7. Stavros K, Motiwala R, Zhou L, Sejdiu F, Shin S. Calciphylaxis in a dialysis patient diagnosed by muscle biopsy. J Clin Neuromuscul Dis. 2014;15(3):108–11.
8. Edelstein CL, Wickham MK, Kirby PA. Systemic calciphylaxis presenting as a painful, proximal myopathy. Postgrad Med J. 1992;68(797):209–11.
9. Flanigan KM, Bromberg MB, Gregory M, Baringer JR, Jones CR, Nester TA, et al. Calciphylaxis mimicking dermatomyositis: ischemic myopathy complicating renal failure. Neurology. 1998;51(6):1634–40.
10. Randall DP, Fisher MA, Thomas C. Rhabdomyolysis as the presenting manifestation of calciphylaxis. Muscle Nerve. 2000;23(2):289–93.
11. De Luca GC, Eggers SD. A rare complication of azotemic hyperparathyroidism: ischemic calcific myopathy. Neurology. 2010;75(21):1942.
12. Garcia-Lozano JA, Ocampo-Candiani J, Martinez-Cabriales SA, Garza-Rodriguez V. An update on calciphylaxis. Am J Clin Dermatol. 2018;19(4):599–608.

Chapter 21
A 54-Year-Old Man with Progressive Lower Limb Weakness and CK Elevation

Lan Zhou

History

A 54-year-old African American man presented to our neuromuscular clinic for evaluation of progressive lower extremity weakness. Two years prior to the presentation, he noticed right leg weakness which gradually progressed and affected his gait with frequent stumbling and tripping. He then developed the weakness in the left leg but less severe. He had several falls and had to use a cane. He had mild chronic low back pain, sometimes shooting towards the legs and feet. He also had intermittent tingling and numbness in the feet. He denied symptoms in the upper limbs. He denied oculobulbar or respiratory weakness. He was evaluated by a local neurologist. Nerve conduction study (NCS) and electromyography (EMG) reportedly showed findings compatible with a chronic active, right > left, L5 and S1 radiculopathies. Lumbosacral (L/S) spine MRI reportedly showed multi-level disc herniation with mild-to-moderate spinal stenosis at L4-L5 and L5-S1. He underwent a successful laminectomy with no clinical benefit. His leg weakness continued to progress to involve the proximal leg muscles. He also noticed atrophy and occasional fasciculations in the right distal leg muscles. He was then found to have an elevated serum creatine kinase (CK) level at 1,475 U/L. A myopathy was suspected. He underwent a right quadriceps muscle biopsy which reportedly showed mixed neurogenic and myopathic changes with no inflammation. He then underwent a left gastrocnemius muscle biopsy which also reportedly showed mixed neurogenic and myopathic changes with no inflammation. He was referred to our clinic with a question whether his symptoms were caused by radiculopathies, a neuropathy, a myopathy, or a combination of these conditions. He had a past medical history of hypertension and L/S spine

L. Zhou (✉)
Departments of Neurology and Pathology, Boston University Medical Center, Boston, MA, USA
e-mail: lanzhou@bu.edu

L. Zhou et al. (eds.), *A Case-Based Guide to Neuromuscular Pathology*,
https://doi.org/10.1007/978-3-030-25682-1_21

degenerative joint disease with L5 and S1 radiculopathies. He took lisinopril for hypertension. He did not have surgeries other than the L/S spine laminectomy. His family history was positive for hypertension. He also reported that his father died of amyotrophic lateral sclerosis (ALS) at age 53 years. He was married with two children. He did not drink alcohol or smoke cigarettes. He worked for a post office.

Physical Examination

His general examination was unremarkable; there was no spine tenderness. Neurological examination showed normal mental status and cranial nerve functions. Motor and sensory examination was normal in the upper extremities. In the lower extremities, tone was normal but atrophy was noted in the right distal leg and bilateral foot muscles with no muscle fasciculations. Weakness was detected in the hip flexors and knee flexors (MRC 4/5 on the right and 4+/5 on the left) as well as the bilateral distal leg and foot muscles with limited foot and toe movement. Pinprick sensation was reduced at the feet, and vibratory sensation was mildly impaired at the toes. Proprioception was intact. Tendon reflexes were 1+ at the right knee, absent at both ankles, and 2+ elsewhere. Toes were downgoing bilaterally. His gait was steppage.

Investigations

NCS of the right upper limb was normal. NCS of the lower limbs showed absent peroneal motor responses, markedly reduced tibial compound motor action potential (CMAP) amplitudes, and normal sural sensory action potential (SNAP) amplitudes. Needle EMG of selected right lower limb muscles showed fibrillation potentials and positive sharp waves as well as reduced recruitment of large-amplitude and long-duration motor unit potentials in the L3-S1 myotomes. The findings indicated a diffuse, chronic active, neurogenic process, compatible with either a motor neuropathy/neuronopathy or a polyradiculopathy. There was no evidence of a myopathy. Blood tests revealed a high serum CK level at 1,643 U/L. Complete blood count, comprehensive metabolic panel, ESR, ANA, RF, C-ANCA, P-ANCA, serum immunofixation, TSH, B12, anti-GM1 antibody, and Lyme serology were all unremarkable. Cerebrospinal fluid (CSF) study was unrevealing. The prior muscle biopsy slides were reviewed.

Muscle Biopsy Findings

The right quadriceps (Fig. 21.1) and left gastrocnemius muscle biopsies showed prominent chronic active neurogenic changes, including many angular atrophic fibers and target fibers, scattered pyknotic nuclear clumps, and grouped atrophy. The

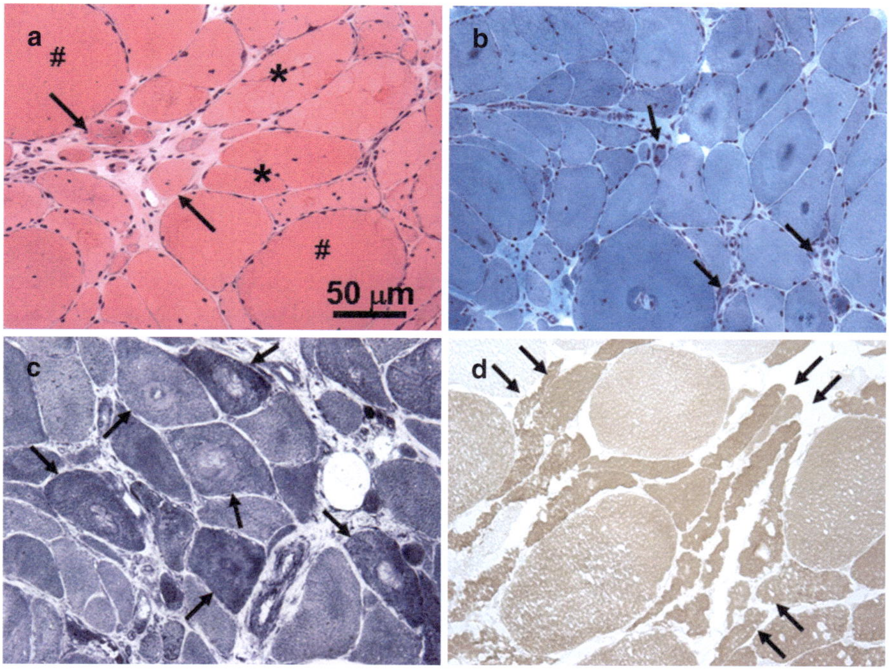

Fig. 21.1 Muscle biopsy sections stained with H&E (**a**) shows markedly increased fiber size variation with a group of atrophic fibers (arrows), some hypertrophic fibers (#), and split fibers (∗) but no inflammation. Gomori trichrome stain (**b**) shows some pyknotic nuclear clumps (arrows), target fibers, and mild endomysial fibrosis but no vacuolar changes. NADH -TR stain (**c**) shows several target fibers (arrows). ATPase pH 9.4 stain (**d**) shows grouped atrophy (arrows) with groups of both type 1 and type 2 atrophic fibers; some atrophic fibers are angulated

biopsies also showed chronic myopathic changes, including markedly increased fiber size variation with many hypertrophic fibers and atrophic fibers, several scattered split fibers, and mild endomysial fibrosis. There was no myofiber necrosis, degeneration, regeneration, or endomysial inflammation to suggest an active myopathic process. The findings are most consistent with a severe, chronic active, neurogenic process with pseudomyopathic changes secondary to long-standing denervation.

Additional Investigation After the Muscle Biopsy Diagnosis

Based on our interpretation of the muscle biopsy abnormalities and a positive family history of ALS, we ordered the Cu/Zn superoxidase dismutase 1 (*SOD1*) gene test, which showed a heterozygous in-frame deletion of GAA at the nucleotide position 481–483, resulting in Glu133del. This is a known mutation causing familial ALS (FALS), which has been reported previously [1] and listed in the ALSOD database (http://alsod.iop.kcl.ac.uk).

Final Diagnosis

Familial ALS Caused by an SOD1 Mutation

Patient Follow-up

The patient was referred to our motor neuron disease clinic for multidisciplinary care. His weakness slowly and continuously progressed over the course of 2 years. He also developed weakness in the upper limbs and respiratory muscles with supine breathing difficulty.

Discussion

ALS, also known as Lou Gehrig's disease, is a degenerative motor neuron disease that affects both upper motor neurons in the motor cortex and lower motor neurons in the brainstem and spinal cord anterior horn. Dysfunction of lower motor neurons causes muscle atrophy, fasciculations, and weakness, while dysfunction of upper motor neurons results in spasticity, weakness, hyperreflexia, and pathological reflexes. Cognitive and behavioral impairment are also common and can be seen in up to 50% of patients with ALS [2].

The estimated prevalence of ALS is 5 in 100,000 people in the United States [3] and 2.6–3.0 in 100,000 people in European populations [2]. It is more common in men than in women with a ratio 1.6 to 1. The majority of the cases are sporadic. The mean age at symptom onset is 56 years in sporadic ALS and 46 years in familial ALS [4]. ALS is debilitating and lethal. The disease is characterized by progressive facial, bulbar, tongue, limb, and respiratory muscle weakness with premature death caused by respiratory failure. The median survival is 2–3 years from symptoms onset. The older age at onset, bulbar onset, cognitive impairment, and certain genotypes are associated with a more rapid disease progression and a shorter lifespan [2, 4, 5].

About 10% of patients with ALS have a family history of the disease. Over two-thirds of FALS and 10% of sporadic ALS can have genetic causes identified [4]. More than 30 genes have been linked to FALS [6, 7]. The most common genetic cause of ALS is a hexanucleotide G4C2 repeat expansion (>30 repeats) in the chromosome 9 open reading frame 72 gene (*C9orf72*), which accounts for 30–40% of FALS, and it also causes frontotemporal dementia [8, 9]. *SOD1* is the first gene that is linked to FALS [10, 11]. SOD1 gene mutations account for about 20% of FALS and up to 7% of sporadic ALS [12–15]. Transactive response DNA binding protein 43 KDa (TDP-43) accumulation is a feature of ALS. It is linked to frontotemporal dementia. Mutations in *TARDBP*, the gene that encodes TDP-43, account for about 5% of FALS. Mutations in the fused in sarcoma gene (*FUS*) also account for about 5% of FALS [4, 6].

The diagnosis of ALS is made based on the clinical features, EMG findings, and absent causative lesions in the brain, spinal cord, or nerve roots. The revised El Escorial criteria are considered the gold standard for the diagnosis of ALS [16]. Genetic testing can help confirm many cases of FALS. A muscle biopsy is not needed. However, as seen in our case, the diagnosis of FALS with *SOD1* gene mutations can be missed or significantly delayed due to the lack of sufficient ALS clinical features at the initial presentation, co-existing spine spondylosis, confusing CK elevation, and ignorance of a positive family history.

Our patient was initially misdiagnosed with L/S polyradiculopathy because his initial symptoms were asymmetrical lower extremity weakness of pure lower motor neuron nature. His initial EMG showed right > left, L5 and S1 radiculopathies, and L/S spine MRI did show disc herniation and spinal stenosis at L4-5 and L5-S1. Radiculopathy from spine degenerative changes is not uncommon at age 50s. However, the scope of his leg weakness cannot not be fully explained by the structural abnormalities of his spine. Worsening of the leg weakness despite a successful laminectomy strongly argues against the L/S radiculopathy being the only or major cause of his leg weakness. It is well known that FALS with *SOD1* gene mutations can present predominantly with lower motor neuron weakness affecting one segment at the early stage [12–14], which can mimic polyradiculopathy. Therefore, making a correct diagnosis at the early stage of the disease can be quite challenging. Frequent neurological follow-up evaluation, careful correlation of clinical presentation with EMG and MRI findings, and obtaining a detailed family history are needed to raise a high clinical suspicion for a FALS. Our patient did not tell his outside neurologist about the family history of ALS. He did not think he had ALS as his disease course was very different from his father's. His father's disease had a rapid progression, and he died of ALS less than 2 years after the symptom onset. Intrafamilial phenotypic heterogeneity is common in FALS causes by an SOD1 mutation. The length of survival is variable.

Our patient was also misdiagnosed with a myopathy because of the CK elevation above 1,000 U/L. The moderate CK elevation led to muscle biopsies, and the chronic myopathic changes on the biopsies misled further. In our patient at age 50s with asymmetrical leg weakness and moderate CK elevation without upper motor neuron signs at the time of evaluation, a myopathy such as inclusion body myositis would be a reasonable consideration. However, it is worth noting that mild and moderate CK elevation can be seen not only in myopathies but also in a variety of motor neuron diseases, including sporadic ALS [17], Kennedy's disease [18, 19], spinal muscular atrophy [20], and post-polio syndrome [21]. The etiology of CK elevation in motor neuron diseases is unclear. It is thought to be related to active denervation, but one study showed that the degree of CK elevation did not correlate with the degree of denervation noted in the EMG study [22]. It is not uncommon for a muscle biopsy to show both neurogenic changes and chronic myopathic changes in a motor neuron disease as seen in our case. The chronic myopathic changes have been reported in several motor neuron diseases, including ALS, spinobulbar muscular atrophy, and post-polio syndrome [19, 23–25]. They are attributed to the longstanding denervation, as chronic denervation can cause pseudomyopathic changes [26]. The neurogenic changes are usually prominent in motor neuron diseases such as ALS and spinobulbar muscular atrophy. These changes may include esterase-positive denervated atrophic fibers, pyknotic nuclear clumps, target or targetoid fibers, grouped atrophy, and rare fiber type grouping. Chronic myopathic changes in ALS and spinobulbar muscular atrophy may include increased fiber size variation with the presence of both atrophic and hypertrophic fibers, increased number of internalized nuclei, split fibers, and endomysial fibrosis [19, 25]. Occasional necrotic fibers, regenerating fibers, and minimal inflammation may also be present [19]. It has been shown that type grouping of normal-sized fibers is common in peripheral neuropathy but rare in motor neuron diseases, and that grouped atrophy in motor neuron diseases or motor neuropathies usually consists of mixed type 1 and type 2 atrophic fibers [27].

Patients with ALS are best managed by ALS clinics which can provide multidisciplinary care. The disease is debilitating and lethal. The treatment goal is to improve quality of life and prolong survival. There are currently two disease-modifying drugs approved by the US Food and Drug Administration (FDA) for ALS, including riluzole and Edaravone. Riluzole, which blocks the release of glutamate, was approved for ALS in 1995. It showed to provide a survival benefit of approximately 3 months [28, 29]. Edaravone, a free radical scavenger, was approved for ALS in 2017. It showed benefit in treating a small subset of patients at an early stage of ALS [30]. The symptomatic management includes rehabilitation, noninvasive ventilation support, swallow evaluation with diet modification or gastrostomy placement, nutritional support, cognitive and behavioral evaluations, and control of pseudobulbar affect, sialorrhea, limb spasticity, depression, fatigue, pain, and muscle cramps.

Pearls

Clinical Pearls

1. ALS is a degenerative motor neuron disease that affects both upper motor neurons and lower motor neurons. Patients with ALS manifest progressive facial, bulbar, tongue, limb, and respiratory muscle weakness with both upper motor neuron and lower motor neuron signs.
2. The majority of ALS cases are sporadic; about 10% are familial. The mean age at symptom onset is 56 years in sporadic ALS and 46 years in familial ALS. Intra-familial phenotypic heterogeneity is common in FALS.
3. Over two-thirds of FALS and 10% of sporadic ALS cases can have genetic causes identified. Among over 30 genes that have been linked to FALS, the *C9orf72* gene mutations with a hexanucleotide G4C2 repeat expansion (>30 repeats) is the most common (accounting for 30–40% of FALS), followed by the *SOD1* (20%), *TARDBP* (5%), and *FUS* (5%) gene mutations.
4. The diagnosis of ALS is made based on clinical features and EMG findings using the revised El Escorial criteria after ruling out ALS mimics. CK can

be mildly or moderately elevated as seen in other motor neuron diseases. Genetic testing can help confirm many cases of FALS.

5. The diagnosis of FALS with *SOD1* gene mutations can be missed or significantly delayed due to the lack of sufficient ALS clinical features at the initial presentation, co-existing spine spondylosis, moderate CK elevation, and ignorance of a positive family history. It may be misdiagnosed with a polyradiculopathy due to co-existing spine spondylosis, or a myopathy due to CK elevation and chronic myopathic changes on muscle biopsy.
6. A muscle biopsy is not needed for the diagnosis of FALS. It may still be performed when the suspicion is not high especially at the early stage of the disease, and when a muscle disease such as inclusion body myositis is of consideration.
7. Patients with ALS are best managed by ALS clinics which can provide multidisciplinary care. Currently, there are two disease-modifying drugs approved by the US FDA for ALS, and they are riluzole and Edaravone.

Pathology Pearls

1. Muscle biopsies in motor neuron diseases commonly show prominent neurogenic changes and chronic myopathic changes. The chronic myopathic changes are most likely secondary to longstanding denervation to represent pseudomyopathic changes.
2. The neurogenic changes in motor neuron disease are chronic active, which may include esterase-positive denervated atrophic fibers, pyknotic nuclear clumps, target or targetoid fibers, grouped atrophy, and rare fiber type grouping.
3. Chronic myopathic changes may include increased fiber size variation with the presence of both atrophic and hypertrophic fibers, increased number of internalized nuclei, split fiber, and endomysial fibrosis. Occasional necrotic fibers, regenerating fibers, and minimal inflammation may also be seen.

References

1. Hosler BA, Nicholson GA, Sapp PC, Chin W, Orrell RW, de Belleroche JS, et al. Three novel mutations and two variants in the gene for Cu/Zn superoxide dismutase in familial amyotrophic lateral sclerosis. Neuromuscul Disord. 1996;6(5):361–6.
2. van Es MA, Hardiman O, Chio A, Al-Chalabi A, Pasterkamp RJ, Veldink JH, et al. Amyotrophic lateral sclerosis. Lancet. 2017;390(10107):2084–98.
3. Mehta P, Kaye W, Bryan L, Larson T, Copeland T, Wu J, et al. Prevalence of amyotrophic lateral sclerosis – United States, 2012–2013. MMWR Surveill Summ. 2016;65(8):1–12.
4. Tiryaki E, Horak HA. ALS and other motor neuron diseases. Continuum (Minneap Minn). 2014;20(5 Peripheral Nervous System Disorders):1185–207.

5. Oskarsson B, Gendron TF, Staff NP. Amyotrophic lateral sclerosis: an update for 2018. Mayo Clin Proc. 2018;93(11):1617–28.
6. Renton AE, Chio A, Traynor BJ. State of play in amyotrophic lateral sclerosis genetics. Nat Neurosci. 2014;17(1):17–23.
7. Mathis S, Goizet C, Soulages A, Vallat JM, Masson GL. Genetics of amyotrophic lateral sclerosis: a review. J Neurol Sci. 2019;399:217–26.
8. DeJesus-Hernandez M, Mackenzie IR, Boeve BF, Boxer AL, Baker M, Rutherford NJ, et al. Expanded GGGGCC hexanucleotide repeat in noncoding region of C9ORF72 causes chromosome 9p-linked FTD and ALS. Neuron. 2011;72(2):245–56.
9. Renton AE, Majounie E, Waite A, Simon-Sanchez J, Rollinson S, Gibbs JR, et al. A hexanucleotide repeat expansion in C9ORF72 is the cause of chromosome 9p21-linked ALS-FTD. Neuron. 2011;72(2):257–68.
10. Rosen DR. Mutations in Cu/Zn superoxide dismutase gene are associated with familial amyotrophic lateral sclerosis. Nature. 1993;364(6435):362.
11. Rosen DR, Siddique T, Patterson D, Figlewicz DA, Sapp P, Hentati A, et al. Mutations in Cu/Zn superoxide dismutase gene are associated with familial amyotrophic lateral sclerosis. Nature. 1993;362(6415):59–62.
12. Andersen PM, Nilsson P, Keranen ML, Forsgren L, Hagglund J, Karlsborg M, et al. Phenotypic heterogeneity in motor neuron disease patients with CuZn-superoxide dismutase mutations in Scandinavia. Brain. 1997;120(Pt 10):1723–37.
13. Cudkowicz ME, McKenna-Yasek D, Sapp PE, Chin W, Geller B, Hayden DL, et al. Epidemiology of mutations in superoxide dismutase in amyotrophic lateral sclerosis. Ann Neurol. 1997;41(2):210–21.
14. Gamez J, Corbera-Bellalta M, Nogales G, Raguer N, Garcia-Arumi E, Badia-Canto M, et al. Mutational analysis of the Cu/Zn superoxide dismutase gene in a Catalan ALS population: should all sporadic ALS cases also be screened for SOD1? J Neurol Sci. 2006;247(1):21–8.
15. Jones CT, Swingler RJ, Simpson SA, Brock DJ. Superoxide dismutase mutations in an unselected cohort of Scottish amyotrophic lateral sclerosis patients. J Med Genet. 1995;32(4):290–2.
16. Makki AA, Benatar M. The electromyographic diagnosis of amyotrophic lateral sclerosis: does the evidence support the El Escorial criteria? Muscle Nerve. 2007;35(5):614–9.
17. Ilzecka J, Stelmasiak Z. Creatine kinase activity in amyotrophic lateral sclerosis patients. Neurol Sci. 2003;24(4):286–7.
18. Lee JH, Shin JH, Park KP, Kim IJ, Kim CM, Lim JG, et al. Phenotypic variability in Kennedy's disease: implication of the early diagnostic features. Acta Neurol Scand. 2005;112(1):57–63.
19. Chahin N, Sorenson EJ. Serum creatine kinase levels in spinobulbar muscular atrophy and amyotrophic lateral sclerosis. Muscle Nerve. 2009;40(1):126–9.
20. Rudnik-Schoneborn S, Lutzenrath S, Borkowska J, Karwanska A, Hausmanowa-Petrusewicz I, Zerres K. Analysis of creatine kinase activity in 504 patients with proximal spinal muscular atrophy types I–III from the point of view of progression and severity. Eur Neurol. 1998;39(3):154–62.
21. Waring WP, Davidoff G, Werner R. Serum creatine kinase in the post-polio population. Am J Phys Med Rehabil. 1989;68(2):86–90.
22. Chahin N, Engel AG. Correlation of muscle biopsy, clinical course, and outcome in PM and sporadic IBM. Neurology. 2008;70(6):418–24.
23. Amrit AN, Anderson MS. Serum creatine phosphokinase in amyotrophic lateral sclerosis. Correlation with sex, duration, and skeletal muscle biopsy. Neurology. 1974;24(9):834–7.
24. Dalakas MC. Morphologic changes in the muscles of patients with postpoliomyelitis neuromuscular symptoms. Neurology. 1988;38(1):99–104.
25. Soraru G, D'Ascenzo C, Polo A, Palmieri A, Baggio L, Vergani L, et al. Spinal and bulbar muscular atrophy: skeletal muscle pathology in male patients and heterozygous females. J Neurol Sci. 2008;264(1–2):100–5.
26. Drachman DB, Murphy SR, Nigam MP, Hills JR. "Myopathic" changes in chronically denervated muscle. Arch Neurol. 1967;16(1):14–24.

27. Baloh RH, Rakowicz W, Gardner R, Pestronk A. Frequent atrophic groups with mixed-type myofibers is distinctive to motor neuron syndromes. Muscle Nerve. 2007;36(1):107–10.
28. Bensimon G, Lacomblez L, Meininger V. A controlled trial of riluzole in amyotrophic lateral sclerosis. ALS/Riluzole Study Group. N Engl J Med. 1994;330(9):585–91.
29. Lacomblez L, Bensimon G, Leigh PN, Guillet P, Meininger V. Dose-ranging study of riluzole in amyotrophic lateral sclerosis. Amyotrophic Lateral Sclerosis/Riluzole Study Group II. Lancet. 1996;347(9013):1425–31.
30. Writing G, Edaravone ALSSG. Safety and efficacy of edaravone in well defined patients with amyotrophic lateral sclerosis: a randomised, double-blind, placebo-controlled trial. Lancet Neurol. 2017;16(7):505–12.

Chapter 22
A 63-Year-Old Man with Progressive Limb Weakness and Slurred Speech

Lan Zhou and Susan C. Shin

History

A 63-year-old Chinese-American man presented with progressive limb weakness and slurred speech over the course of 4 years. The patient first noticed leg weakness with difficulty climbing stairs. The symptom gradually worsened, and he also developed difficulty holding arms up or carrying heavy objects. His hand grip also appeared weak. His speech became slurred. The weakness was constant and not fatigable. He also reported morning stiffness in his fingers and toes sometimes. He denied double vision, droopy eyelids, or trouble swallowing or breathing. He reported no muscle twitching or cramping. He denied pain, numbness, or sphincteric dysfunction. He denied fevers, malaise, appetite changes, or weight loss. He reported a normal developmental history. He had a past medical history of hypertension and chronic obstructive pulmonary disease. His medications included amlodipine, advair, and spiriva. He denied any family history of neurologic diseases. He was married with three children. He had smoked cigarettes for many years but did not drink alcohol.

L. Zhou (✉)
Departments of Neurology and Pathology, Boston University Medical Center,
Boston, MA, USA
e-mail: lanzhou@bu.edu

S. C. Shin
Department of Neurology, Icahn School of Medicine at Mount Sinai, New York, NY, USA
e-mail: susan.shin@mssm.edu

L. Zhou et al. (eds.), *A Case-Based Guide to Neuromuscular Pathology*,
https://doi.org/10.1007/978-3-030-25682-1_22

Physical Examination

His general examination was significant for mild spine scoliosis but no tenderness. There was no breast enlargement. Neurological examination showed weakness in the bilateral orbicularis oculi, orbicularis oris, and buccinators (MRC: 4/5). His soft palate elevated symmetrically, but his speech was slightly nasal. His tongue protruded midline with atrophy and weakness (4/5) but no obvious fasciculations. Motor examination of his limbs showed normal tone and bulk. Weakness was detected in the bilateral deltoid (right 4-, left 4), biceps (right 5-, left 4+), triceps (right 4, left 3), wrist extensors (right 5-, left 4), finger extensors (right 4, left 4), interossei (right 4, left 4), hip flexors (right 4, left 4), and foot plantar flexors (right 4+, left 4+). There were no muscle fasciculations. He had difficulty getting up from a chair without his hands to push the chair. Pinprick sensation was reduced from the toes to above the ankles. Vibratory sensation was impaired at the toes and ankles. Joint position sense was intact. Deep tendon reflexes were diffusely absent. Toes were downgoing bilaterally. Coordination testing was normal. Gait was steady; he was able to walk on his heels but not on his toes or in tandem.

Investigations

Complete blood count, comprehensive metabolic panel, HbA1C, Vitamin B12, TSH, free T4, ANA, ENA, serum immunofixation, myositis antibody panel, and paraneoplastic antibody panel were all unremarkable. Creatine kinase (CK) level was elevated at 662 U/L (normal: 55–170). Brain MRI with and without contrast was normal. Whole spine MRI showed multi-level disc protrusions with no significant cord or root compression. Nerve conduction study (NCS) and electromyography (EMG) showed widespread mild active denervation changes in the forms of fibrillation potentials and positive sharp waves, and prominent chronic denervation-reinnervation changes with reduced recruitment of motor unit potentials which were mostly of large amplitudes and broad durations. It also showed evidence of a length-dependent sensory axonal loss with reduced sensory nerve action potential (SNAP) amplitudes. The findings are consistent with a severe, chronic active, motor greater than sensory, axonal polyneuropathy, but more suggestive of a motor neuron disease superimposed by a sensory axonal polyneuropathy. A combined left sural nerve and gastrocnemius muscle biopsy was performed.

Muscle and Nerve Biopsy Findings

The left sural nerve biopsy (Fig. 22.1) showed a mild-to-moderate depopulation of myelinated nerve fibers, more affecting large myelinated fibers. There were no myelin ovoids, regenerating clusters, large thinly-myelinated fibers, onion bulbs,

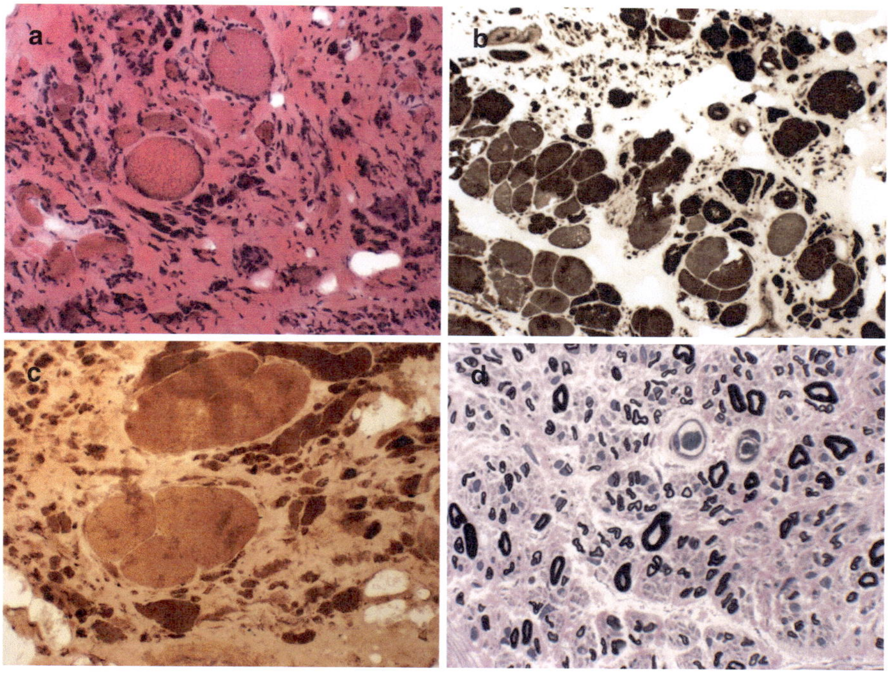

Fig. 22.1 H&E stained muscle biopsy section (**a**) shows striking endomysial fibrosis, abundant severely atrophic fibers and pyknotic nuclear clumps, and a few hypertrophic fibers. A split fiber is also shown. ATPase pH 9.4 stain (**b**) shows grouped atrophy and fiber type grouping. Esterase stain (**c**) shows groups of severely atrophic fibers and two split hypertrophic fibers. Toluidine blue stained resin embedded sural nerve plastic section (**d**) shows mild-to-moderate depopulation of myelinated nerve fibers, more affecting large myelinated fibers, with no myelin ovoids, regenerating clusters, large thinly-myelinated fibers, or onion bulbs

inflammation, or amyloid deposition. The findings are consistent with a mild-to-moderate chronic axonal neuropathy. The left gastrocnemius muscle biopsy (Fig. 22.1) showed severe chronic myopathic changes and some neurogenic changes with abundant severely atrophic fibers scattered and in groups, a few hypertrophic fibers, a few split fibers, fiber type grouping, and extensive endomysial fibrosis. There was no myofiber necrosis or inflammation.

Additional Investigation After the Muscle and Nerve Biopsy Diagnosis

Based on the predominant motor weakness involving the facial, bulbar, and limb muscles, the chronicity of the neurogenic changes on needle EMG, and the nerve and muscle biopsy findings, a motor neuron disease, spinobulbar muscular atrophy (Kennedy's disease), was strongly suspected. The chronic myopathic changes on muscle biopsy were felt to represent pseudomyothic changes. The subsequent gene test showed an abnormal expansion of the CAG tandem repeat (47 CAG repeats) (normal: 11–33; borderline: 34–39) in the androgen receptor gene, confirming the diagnosis of Kennedy's disease.

Final Diagnosis

Kennedy's disease

Patient Follow-up

The patient was referred to a motor neuron disease clinic for multidisciplinary care. His weakness slowly progressed over the course of 2 years.

Discussion

Kennedy's disease, also known as spinobulbar muscular atrophy, is a rare X-linked recessive hereditary motor neuron disease [1]. It is caused by an expansion of the CAG tandem repeat in the androgen receptor gene [2]. The disease affects lower motor neurons in the brainstem and spinal cord with resultant slowly progressive facial, bulbar, and limb weakness [3]. In addition to the weakness, patients may also show evidence of sensory neuropathy and signs of androgen deficiency such as poor sexual function, reduced fertility, and gynecomastia [3, 4].

The mean age at onset is 40s [5, 6]. There is a wide range of age at symptom onset, which inversely correlates with the size of the CAG repeat expansion [7, 8]. The disease onset is insidious. The initial symptom in a majority of the patients is caused by proximal leg weakness with difficulty getting up from a low chair or difficulty climbing stairs. This is followed by bulbar, facial, and other limb muscle weakness that manifests dysarthria, dysphagia, and weakness in the upper limbs. Patients may note fasciculations and cramping in the affected muscles as well as postural hand or leg tremors. They may also report sexual dysfunction and reduced fertility. Cardiac and respiratory muscles are usually not affected. Besides dysarthria, muscle atrophy, and weakness, examination often detects tongue atrophy and fasciculations, quivering chin (perioral fasciculations-myokymia), diffusely diminished tendon reflexes, and gynecomastia. It is also not uncommon to detect asympatomatic distal sensory loss as seen in our patient. It has been shown that bulbar symptoms, gynecomastia, and insulin resistance, but not the disease progression rate, correlate with the length of the CAG repeat [5, 9]. Serum CK level is mildly or moderately elevated from 200 s to 2,000 s U/L in a majority of the patients, and CK elevation is also seen in other motor neuron diseases such as amyotrophic lateral sclerosis (ALS), spinal muscular atrophy (SMA), and post-polio syndrome [10–13]. CK elevation is more significant in Kennedy's disease than in ALS [10], which may lead to a misdiagnosis of a primary myopathy. The etiology of CK elevation in motor neuron diseases is not fully understood. EMG in Kennedy's disease typically shows diffuse active denervation changes including fibrillations and positive sharp waves, and more prominent chronic denervation-reinnervation changes including reduced recruitment and giant motor unit potentials [14]. In most of the patients with Kennedy's disease, including our patient, NCS shows a sensory neuropathy [14], a feature that distinguishes Kennedy's disease from other motor neuron diseases such as ALS, primary muscular atrophy, and adult-onset spinal muscular atrophy (SMA). The abnormality is caused primarily by distally accentuated sensory axonopathy with dorsal root ganglion cells less affected [15]. Kennedy's disease does not affect upper motor neurons with no upper motor neuron signs, another useful feature that differentiates Kennedy's disease from ALS.

The diagnosis of Kennedy's disease is made by genetic testing, which is commercially available. The disease diagnosis, however, is often delayed by several years [6] due to the insidious onset, slow progression of weakness, co-existing sensory neuropathy, CK elevation, lack of gynecomastia or a positive family history in some patients, and lack of awareness. Although a muscle biopsy is not needed for the diagnosis of Kennedy's disease, it is sometimes done before a high clinical suspicion for Kennedy's disease is raised to rule out other disorders which can affect both motor and sensory nerves/neurons. As illustrated here, a sural nerve biopsy in Kennedy's disease shows chronic axonal neuropathy, consistent with the findings by another study [15]. A muscle biopsy in Kennedy's disease can be difficult to interpret as seen in our case [4]. Biopsy of a muscle with relatively preserved strength or mild weakness often shows prominent neurogenic changes, such as esterase-positive denervated fibers, pyknotic nuclear clumps, target or targetoid fibers, grouped atrophy, and rare fiber type grouping. Biopsy of a muscle with significant weakness usually shows chronic myopathic changes in addition to the neurogenic changes, such as increased fiber size variation, increased number of internalized nuclei, fiber splitting, and endomysial fibrosis [10, 16]. Occasional necrotic fibers, regenerating fibers, rimmed vacuoles, and minimal inflammation may also be seen [10]. The chronic myopathic changes have been reported in other motor neuron diseases, such as ALS and post-polio syndrome [17, 18]. They are attributed to long-standing denervation to represent pseudomyopathic changes [19]. In Kennedy's disease, the accumulation of mutant androgen receptor protein may also contribute to the myopathic changes [16]. It has been shown that type grouping of normal-sized fibers is common in peripheral neuropathy but rare in motor neuron diseases, and that grouped atrophy in motor neuron diseases or motor neuropathies usually consists of mixed type 1 and type 2 atrophic fibers [20].

The disease progression in Kennedy's disease is slow as compared with other motor neuron diseases such as ALS. The median age of using a wheelchair is 60 years [5], and the lifespan is not significantly affected [7]. Due to the bulbar involvement, the risk of chocking and aspiration pneumonia is high. Currently, there is no effective disease-modifying therapy. The management is mainly supportive to prevent falls and aspiration pneumonia by rehabilitation and swallow evaluation with diet modification. Genetic counseling should be provided.

The exact pathogenic mechanism of the CAG repeat expansion in the androgen receptor gene remains elusive. The available evidence supports that the neurodegeneration is caused by the androgen-dependent gain of toxic functions [21, 22]. Upon ligand binding, the mutant androgen receptor proteins translocate from cytoplasm to nucleus causing toxic aggregations and cell dysfunction [22]. The CAG repeat encodes a polyglutamine tract. There are widespread nuclear and cytoplasmic inclusions containing mutant polyglutamine androgen receptor in patients with Kennedy's disease [23]. Suppressing peripheral and muscle expression of mutant polyglutamine androgen receptor has been shown effective in treating a mouse model of Kennedy's disease [24, 25]. Clinical trials in human patients with Kennedy's disease have been targeting the androgen receptor ligand to reduce its binding to the receptor and subsequent toxicity. Leuprorelin, but not dustasteride, showed a mild benefit in delaying the functional decline [26, 27]. Clenbuterol, a β2-adrenoceptor agonist, also appeared beneficial in a pilot study [28]. Future therapy development may also target the CAG repeat expansion.

Pearls

Clinical Pearls

1. Kennedy's disease is a rare X-linked recessive hereditary motor neuron disease that is caused by the CAG repeat expansion (>39 repeats) in the androgen receptor gene.
2. Kennedy's disease affects lower motor neurons in the brainstem and spinal cord. It manifests slowly progressive facial, bulbar, and limb weakness. None-motor manifestations include poor sexual function, reduced fertility, and gynecomastia.
3. Kennedy's disease affects adult males with the age at onset and the disease symptoms correlating with the length of the CAG repeats.
4. CK is usually mildly or moderately elevated. EMG typically shows diffuse active denervation changes and more prominent chronic reinnervation changes. NCS commonly shows distal sensory neuropathy.
5. The diagnosis of Kennedy's disease is made by genetic testing with no need for a muscle or a nerve biopsy. A muscle and nerve biopsy may be occasionally performed if the awareness or suspicion is not high or if the other diseases which can cause both motor and sensory neuropathy/neuronopathy need to be ruled out.
6. The progression of Kennedy's disease is slow. The median age of using a wheelchair is 60 years, and the lifespan is not significantly affected.

7. There is no effective disease-modifying therapy for Kennedy's disease currently. The management is mainly supportive to prevent falls and aspiration pneumonia.

Pathology Pearls

1. A sural nerve biopsy in Kennedy's disease usually shows a chronic axonal neuropathy with reduced myelinated axon density but no demyelination or inflammation.
2. A muscle biopsy in Kennedy's disease often shows mixed neurogenic and myopathic changes.
3. The neurogenic changes are chronic active, which may include esterase-positive denervated atrophic fibers, pyknotic nuclear clumps, target or targetoid fibers, grouped atrophy, and rare fiber type grouping.
4. Chronic myopathic changes are more prominent in muscles with significant weakness. They are most likely to represent pseudomyopathic changes secondary to the long-standing denervation. These changes may include increased fiber size variation, increased number of internalized nuclei, fiber splitting, and endomysial fibrosis. Occasional necrotic fibers, regenerating fibers, rimmed vacuoles, and minimal inflammation may also be seen.

References

1. Kennedy WR, Alter M, Sung JH. Progressive proximal spinal and bulbar muscular atrophy of late onset. A sex-linked recessive trait. Neurology. 1968;18(7):671–80.
2. La Spada AR, Wilson EM, Lubahn DB, Harding AE, Fischbeck KH. Androgen receptor gene mutations in X-linked spinal and bulbar muscular atrophy. Nature. 1991;352(6330):77–9.
3. Breza M, Koutsis G. Kennedy's disease (spinal and bulbar muscular atrophy): a clinically oriented review of a rare disease. J Neurol. 2019;266(3):565–73.
4. Jokela ME, Udd B. Diagnostic clinical, electrodiagnostic and muscle pathology features of spinal and bulbar muscular atrophy. J Mol Neurosci. 2016;58(3):330–4.
5. Atsuta N, Watanabe H, Ito M, Banno H, Suzuki K, Katsuno M, et al. Natural history of spinal and bulbar muscular atrophy (SBMA): a study of 223 Japanese patients. Brain. 2006;129(Pt 6):1446–55.
6. Rhodes LE, Freeman BK, Auh S, Kokkinis AD, La Pean A, Chen C, et al. Clinical features of spinal and bulbar muscular atrophy. Brain. 2009;132(Pt 12):3242–51.
7. Finsterer J, Soraru G. Onset manifestations of spinal and bulbar muscular atrophy (Kennedy's disease). J Mol Neurosci. 2016;58(3):321–9.
8. Igarashi S, Tanno Y, Onodera O, Yamazaki M, Sato S, Ishikawa A, et al. Strong correlation between the number of CAG repeats in androgen receptor genes and the clinical onset of features of spinal and bulbar muscular atrophy. Neurology. 1992;42(12):2300–2.
9. Nakatsuji H, Araki A, Hashizume A, Hijikata Y, Yamada S, Inagaki T, et al. Correlation of insulin resistance and motor function in spinal and bulbar muscular atrophy. J Neurol. 2017;264(5):839–47.

10. Chahin N, Sorenson EJ. Serum creatine kinase levels in spinobulbar muscular atrophy and amyotrophic lateral sclerosis. Muscle Nerve. 2009;40(1):126–9.
11. Ilzecka J, Stelmasiak Z. Creatine kinase activity in amyotrophic lateral sclerosis patients. Neurol Sci. 2003;24(4):286–7.
12. Rudnik-Schoneborn S, Lutzenrath S, Borkowska J, Karwanska A, Hausmanowa-Petrusewicz I, Zerres K. Analysis of creatine kinase activity in 504 patients with proximal spinal muscular atrophy types I-III from the point of view of progression and severity. Eur Neurol. 1998;39(3):154–62.
13. Waring WP, Davidoff G, Werner R. Serum creatine kinase in the post-polio population. Am J Phys Med Rehabil. 1989;68(2):86–90.
14. Ferrante MA, Wilbourn AJ. The characteristic electrodiagnostic features of Kennedy's disease. Muscle Nerve. 1997;20(3):323–9.
15. Sobue G, Hashizume Y, Mukai E, Hirayama M, Mitsuma T, Takahashi A. X-linked recessive bulbospinal neuronopathy. A clinicopathological study. Brain. 1989;112(Pt 1):209–32.
16. Soraru G, D'Ascenzo C, Polo A, Palmieri A, Baggio L, Vergani L, et al. Spinal and bulbar muscular atrophy: skeletal muscle pathology in male patients and heterozygous females. J Neurol Sci. 2008;264(1–2):100–5.
17. Amrit AN, Anderson MS. Serum creatine phosphokinase in amyotrophic lateral sclerosis. Correlation with sex, duration, and skeletal muscle biopsy. Neurology. 1974;24(9):834–7.
18. Dalakas MC. Morphologic changes in the muscles of patients with postpoliomyelitis neuromuscular symptoms. Neurology. 1988;38(1):99–104.
19. Drachman DB, Murphy SR, Nigam MP, Hills JR. "Myopathic" changes in chronically denervated muscle. Arch Neurol. 1967;16(1):14–24.
20. Baloh RH, Rakowicz W, Gardner R, Pestronk A. Frequent atrophic groups with mixed-type myofibers is distinctive to motor neuron syndromes. Muscle Nerve. 2007;36(1):107–10.
21. Grunseich C, Fischbeck KH. Spinal and bulbar muscular atrophy. Neurol Clin. 2015;33(4):847–54.
22. Li M, Miwa S, Kobayashi Y, Merry DE, Yamamoto M, Tanaka F, et al. Nuclear inclusions of the androgen receptor protein in spinal and bulbar muscular atrophy. Ann Neurol. 1998;44(2):249–54.
23. Adachi H, Katsuno M, Minamiyama M, Waza M, Sang C, Nakagomi Y, et al. Widespread nuclear and cytoplasmic accumulation of mutant androgen receptor in SBMA patients. Brain. 2005;128(Pt 3):659–70.
24. Cortes CJ, Ling SC, Guo LT, Hung G, Tsunemi T, Ly L, et al. Muscle expression of mutant androgen receptor accounts for systemic and motor neuron disease phenotypes in spinal and bulbar muscular atrophy. Neuron. 2014;82(2):295–307.
25. Lieberman AP, Yu Z, Murray S, Peralta R, Low A, Guo S, et al. Peripheral androgen receptor gene suppression rescues disease in mouse models of spinal and bulbar muscular atrophy. Cell Rep. 2014;7(3):774–84.
26. Fernandez-Rhodes LE, Kokkinis AD, White MJ, Watts CA, Auh S, Jeffries NO, et al. Efficacy and safety of dutasteride in patients with spinal and bulbar muscular atrophy: a randomised placebo-controlled trial. Lancet Neurol. 2011;10(2):140–7.
27. Hashizume A, Katsuno M, Suzuki K, Hirakawa A, Hijikata Y, Yamada S, et al. Long-term treatment with leuprorelin for spinal and bulbar muscular atrophy: natural history-controlled study. J Neurol Neurosurg Psychiatry. 2017;88(12):1026–32.
28. Querin G, D'Ascenzo C, Peterle E, Ermani M, Bello L, Melacini P, et al. Pilot trial of clenbuterol in spinal and bulbar muscular atrophy. Neurology. 2013;80(23):2095–8.

Chapter 23
A 6-Year-Old Girl with Muscle Pain and Swelling in the Thighs

Diana P. Castro, Chunyu Cai, and Dustin Jacob Paul

History

A 6-year-old girl who was previously healthy. She developed muscle pain and swelling in her thighs. Her mother reported that for the last 6 months, her daughter developed episodes of muscle swelling and pain in her thighs whenever she exercised or walked more than 30 minutes. Episodes were always triggered by physical activity. Pain was partially controlled with NSAIDs or Acetaminophen. She was previously seen in the emergency department for bilateral thigh pain and fatigue. Her CK was 40,000 U/L with elevated liver function tests and positive red blood cells in urinalysis examination. Rheumatology evaluated the patient and subsequently referred her to our neuromuscular clinic for further assessment.

Physical Examination

The patient was alert and awake with normal speech for her age. Cranial nerves were intact and muscle tone was normal. Strength was normal (MRC: 5/5), except

D. P. Castro (✉)
Department of Neurology and Neurotherapeutics, University of Texas Southwestern Medical Center, Children's Medical Center of Dallas, Dallas, TX, USA
e-mail: diana.castro@utsuthwestern.edu

C. Cai
Department of Pathology, University of Texas Southwestern Medical Center, Dallas, TX, USA
e-mail: chunyu.cai@utsouthwestern.edu

D. Jacob Paul
Department of Neurology and Neurotherapeutics, University of Texas Southwestern Medical Center, Dallas, TX, USA
e-mail: dustin.paul@utsouthwestern.edu

L. Zhou et al. (eds.), *A Case-Based Guide to Neuromuscular Pathology*,
https://doi.org/10.1007/978-3-030-25682-1_23

for minimal hip flexor weakness (5−/5). Deep tendon reflexes were 2+, except for 1+ at the ankle. Her gait, coordination and sensory exam were normal. The patient reported mild tenderness on palpation of her quadriceps.

Investigations

Her serum creatine kinase (CK) level was initially 40,000 U/L, but at the time of muscle biopsy it was 137. Her hip and lower extremity MRI with and without contrast showed no significant myotendinous signal abnormality identified in the pelvis or proximal lower extremities. Brain MRI with and without contrast was reported normal. A left quadriceps muscle biopsy was performed.

Muscle Biopsy Findings

The left quadriceps muscle biopsy showed the presence of intensely basophilic macrophages in the perimysium and endomysium connective tissue (Fig. 23.1a). The macrophages were strongly positive for nonspecific esterase stain (Fig. 23.1b) and acid phosphatase (Fig. 23.1c) stains on cryostat sections. The granules within macrophages were positive for periodic acid Schiff (PAS) stain (Fig. 23.1d) and for immunostain of the macrophage marker CD68 (Fig. 23.1e). Morin stain showed strong green fluorescent signal in these macrophages (Fig. 23.1f), which confirmed the presence of aluminum in the macrophages. Electron microscopy (EM) also demonstrated spiculated electron dense inclusions characteristic of aluminum salt (Fig. 23.1g, h). The findings were diagnostic for macrophagic myofasciitis.

Final Diagnosis

Macrophagic Myofascitis

Patient Follow-up

The patient was started on prednisone 1 mg/kg/day for 2 months, followed by a slow tapering schedule to be weaned off. She had dramatic improvement of her symptoms. Unfortunately, she had recurrent episodes of swelling and muscle pain a year after steroids were weaned off. She was re-started on steroid therapy with a partial control of her symptoms. CK level had been decreasing progressively.

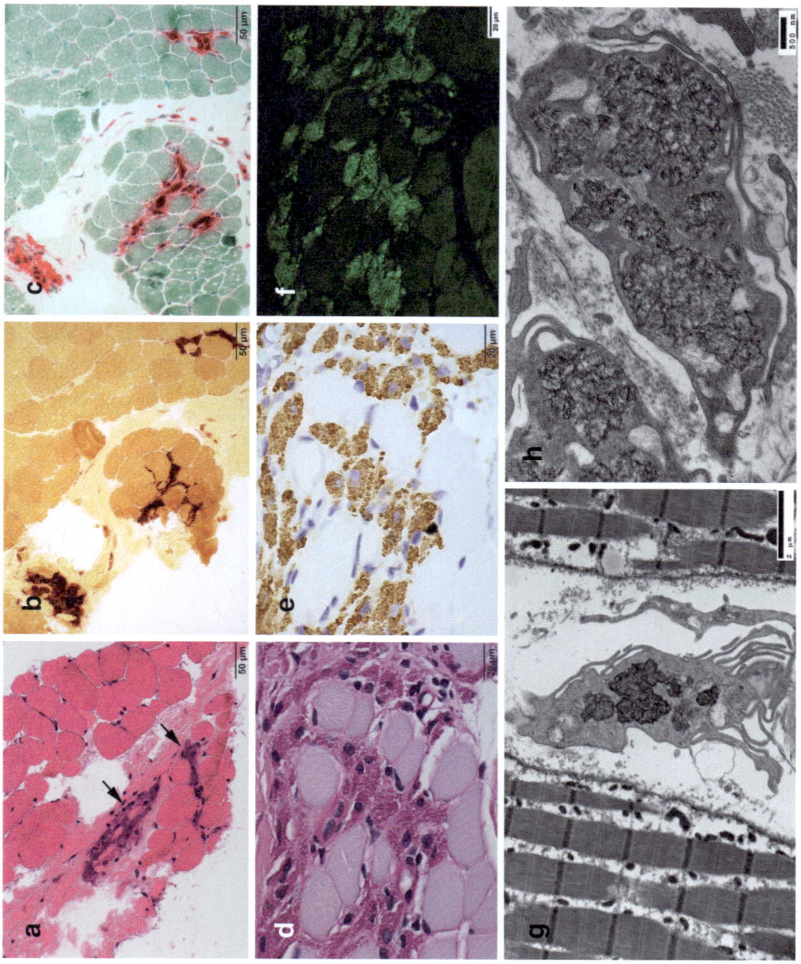

Fig. 23.1 Quadriceps muscle biopsy from this patient. (**a**) H&E stain, arrows point to the macrophages in perimysium and endomysia connective tissue with granular basophilic cytoplasm. (**b**) Nonspecific esterase stain, (**c**) Acid phosphatase stain, (**d**) PAS stain, (**e**) CD68 immunostain, (**f**) Morin stain, (**g–h**) EM images of macrophages containing spiculated inclusions. (**a–c** were from cryostat sections. **d–f** were from FFPE sections. **g–h** were EM images)

Discussion

Macrophagic myofasciitis is an inflammatory condition associated with aluminum containing vaccines, including DTaP, hepatitis A(HepA), HepB, human papilloma virus (HPV), HIB, and pneumococcal conjugate vaccine (PCV) [1]. The lesion of MMF is restricted to the vaccine injection sites, namely the quadriceps muscle of children and deltoid muscle of adults. Pathologically, the characteristic finding in muscle biopsy is the presence of macrophages that contain aluminum salt derived from aluminum adjuvant-containing vaccines [2]. These macrophages tend to aggregate in the perimysium (Fig. 23.2a) but do not form multinucleated giant cells. A lymphocytic component may be present within the aggregate (Fig. 23.2b, arrow). In cases where the macrophages infiltrate the endomysial compartment, they percolate through the interstitial connective tissue without causing obvious myofiber damage or myofiber MHC1 upregulation (Fig. 23.2c). Morin compound (2-(2,4-dihydroxyphenyl)-3,5,7-trihydroxychromen-4-one) is a flavonoid that forms a green-blue fluorescent complex with aluminum [3]. Morin fluorescence reactivity is strongly positive in the aluminum particles in the cytoplasm of the basophilic

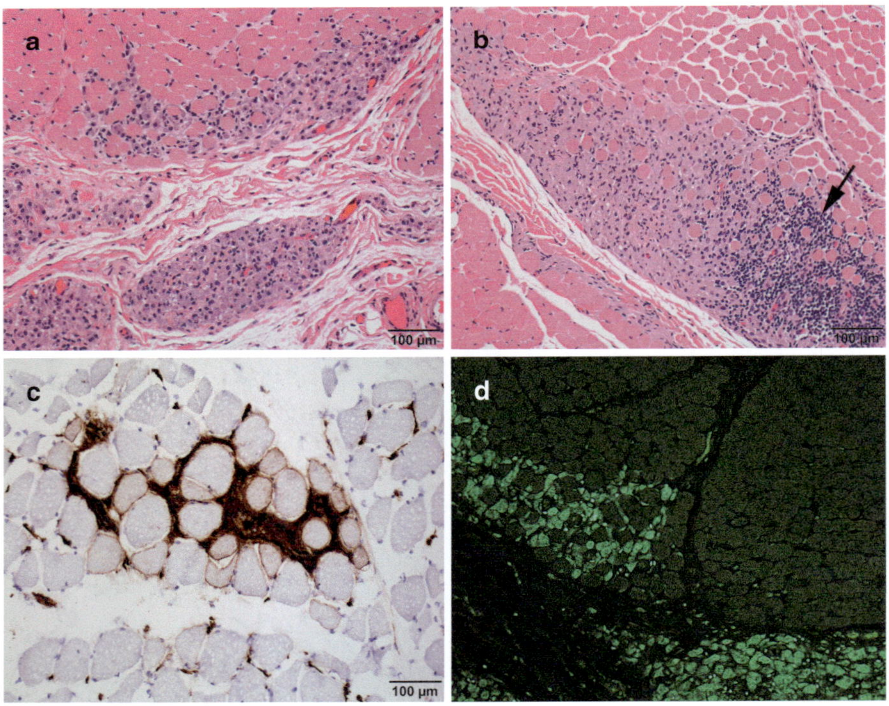

Fig. 23.2 Other examples of MMF. (**a**): Macrophage aggregates in perimysium with extension into endomysium. (**b**): Lymphocytic inflammation (arrow) can be present within the macrophage aggregate. (**c**) MHC class 1 immunostaining is positive in the macrophages but there is minimal myofiber upregulation. Necrotic or regenerating fibers are usually absent. (**d**) Morin stain reactivity is restricted to the cytoplasm of macrophages, not in myofibers or connective tissue

macrophages, weakly positively in some nuclei (likely due to the presence of zinc finger transcription factors), but not in myofibers or connective tissue (Fig. 23.1f, Fig. 23.2d). Morin stain is highly specific for MMF, and is negative in granulomatous myositis, sarcoidosis, or inflammatory myositis with abundant macrophages [4].

In children younger than 3 year of age, MMF is often an incidental finding in a muscle biopsy and may not have clinical significance. Older children and adults with MMF may present with chronic fatigue and arthromyalgias. Usually there is a slow development of symptoms over several months to years. In the adult population, the average delay between the last vaccination and biopsy is 4–5 years [5]. Therefore, a "recent" vaccination history may not be present. Diffuse myalgias are the cardinal feature usually starting in the distal limbs progressing over the whole body. On examination, patients exhibit a few or no tender point sites and normal muscle strength. Spinal pain is also frequently observed. Patients usually report diffuse arthromyalgias with pain exacerbated by activity. The second cardinal feature is fatigue which may precede pain by several months. Some patients may have cognitive dysfunction with dysexecutive syndrome, memory impairment, and sometimes psychiatric complaints consistent with mood disorders. However, a causal link between central nervous system symptoms and MMF has not been widely accepted [6]. CK levels may be elevated at onset but usually normal at time of muscle biopsy. Persistently elevated CK levels should prompt evaluation for other diagnosis. Differential diagnosis consists of inflammatory myopathies, metabolic myopathies, and limb-girdle muscular dystrophies. Diagnosis is achieved by muscle biopsy confirming the presence of aluminum-containing macrophages within the perimysium or endomysium. Treatment generally involves immunosuppression and prognosis is good.

Pearls

Clinical Pearls

1. The main clinical symptoms of MMF are diffuse arthromyalgia and fatigue.
2. The delay between vaccination and muscle biopsy can be many years. A "recent" vaccination history is not required for the diagnosis.
3. The main treatment is steroid therapy.

Pathology Pearls

1. The hallmark of MMF pathology is the presence of macrophages with intensely basophilic granular cytoplasm containing aluminum salt.
2. The presence of aluminum salt can be confirmed by positive cytoplasmic reactivity on a Morin stain or identification of spiculated electron dense inclusions within the cytoplasm of macrophages on EM.

References

1. Gherardi RK, Coquet M, Cherin P, Authier FJ, Laforet P, Belec L, et al. Macrophagic myofasciitis: an emerging entity. Groupe d'Etudes et Recherche sur les Maladies Musculaires Acquises et Dysimmunitaires (GERMMAD) de l'Association Francaise contre les Myopathies (AFM). Lancet (London, England). 1998;352(9125):347–52.
2. Gherardi RK, Coquet M, Cherin P, Belec L, Moretto P, Dreyfus PA, et al. Macrophagic myofasciitis lesions assess long-term persistence of vaccine-derived aluminium hydroxide in muscle. Brain J Neurol. 2001;124(Pt 9):1821–31.
3. Malinin GI, Malinin TI. Rapid microscopic detection of malaria parasites permanently fluorochrome stained in blood smears with aluminum and morin. Am J Clin Pathol. 1991;95(3):424–7.
4. Chkheidze R, Burns DK, White CL, Castro D, Fuller J, Cai C. Morin stain detects aluminum-containing macrophages in macrophagic myofasciitis and vaccination granuloma with high sensitivity and specificity. J Neuropathol Exp Neurol. 2017;76(4):323–31.
5. Rigolet M, Aouizerate J, Couette M, Ragunathan-Thangarajah N, Aoun-Sebaiti M, Gherardi RK, et al. Clinical features in patients with long-lasting macrophagic myofasciitis. Front Neurol. 2014;5:230.
6. Van Der Gucht A, Aoun Sebaiti M, Guedj E, Aouizerate J, Yara S, Gherardi R, et al. Brain FDG-PET metabolic abnormalities in patients with long-lasting macrophagic myofasciitis. J Nucl Med. 2017;58(3):492–8.

Chapter 24
A 4-Year-Old Boy with Progressive Weakness, Difficulty Walking and Running, and Increased Falls

Diana P. Castro, Chunyu Cai, and Dustin Jacob Paul

History

A 4-year-old boy was brought to our clinic for evaluation of progressive weakness, difficulty walking and running, and increased falls. His mother reported that he was "clumsy", and had difficulties climbing stairs and rising from a sitting position. The patient was born full term, and there were no complications during pregnancy or delivery. His gross motor development was delayed. He sat without assistance at 15 months and walked independently at 19 months of age.

His family history was negative for neuromuscular diseases.

Physical Examination

The patient was alert, awake and oriented to person, place, and time. Cranial nerves were intact. His general examination was notable for macroglossia and large calves. Muscle tone was decreased in the lower extremities. Weakness was detected in the

D. P. Castro (✉)
Department of Neurology and Neurotherapeutics, University of Texas Southwestern Medical Center, Children's Medical Center of Dallas, Dallas, TX, USA
e-mail: diana.castro@utsuthwestern.edu

C. Cai
Department of Pathology, University of Texas Southwestern Medical Center, Dallas, TX, USA
e-mail: chunyu.cai@utsouthwestern.edu

D. Jacob Paul
Department of Neurology and Neurotherapeutics, University of Texas Southwestern Medical Center, Dallas, TX, USA
e-mail: dustin.paul@utsouthwestern.edu

L. Zhou et al. (eds.), *A Case-Based Guide to Neuromuscular Pathology*,
https://doi.org/10.1007/978-3-030-25682-1_24

proximal limb muscles, more affecting the legs than the arms. His gait examination showed exaggerated lordosis, slow and waddling gait. He was unable to run or climb stairs without holding a rail and his Gower's sign was positive. Deep tendon reflexes were 1+ throughout and his toes were down going bilaterally. Sensory examination, coordination testing, and cerebellar function were normal. Achilles tendons were tight bilaterally.

Investigations

His serum creatine kinase (CK) level was markedly increased at 17,000 U/L (normal: 50–350). The dystrophin gene test showed a DNA sequence variant of unclear significance, which was described as transition A > G (IVS51 + 10) in the dystrophin gene. A quadriceps muscle biopsy was performed for further evaluation.

Biopsy Findings

The muscle biopsy showed a chronic active myopathy (Fig. 24.1a). Features of chronicity include marked fiber size variation, fatty replacement of perimysium, endomysial fibrosis, frequent internalized nuclei, split fibers, and fibers with abnormal internal architecture. Active myopathic changes include scattered necrotic and regenerating fibers. Immunohistochemical staining for dystrophin epitopes (rod domain, carboxy terminus and amino terminus) showed an absence of sarcolemma reactivity in almost all areas of the biopsy (Fig. 24.1b), except for rare revertant fibers with partially restored carboxy terminus expression (Fig. 24.1c). Immunostaining for alpha-dystroglycan was also attenuated (Fig. 24.1d). Immunostaining for sarcoglycans (alpha, beta, gamma and delta) were relatively preserved. The findings are supportive of Duchenne muscular dystrophy (DMD).

Final Diagnosis

Duchenne Muscular Dystrophy

Patient Follow-up

After the diagnosis of DMD was made, the patient was started on Prednisone 0.75 mg/kg/day and a proton pump inhibitor for GI prophylaxis. The patient was also evaluated and followed by our cardiology and pulmonary team. He continued to deteriorate over the years and lost ambulation by 10 years of age after a fall and

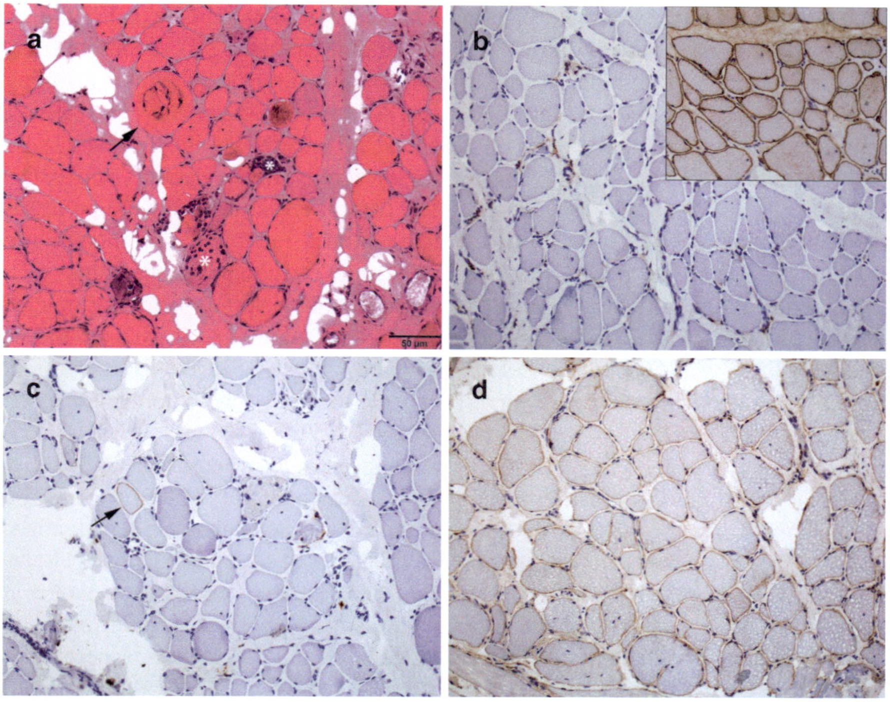

Fig. 24.1 Duchenne muscular dystrophy. (**a**) H&E shows dystrophic changes (asterisks indicate necrotic fibers, arrow indicates myofiber with abnormal internal architecture). (**b**) Immunostaining for dystrophin N terminus (DYS3) shows absent sarcolemma reactivity (Inset shows spectrin positive control). (**c**) Immunostaining for dystrophin C terminus (DYS2) shows rare revertant fiber (arrow). (**d**) Immunostaining for alpha-dystroglycan shows attenuated sarcolemma reactivity. (All images are taken at the same magnification)

subsequent femur fracture. He was unable to stand to bear weight, with or without assistance. He was unable to go from a supine to a sitting position without assistance and required pillows for support when pulled to sit. He could assist with dressing himself, brushing his teeth, and feeding himself independently. The patient developed progressive upper extremity weakness at age 16 years. He also developed obstructive sleep apnea and restrictive lung disease, requiring non-invasive ventilation overnight. He had dilated cardiomyopathy. Echocardiogram showed normal ventricular systolic function and under filled ventricles. He took Lisinopril, Carvedilol and Spironolactone. He had a hiatal hernia and required a GT and Nissen. He had not developed neuromuscular scoliosis.

Discussion

DMD is an X-linked recessive disease caused by mutations in the dystrophin gene with an incidence of 1 in 3,500–5,000 live birth males [1–3]. Dystrophin is an intracellular cytoskeletal protein that stabilizes the plasma membrane and stabilizes the dystrophin glycoprotein complex, preventing degradation of the muscle fiber. Loss of these membrane proteins causes degeneration of the muscle fibers resulting in elevated CK level and muscle weakness. DMD is characterized by progressive muscle weakness and degeneration of skeletal and cardiac muscles. Weakness starts at the hip and progresses to involve the whole lower extremities. Patients stop ambulating between 10 and 15 years of age. Then, truncal weakness followed by upper extremity weakness develops. Physical examination is notable for proximal more than distal weakness, hypotonia, decreased reflexes, abnormal waddling gait, increased lordosis, difficulty running and jumping, calf pseudohypertrophy, macroglossia, and positive Gowers' sign. Duchenne boys usually present with symptoms around age 2–5 years, become wheelchair bound by age 12–15 years, and die around age 30 years due to cardiac or respiratory muscle weakness and complications [4]. Our patient had a typical presentation of DMD.

Differential diagnosis includes limb-girdle muscular dystrophy, Emery-Dreifuss muscular dystrophy, spinal muscular atrophy, mitochondrial or other metabolic myopathies. Once the clinical features are apparent to help narrow the diagnosis, genetic testing is performed looking for deletions, duplications or sequence alterations in the dystrophin gene. In a small percentage of patients, no known pathogenic variants can be found as seen in our patient, whose dystrophin gene test only showed a DNA sequence variant of unclear significance, a muscle biopsy is necessary. Biopsy shows chronic active myopathy with near complete absence of dystrophin protein expression by immunohistochemistry (IHC), which confirms the diagnosis of DMD. This case illustrates the shift in diagnostic paradigm for muscular dystrophies in the genetic era. Clinically prototypical cases of dystrophies are usually diagnosed by paneled genetic analysis. The pathologists nowadays are more likely to encounter muscle biopsies from patients whose initial genetic testing did not match the clinical impression, or genetic testing identified a variant of uncertain significance, or the patient had late onset or unusual clinical features that mimic acquired myopathies. The hallmarks of muscular dystrophy are chronic myopathic changes, which are sometimes referred to as "dystrophic" changes. Those changes, however, are nonspecific and do not distinguish dystrophy subclasses. Immunohistochemical stains can serve as surrogate markers for some underlying mutations when the mutations result in loss of normal protein expression. We typically perform an IHC panel including beta-spectrin (sarcolemma integrity control), dystrophin epitopes (rod domain, carboxy terminus and amino terminus), sarcoglycans (alpha, beta, gamma and delta), caveolin-3, dysferlin, merosin (80 KDa and 300 KDa), alpha-dystroglycan, collagen IV, collagen VI and emerin, on any pediatric muscle specimen with chronic myopathic changes.

DMD management involves a multidisciplinary approach involving experts in different medial fields, including neurology, cardiology, pulmonology, orthopedic surgery, endocrinology, dietitian, physical and occupational therapies. Glucocorticoids are the mainstay of the treatment in DMD to maintain the motor strength and to delay the loss of ambulation [5, 6]. The only FDA approved medication is Exondys, an antisense oligonucleotide for exon 51 skipping. This therapy is applicable to only 13% of patients with DMD [2–4]. Therapeutic approaches that are currently under exploration include gene transfer (micro-dystrophin), exon skipping, trans-splicing, genome editing, stop codon read-through and cell replacement therapy [7, 8].

Pearls

Clinical Pearls

1. DMD is an X-linked recessive disease affecting skeletal and cardiac muscles. Patients with DMD usually present with symptoms around age 2–5 years, become wheelchair bound by age 12–15 years, and die around age 30 years due to cardiac or respiratory weakness and complications.
2. DMD should be suspected in males with proximal limb weakness at age 2–5 years and marked CK elevation.
3. A muscle biopsy can be spared in many patients with DMD because the disease can be diagnosed by the dystrophin gene test. However, a muscle biopsy with dystrophin immunostaining is still useful in patients with DMD phenotype but no known pathological dystrophin gene mutations.
4. DMD management involves a multidisciplinary team approach.
5. Glucocorticoids are the mainstay of treatment in DMD, and the only FDA approved medication is Exondys 51, an antisense oligonucleotide for exon 51 skipping, which is applicable to only 13% of patients with DMD.

Pathology Pearls

1. The muscle pathology hallmarks of a muscular dystrophy are chronic myopathic changes.
2. An immunostaining panel can help confirm or narrow down possible underlining genetic defects and should be performed on any pediatric muscle biopsy with chronic myopathic changes.

References

1. Darras BT, Urion DK, Ghosh PS. Dystrophinopathies. 2000 Sep 5 [Updated 2018 Apr 26]. In: Adam MP, Ardinger HH, Pagon RA, et al., editors. GeneReviews® [Internet]. Seattle (WA): University of Washington, Seattle; 1993–2019. www.ncbi.nlm.nih.gov/books/NBK1119. Accessed 31 May 2019.
2. Aartsma-Rus A, Van Deutekom JC, Fokkema IF, Van Ommen GJ, Den Dunnen JT. Entries in the Leiden Duchenne muscular dystrophy mutation database: an overview of mutation types and paradoxical cases that confirm the reading-frame rule. Muscle Nerve. 2006;34(2):135.

3. Romitti PA, Zhu Y, Puzhankara S, James KA, Nabukera SK, Zamba GK, Ciafaloni E, Cunniff C, Druschel CM, Mathews KD, Matthews DJ, Meaney FJ, Andrews JG, Conway KM, Fox DJ, Street N, Adams MM, Bolen J, MD STARnet. Prevalence of Duchenne and Becker muscular dystrophies in the United States. Pediatrics. 2015;135(3):513. Epub 2015 Feb 16
4. Birnkrant DJ, Bushby K, Bann CM, Apkon SD, Blackwell A, Brumbaugh D, Case LE, Clemens PR, Hadjiyannakis S, Pandya S, Street N, Tomezsko J, Wagner KR, Ward LM, Weber DR, DMD Care Considerations Working Group. Diagnosis and management of Duchenne muscular dystrophy, part 1: diagnosis, and neuromuscular, rehabilitation, endocrine, and gastrointestinal and nutritional management. Lancet Neurol. 2018;17(3):251. Epub 2018 Feb 3
5. Bushby K, Finkel R, Birnkrant DJ, Case LE, Clemens PR, Cripe L, et al. Diagnosis and management of Duchenne muscular dystrophy, part 2: implementation of multidisciplinary care. Lancet Neurol. 2010;9(2):177–89.
6. Bushby K, Finkel R, Birnkrant DJ, Case LE, Clemens PR, Cripe L, et al. Diagnosis and management of Duchenne muscular dystrophy, part 1: diagnosis, and pharmacological and psychosocial management. Lancet Neurol. 2010;9(1):77–93.
7. Yokota T, Maruyama R, Rodrigues M, Yokota T, Walker JM. An overview of recent advances and clinical applications of exon skipping and splice modulation for muscular dystrophy and various genetic disorders. Exon skipping and inclusion therapies: methods and protocols exon skipping and inclusion therapies. 09/01/2018.1828:31–55.
8. Shieh PB. Emerging strategies in the treatment of Duchenne muscular dystrophy. Neurotherapeutics. 2018;15(4):840–8.

Chapter 25
A 2-Year-Old Girl with Hypotonia Since Birth and Delayed Motor and Speech Development

Diana P. Castro, Chunyu Cai, and Dustin Jacob Paul

History

A 2-year-old girl presented with hypotonia since birth. Pregnancy course was uncomplicated, except for decreased fetal movements. The patient was born at full term via caesarean section due to previous C-section. At delivery, infant did not require resuscitation but had poor latch so could not be breast fed and was eventually bottle fed. Her motor development was delayed with rolling over at 9 months, sitting with support at 6 months and independently at 9 months. She had never crawled or pulled to stand, and only stood with a kid walk device. She developed pincer grasp at 9 months of age. At the age of 2 years she was able to feed herself independently using a fork and spoon and used a sippy cup for drinking. She could not dress herself, but she tried to help her mother with clothing and brushed her teeth with assistance. She did hold a crayon and color. She did indicate when she needed to use the bathroom, but occasionally had urinary incontinence. She was social and enjoyed interacting and playing with siblings.

D. P. Castro (✉)
Department of Neurology and Neurotherapeutics, University of Texas Southwestern Medical Center, Children's Medical Center of Dallas, Dallas, TX, USA
e-mail: diana.castro@utsuthwestern.edu

C. Cai
Department of Pathology, University of Texas Southwestern Medical Center, Dallas, TX, USA
e-mail: chunyu.cai@utsouthwestern.edu

D. Jacob Paul
Department of Neurology and Neurotherapeutics, University of Texas Southwestern Medical Center, Dallas, TX, USA
e-mail: dustin.paul@utsouthwestern.edu

L. Zhou et al. (eds.), *A Case-Based Guide to Neuromuscular Pathology*,
https://doi.org/10.1007/978-3-030-25682-1_25

Her speech was delayed with only 20 words at 2 years of age and did not use phrases. She did use sign language for some communication and parents thought that she understood what they said to her. Family history was negative for any neurologic disorders.

Physical Examination

The patient was alert and interactive. Her speech was delayed but was able to understand everything with hypophonic speech. She had long elongated myopathic facies with high arched palate. Cranial nerves were notable for facial weakness, poor facial expression, and inability to close eyelids fully. During the examination her mouth was open with tongue protruding. Her muscle tone and bulk were decreased in the upper and lower extremities. Motor exam was limited due to patient's age. She was unable to go from supine to sitting independently and was unable to bear weight on her legs. She was unable to roll over from front to back or back to front. When sitting up she could hold her head up steadily, but her head did not tilt forward. Her arms could abduct to about 90 degrees, she flexed at elbows and she had a weak hand grasp bilaterally. Her hands had hyper extensible joints. Her right leg was minimally antigravity but not her left leg. But her lower extremities moved in the same plane of the bed.

Investigations

Her creatine kinase level was 325 IU/L (normal: 50–350). Her brain MRI showed extensive increased T2 signal throughout the supratentorial white matter. A left quadriceps muscle biopsy was performed.

Muscle Biopsy Findings

The left quadriceps muscle biopsy from the patient showed an end-stage muscle with prominent fatty replacement and sparse remaining myofibers (Fig. 25.1a). The remaining myofibers showed chronic myopathic changes and marked interstitial fibrosis. A muscular dystrophy immunostaining panel demonstrated intact sarcolemmal dystrophin epitopes (rod domain, carboxy terminus and amino terminus), sarcoglycans (alpha, beta, gamma and delta), caveolin-3, dysferlin, α-dystroglycan, collagen IV, collagen VI, and nuclear emerin reactivity (representative images for α-dystroglycan and dystrophin carboxy terminus were shown in Fig. 25.1b, c, respectively), but complete absence of both the merosin 80 kD C-terminal

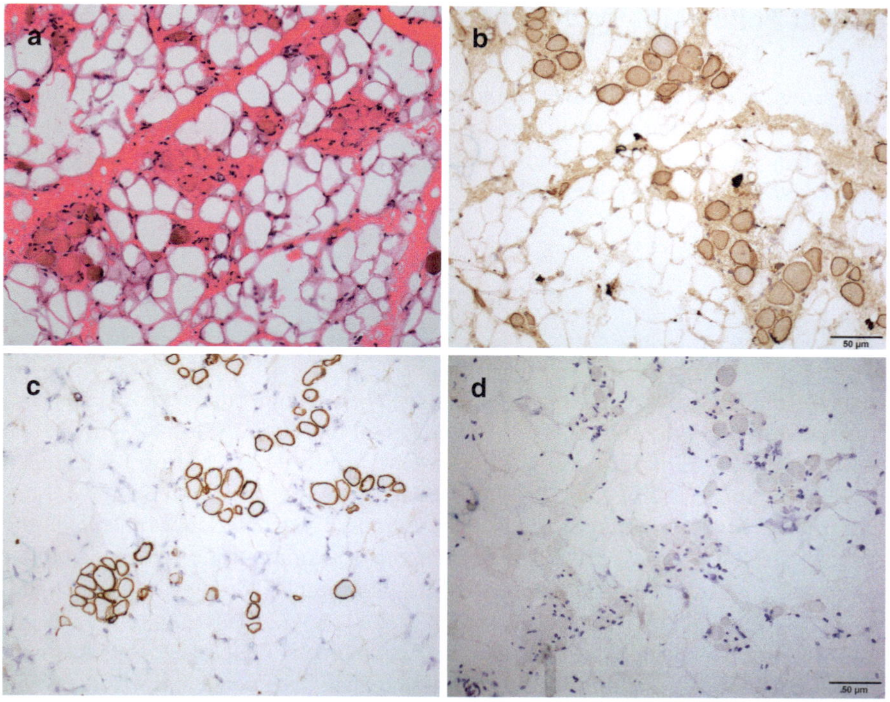

Fig. 25.1 Muscle pathology in merosin deficiency. (**a**) H&E stained cryostat section shows an end stage muscle with few remaining fibers. Immunostaining shows intact alpha-dystroglycan (**b**) and dystrophin (**c**, DYS2 epitope) sarcolemmal reactivity, but complete absence of merosin (**d**, 80kD epitope)

(Fig. 25.1d) and 300 kD N-terminal epitopes reactivity. These findings are diagnostic for a merosin deficient congenital muscular dystrophy.

Additional Investigation After the Muscle Biopsy Diagnosis

Her genetic testing revealed an abnormality in the *LAMA2* gene, described as an heterozygous mutation in exon 2 with sequence variant defined as c.268delA (p.Ser90Alafs∗35) and deletion of exon 4-41 with approximate genomic locations 129, 397, 936 in intron 3 and 129, 753, 986 in intron 4.

Final Diagnosis

Merosin (laminin α2-chain) Deficient Congenital Muscular Dystrophy (MDC1A)

Patient Follow-up

The patient is currently followed at the pediatric neuromuscular clinic. A multidisciplinary clinic including neurology, pulmonology and neuromuscular therapists follow her on a regular basis. Her development is very slow. She is non-ambulatory and is developing thoracic scoliosis.

Discussion

Merosin deficient congenital muscular dystrophy is an autosomal recessive disease. It is one of the most common forms of congenital muscular dystrophy (CMD) and represents 10–40% of all cases in different CMD series [1–3]. Merosin is encoded by *laminin alpha 2 chain gene (LAMA2)* and is the predominant homologue of laminin α chain in the basal lamina of skeletal muscle fibers and Schwann cells in the nervous systems [4]. In skeletal muscle, merosin is a component of the extracellular matrix and connects to the sarcolemmal dystrophin complex through α-dystroglycan; its absence leads to myofiber degeneration. There is a wide spectrum of the disease with varying amounts of complete or partial merosin deficiency. Patients with MDC1A usually present at birth or early infancy with hypotonia and weakness [5]. Usually there are respiratory and feeding difficulties. Ophthalmoparesis particularly in upper gaze is common. There is elevation of CK level up to 10x the normal value. Increased T2 signal intensity in the white matter can be found on brain MRI, which is thought to be from abnormal myelination. Epilepsy can be present in 20% of patients and most patients are cognitively intact. Since laminin α2 is also present in Schwann cells, some patients develop a peripheral neuropathy. There is cardiac involvement in approximately 30% of the patients. Differential diagnosis consists of congenital myopathies and congenital myasthenic syndrome given the vertical gaze palsies as well as congenital muscular dystrophy.

The initial workup includes serum CK and brain MRI. Muscle biopsy is useful to differentiate merosin deficient congenital muscular dystrophy from other chronic active myopathies with similar clinical presentations. A specific genetic diagnosis relies on the gene mutation analysis. Muscle pathology of merosin deficient congenital muscular dystrophy is characterized by a complete or a partial deficiency of merosin with dystrophic characteristics, including myofiber necrosis, degeneration, regeneration, endomysial inflammation, and fibrofatty tissue replacement. The dystrophic changes alone do not differentiate different types of muscular dystrophies or other chronic active myopathies. An immunostaining panel encompassing the most common muscular dystrophy related proteins including merosin, α-dystroglycan, collagen IV, collagen VI, dystrophin epitopes, sarcoglycans, caveolin-3, dysferlin, and emerin should be performed. Merosin detection needs the use of two antibodies, the Millipore MAB1922 antibody to recognize the N-terminal of the 80-kDa protein fragment and the Leica/Novacastra NCL-MEROSIN antibody to recognize the C-terminal 300 kDa fragment. This aids in the cases of partial merosin deficiencies.

Management is multidisciplinary and includes neurology, cardiology, pulmonology and orthopedics similar to many of the congenital muscular dystrophies. The therapies using combinatorial approach of both protein therapy and gene therapy are currently being studied [6].

Pearls

Clinical Pearls

1. MDC1A should be suspected in patients with weakness, hypotonia and gaze palsies.
2. Brain MRI T2 white matter hyperintensities can be seen due to dysmyelination.
3. Patients can develop polyneuropathy due to myelination involvement.
4. Patients are cognitively intact and only 20% may develop seizures.

Pathology Pearls

1. Merosin deficiency is a common form of CMD and should be evaluated by immunohistochemistry on any pediatric muscle biopsy with chronic active myopathic changes.
2. Histology alone is nonspecific and usually does not distinguish among different types of muscular dystrophy or acquired chronic myopathies. An immunostaining panel encompassing the most common muscular dystrophy related proteins including merosin, α-dystroglycan, collagen IV, collagen VI, dystrophin epitopes, sarcoglycans, caveolin-3, dysferlin, and emerin should be performed.
3. Complete merosin deficiency leads to presentation at birth and a complete absence of both 80kD and 300kD epitope reactivity on immunohistochemistry; these cases are referred to as "merosin negative congenital muscular dystrophy".
4. Patients with a partial merosin deficiency may present in childhood or early adulthood. Muscle biopsies show partial reduction or focal loss of merosin. The antibody that detects the C-terminal 300 kD fragment is more sensitive than the antibody that detects the 80 kD N-terminal epitope [7].

References

1. Clement EM, Feng L, Mein R, Sewry CA, Robb SA, Manzur AY, et al. Relative frequency of congenital muscular dystrophy subtypes: analysis of the UK diagnostic service 2001–2008. Neuromuscul Disord. 2012;22(6):522–7.
2. Gilbreath HR, Castro D, Iannaccone ST. Congenital myopathies and muscular dystrophies. Neurol Clin. 2014;32(3):689–703, viii
3. Geranmayeh F, Clement E, Feng LH, Sewry C, Pagan J, Mein R, et al. Genotype-phenotype correlation in a large population of muscular dystrophy patients with LAMA2 mutations. Neuromuscul Disord. 2010;20(4):241–50.
4. Sunada Y, Edgar TS, Lotz BP, Rust RS, Campbell KP. Merosin-negative congenital muscular dystrophy associated with extensive brain abnormalities. Neurology. 1995;45(11):2084–9.
5. Iannaccone ST, Castro D. Congenital muscular dystrophies and congenital myopathies. Continuum (Minneap Minn). 2013;19(6 Muscle Disease):1509–34.
6. Durbeej M. Laminin-alpha2 chain-deficient congenital muscular dystrophy: pathophysiology and development of treatment. Curr Top Membr. 2015;76:31–60.
7. Dubowitz V, Sewry CA, Lane RJM. Muscle biopsy: a practical approach. 3rd ed. Great Britain: Saunders Elsevier; 2007. xiii, 611 p.

Chapter 26
An 8-year-old boy with delayed motor milestones and proximal leg muscle weakness

Partha S. Ghosh and Hart G. W. Lidov

History

An 8-year-old boy presented to the neuromuscular clinic for muscle weakness. He was born at term without complications; his fetal movements were normal. He walked at 15 months; his parents felt that he always had an abnormal gait. He was slower compared to other children in running. He needed to hold on the railing while climbing stairs. He could not get up from the sitting position without support. His weakness remained stable over the years. There was no history of upper limb weakness, ptosis, or dysphagia. He had autism spectrum disorder and anxiety disorder. He also had moderate persistent asthma. There was no family history of neuromuscular disorders.

Physical Examination

On neurological examination there was no ptosis, ophthalmoparesis or facial weakness. He had proximal upper limb weakness (deltoid and triceps 4+/5 MRC grade) and proximal lower limb weakness (iliopsoas 4+/5, gluteus medius and maximus 4/5, quadriceps 5−/5). Tendon reflexes were normal. He had modified Gowers sign;

P. S. Ghosh (✉)
Department of Neurology, Boston Children's Hospital,
Boston, MA, USA
e-mail: partha.ghosh@childrens.harvard.edu

H. G. W. Lidov
Department of Pathology, Boston Children's Hospital, Boston, MA, USA
e-mail: hart.lidov@childrens.harvard.edu

L. Zhou et al. (eds.), *A Case-Based Guide to Neuromuscular Pathology*,
https://doi.org/10.1007/978-3-030-25682-1_26

waddling noted during running. There was no calf hypertrophy or joint contractures. Sensory and cerebellar examinations were normal.

Investigations

He had normal serum creatine kinase (89 U/L), lactate, thyroid functions, total and free carnitine, and acylcarnitine. EMG was not performed. A right quadriceps muscle biopsy was performed.

Muscle Biopsy Findings

Muscle biopsy of the right quadriceps muscle (Fig. 26.1a) showed moderate fiber size variation with preponderance of type I fibers, increased internal nuclei with nuclei more towards the center of the fibers. NADH-TR histochemical stain (Fig. 26.1b) revealed a variety of changes in scattered fibers including cleared out central areas, increased staining in a central dot-like pattern and scattered fibers with radial strand-like abnormalities. There was a mild increase in endomysial connective tissue. Overall features were consistent with congenital myopathy, most likely centronuclear myopathy (CNM).

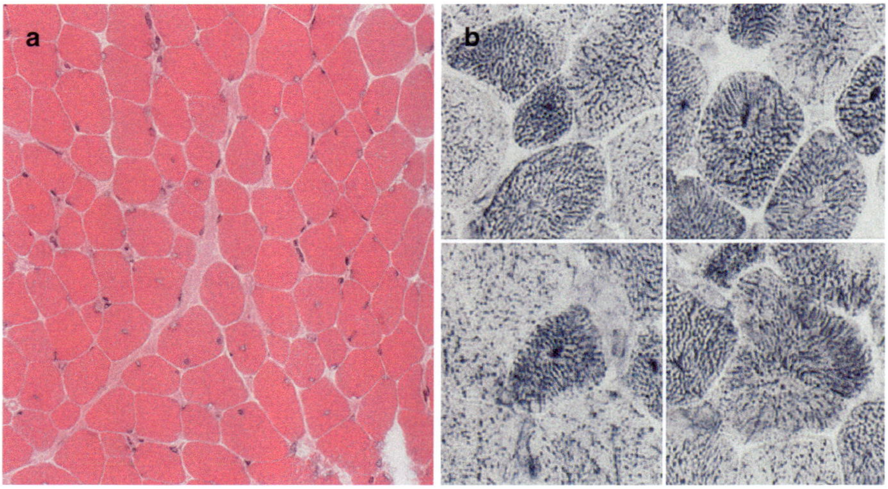

Fig. 26.1 Muscle biopsy findings of the right quadriceps muscle. (**a**) H&E showing excessive variation in fiber diameter, and increased numbers of fibers with centrally placed nuclei. (**b**) NADH-TR histochemistry showing four fibers had central nuclei and exhibit the typical radial distribution pattern

Additional Investigation After Muscle Biopsy Diagnosis

Next generation sequence panel showed that he had a heterozygous de novo mutation of the Dynamin 2 (*DNM2*) gene (c.1393C > T, p.Arg465Trp) which is a known pathogenic mutation.

Final Diagnosis

Autosomal dominant centronuclear myopathy from a de novo *DNM2* mutation

Patient Follow-up

At the time of last follow-up, 1 year from the initial diagnosis, there was no progression of his muscle weakness. He was getting regular physical therapy and did not require assistive devices for ambulation. He was followed in pulmonary clinic for his asthma and there was no concern for respiratory muscle weakness.

Discussion

The child in this vignette presented with proximal lower limb weakness from early childhood. Pertinent negatives were absence of family history, ocular/bulbar findings, facial or neck muscle weakness, calf hypertrophy, and joint contractures.

Though anterior horn cell disorders (spinal muscular atrophy) and radiculoneuropathies could present with proximal limb weakness, retained tendon reflexes were against those diagnoses. Neuromuscular junction disorders seemed unlikely due to absence of ocular-bulbar involvement and lack of diurnal variation of symptoms. Myopathy was the most likely possibility in this case. Chronic course and early onset of symptoms suggested a genetic myopathy. In a boy with autism spectrum disorder and myopathy, dystrophinopathy (Duchenne and Becker muscular dystrophy) should be considered. Nonprogressive course, absence of calf hypertrophy and normal CK were against dystrophinopathy.

The investigative approach in a child with myopathy includes measurement of serum CK, EMG, muscle ultrasound or muscle MRI, muscle biopsy and finally genetic testing [1, 2]. Normal CK in our patient ruled out most of the muscular dystrophies. Congenital myopathies can have normal CK. EMG can further differentiate myopathy from a neurogenic process. EMG was however, not performed in this patient. A muscle biopsy was considered as the next step in this case which showed features of CNM. Next generation sequencing confirmed the final diagnosis of CNM due to *DNM2* mutation.

Centronuclear myopathies are a group of clinical and genetically heterogeneous entity characterized by the presence of centralized nuclei in majority of the muscle fibers [3]. Additional histologic features include hypotrophy of the type I fibers and characteristic patterns of disorganization of oxidative enzymes [4]. Clinically, there is a wide spectrum of severity ranging from severe neonatal presentation to more mild adult disease [5, 6]. Ophthalmoparesis is commonly encountered which may help to differentiate CNM from other congenital myopathies [7]. Mutations in at least eight genes are described as causes of CNM: *MTM1, DNM2, BIN1, RYR1, TTN, MTMR14, SPEG,* and *CCDC78* [8, 9]. Based on the inheritance pattern, CNM can be divided into the following groups: (1) X-lined recessive due to mutation of myotubularin gene-*MTM1* (mytotubular myopathy) which has a severe neonatal presentation with profound hypotonia and respiratory failure [10]; (2) autosomal dominant caused by mutation of *DNM2* gene causing a milder phenotype [11]; and (3) autosomal recessive form which is of intermediate severity caused by mutations of amphiphysin 2 *(BIN1)* and ryanodine receptor *(RYR1)* genes respectively [8, 9]. Heterozygous variants in *CCDC78* and *MTMR14* genes are associated with autosomal dominant early-onset centronuclear myopathy [12, 13]. Recently mutations in *TTN* and *SPEG* are considered as additional cases of autosomal recessive CNM [14, 15].

Mutations in *DNM2* gene account for about 50% of cases of CNM [4]. A wide spectrum of clinical severity has been described in *DNM2*-related CNM varying from severe disease with neonatal onset to a milder disease with adult onset [11, 16, 17] Facial weakness, bilateral ptosis and ophthalmoparesis are common manifestations along with distal muscle atrophy, finger and ankle contractures and pes cavus [18]. However, the child described in this vignette had proximal muscle weakness without other features. There are only a few cases of *DNM2*-CNM presenting as late-onset dilated cardiomyopathy, ventricular septal defect or valvular irregularities and non-life-threatening arrhythmias [6, 18]. Cognitive impairment has been rarely reported in this condition, only in two families carrying the E368Q and R465W mutations and in one additional patient also showing the R465W mutation [17, 19]. Our patient had R465W mutation and had autism spectrum disorder.

Muscle imaging in *DNM2* related myopathy shows a characteristic pattern with early involvement of the following muscles: medial gastrocnemius and soleus in the lower leg, adductor longus and hamstrings in the thighs, and gluteus minimus in the pelvis [18–20].

Histopathological hallmarks on muscle biopsy in *DNM2*-related CNM are (1) hypotrophy and predominance of type I fibers, (2) radial arrangement of sarcoplasmic strands and (3) centrally located nuclei [4].

To date, 19 different *DNM2* mutations have been reported in approximately 100 families [6]. Mutations affecting the middle domain (MD) are generally associated with a milder clinical course [11, 20] whereas those associated with mutations affecting the pleckstrin-homology (PH) and GTPase effector (GED) domains of *DNM2* are frequently associated with a severe phenotype [6, 16]. It has been found that *DNM2* mutations affecting the PH domain have also been associated with dominant intermediate Charcot Marie Tooth Disease [21], and in an axonal variant of the same group of disorders, CMT2M [22]. The majority of patients with *DNM2* mutations are sporadic cases with de novo dominant heterozygous mutations [6]. Mutational hot spots for *DNM2* related CNM myopathy involve two adjacent amino acids, Glu368 and Arg369, encoded on exon 8, and a single amino acid Arg465, encoded on exon 11 [6], the latter was found in our case.

There is no specific cure for *DNM2* related CNM. There are case reports of some patients with improvement with neuromuscular junction augmentation therapy (pyridostigmine) [23]. Allele-specific siRNA sequences have been recently shown to achieve functional restoration in patient-derived fibroblasts and murine *DNM2*-mRNA harboring p.R465W mutation (most commonly encountered mutation) which can pave the path for future gene-based therapies [24].

Pearls

Clinical Pearls

1. CNM should be considered in a child with limb girdle pattern of weakness, relatively non-progressive course, and ophthalmoparesis.
2. CK is usually normal.
3. CNM is clinically and genetically heterogeneous; *DNM2* mutations are the most common cause of autosomal dominant CNM.

Pathology Pearls

1. Muscle biopsy shows characteristic findings in CNM, including the presence of centralized nuclei, specific patterns of disorganization in oxidative stains (e.g. radial arrangement of sarcoplasmic strands in *DNM2*-CNM), and type I fiber abundance and hypotrophy.

References

1. Barohn RJ, Dimachkie MM, Jackson CE. A pattern recognition approach to patients with a suspected myopathy. Neurol Clin. 2014;32:569–93.
2. Al-Ghamdi F, Darras BT, Ghosh PS. Spectrum of neuromuscular disorders with HyperCKemia from a tertiary care pediatric neuromuscular center. J Child Neurol. 2018;33:389–96.
3. Zanoteli E, Oliveira AS, Schmidt B, Gabbai AA. Centronuclear myopathy: clinical aspects of ten Brazilian patients with childhood onset. J Neurol Sci. 1998;158:76–82.
4. Romero NB. Centronuclear myopathies: a widening concept. Neuromuscul Disord. 2010;20:223–8.
5. Bevilacqua JA, Monnier N, Bitoun M, Eymard B, Ferreiro A, Monges S, et al. Recessive RYR1 mutations cause unusual congenital myopathy with prominent nuclear internalization and large areas of myofibrillar disorganization. Neuropathol Appl Neurobiol. 2011;37:271–84.

6. Böhm J, Biancalana V, Dechene ET, Bitoun M, Pierson CR, Schaefer E, et al. Mutation spectrum in the large GTPase dynamin 2, and genotype-phenotype correlation in autosomal dominant centronuclear myopathy. Hum Mutat. 2012;33:949–59.
7. North KN, Wang CH, Clarke N, Jungbluth H, Vainzof M, Dowling JJ, et al. Approach to the diagnosis of congenital myopathies. Neuromuscul Disord. 2014;24:97–116.
8. Jungbluth H, Treves S, Zorzato F, Sarkozy A, Ochala J, Sewry C, et al. Congenital myopathies: disorders of excitation-contraction coupling and muscle contraction. Nat Rev Neurol. 2018;14:151–67.
9. Gonorazky HD, Bönnemann CG, Dowling JJ. The genetics of congenital myopathies. Handb Clin Neurol. 2018;148:549–64.
10. Laporte J, Hu LJ, Kretz C, Mandel JL, Kioschis P, Coy JF, et al. A gene mutated in X-linked myotubular myopathy defines a new putative tyrosine phosphatase family conserved in yeast. Nat Genet. 1996;13:175–82.
11. Bitoun M, Maugenre S, Jeannet PY, Lacène E, Ferrer X, Laforêt P, et al. Mutations in dynamin 2 cause dominant centronuclear myopathy. Nat Genet. 2005;37:1207–9.
12. Tosch V, Rohde HM, Tronchère H, Zanoteli E, Monroy N, Kretz C, et al. A novel PtdIns3P and PtdIns(3,5)P2 phosphatase with an inactivating variant in centronuclear myopathy. Hum Mol Genet. 2006;15:3098–106.
13. Majczenko K, Davidson AE, Camelo-Piragua S, Agrawal PB, Manfready RA, Li X, et al. Dominant mutation of CCDC78 in a unique congenital myopathy with prominent internal nuclei and atypical cores. Am J Hum Genet. 2012;91:365–71.
14. Ceyhan-Birsoy O, Agrawal PB, Hidalgo C, Schmitz-Abe K, DeChene ET, Swanson LC, et al. Recessive truncating *titin* gene, TTN, mutations presenting as centronuclear myopathy. Neurology. 2013;81:1205–14.
15. Agrawal PB, Pierson CR, Joshi M, Liu X, Ravenscroft G, Moghadaszadeh B, et al. SPEG interacts with myotubularin, and its deficiency causes centronuclear myopathy with dilated cardiomyopathy. Am J Hum Genet. 2014;95:218–26.
16. Bitoun M, Bevilacqua JA, Prudhon B, Maugenre S, Taratuto AL, Monges S, et al. Dynamin 2 mutations cause sporadic centronuclear myopathy with neonatal onset. Ann Neurol. 2007;62:666–70.
17. Hanisch F, Müller T, Dietz A, Bitoun M, Kress W, Weis J, et al. Phenotype variability and histopathological findings in centronuclear myopathy due to DNM2 mutations. J Neurol. 2011;258:1085–90.
18. Susman RD, Quijano-Roy S, Yang N, Webster R, Clarke NF, Dowling J, et al. Expanding the clinical, pathological and MRI phenotype of DNM2-related centronuclear myopathy. Neuromuscul Disord. 2010;20:229–37.
19. Catteruccia M, Fattori F, Codemo V, Ruggiero L, Maggi L, Tasca G, et al. Centronuclear myopathy related to dynamin 2 mutations: clinical, morphological, muscle imaging and genetic features of an Italian cohort. Neuromuscul Disord. 2013;23:229–38.
20. Schessl J, Medne L, Hu Y, Zou Y, Brown MJ, Huse JT, et al. MRI in DNM2-related centronuclear myopathy: evidence for highly selective muscle involvement. Neuromuscul Disord. 2007;17:28–32.
21. Züchner S, Noureddine M, Kennerson M, Verhoeven K, Claeys K, De Jonghe P, et al. Mutations in the pleckstrin homology domain of dynamin 2 cause dominant intermediate Charcot–Marie–tooth disease. Nat Genet. 2005;37:289–94.
22. Bitoun M, Stojkovic T, Prudhon B, Maurage CA, Latour P, Vermersch P, et al. A novel mutation in the dynamin 2 gene in a Charcot–Marie–tooth type 2 patient: clinical and pathological findings. Neuromuscul Disord. 2008;18:334–8.
23. Gibbs EM, Clarke NF, Rose K, Oates EC, Webster R, Feldman EL, et al. Neuromuscular junction abnormalities in DNM2-related centronuclear myopathy. J Mol Med (Berl). 2013;91:727–37.
24. Trochet D, Prudhon B, Beuvin M, Peccate C, Lorain S, Julien L, et al. Allele-specific silencing therapy for dynamin 2-related dominant centronuclear myopathy. Mol Med. 2018;10:239–53.

Chapter 27
A 6-Year-Old-Boy with Proximal Leg Muscle Weakness and Facial Weakness

Partha S. Ghosh and Hart G. W. Lidov

History

A 6-year-old-boy presented to the neuromuscular clinic for muscle weakness. He was born at term gestation without complications; fetal movements were normal. He walked at 16 months. Parents first noticed waddling gait when he was 3 years old. He would trip and fall often and needed to hold on the railing while climbing stairs. He had easy fatigability but there was no diurnal variation of his symptoms. He had nasal dysarthria and underwent surgery for velopharyngeal insufficiency. There was no history of ptosis, ophthalmoparesis, dysphagia, or recurrent respiratory tract infections. His cognitive functions were normal. Parents were of Caucasian descent and he was younger of three siblings. There was no family history of neuromuscular disorders.

Physical Examination

On neurological examination he had nasal dysarthria, open mouth suggestive of lower bifacial weakness; there was no ptosis or ophthalmoparesis. He had mild generalized hypotonia. He had neck flexor weakness (MRC grade 4+/5), proximal upper limb weakness (deltoid 4+), and proximal lower limb weakness (iliopsoas

P. S. Ghosh (✉)
Department of Neurology, Boston Children's Hospital, Boston, MA, USA
e-mail: partha.ghosh@childrens.harvard.edu

H. G. W. Lidov
Department of Pathology, Boston Children's Hospital, Boston, MA, USA
e-mail: hart.lidov@childrens.harvard.edu

L. Zhou et al. (eds.), *A Case-Based Guide to Neuromuscular Pathology*,
https://doi.org/10.1007/978-3-030-25682-1_27

4+/5, gluteus medius and maximus 4/5). He had pectus excavatum and mild scapular winging. Tendon reflexes were diminished at the knees only. He had modified Gowers sign and mild waddling gait. There was no calf hypertrophy or joint contractures. Sensory and cerebellar examinations were normal.

Investigations

He had normal serum creatine kinase, lactate, thyroid functions, total and free carnitine, acylcarnitine, and urine organic acid. MRI brain and spine were normal. Nerve conduction study (NCS) showed normal sensory and motor responses in the upper and lower limbs. Needle electromyography (EMG) did not show increased insertional activity or spontaneous discharges. Voluntary motor unit potentials were normal though the activation was poor due to sedated study. A left quadriceps muscle biopsy was performed.

Muscle Biopsy Findings

Muscle biopsy of the left quadriceps muscle showed excessive fiber size variation with preponderance of type 1 fibers which were hypotrophic and abundant (Fig. 27.1a). Nemaline rods were present in the sarcoplasm of predominantly type I fibers (Fig. 27.1b). There was a mild increase in endomysial connective tissue. Overall features were consistent with nemaline myopathy (NM).

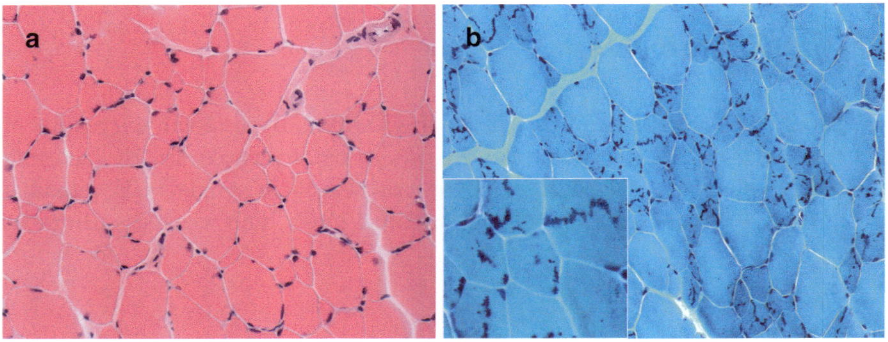

Fig. 27.1 Muscle biopsy findings of the left quadriceps. (**a**) H&E showing excessive variation of fiber diameters and mild increase in endomysial connective tissue. ATPase histochemistry (not shown) demonstrates that the majority of hypotrophic fibers are Type I. (**b**) Gomori Trichrome stain demonstrating nemaline rods in many fibers, predominantly in the small Type I fibers. Insert shows rods at a higher magnification

Additional Investigation After the Muscle Biopsy Diagnosis

Next generation sequence panel showed 2 novel frameshift mutations of the nebulin (*NEB*) gene which were predicted to be pathogenic: maternally inherited c.5244_5254delCTACACTGAAAlnsG,p.Tyr1749Asnfs∗23 and paternally inherited c.24770_24771dupTT,p.Ser8258Leufs∗10.

Final Diagnosis

Autosomal recessive nemaline myopathy from *NEB* mutations (compound heterozygous)

Patient Follow-Up

At the time of last follow-up 1.5 years from the initial diagnosis, there is no progression of his muscle weakness. He had negative cardiology and pulmonary evaluations. He was getting regular physical therapy and did not require assistive devices for ambulation.

Discussion

The child in this vignette presented with proximal lower limb weakness since early childhood. In addition to proximal limb weakness he had neck flexor weakness, facial weakness, nasal dysarthria, mild scapular winging and reduced tendon reflexes at the knees. Pertinent negatives were absence of family history, diurnal variation of symptoms, ocular findings, calf hypertrophy, joint contractures, and normal sensory examination.

The differential diagnosis for this presentation was broad and involves different parts of the lower motor unit. Anterior horn cell disorders particularly spinal muscular atrophy (SMA) type 3 was a consideration in this case due to proximal weakness and reduced knee reflexes. The non-progressive course and lack of diffuse hypo/areflexia argued against the possibility of diffuse polyradiculopathy. Peripheral neuropathies seemed unlikely given lack of distal weakness and sensory findings. Presence of fatigue, facial weakness, and nasal dysarthria might suggest the possibility of a neuromuscular junction (NMJ) disorder. Early onset presentation and chronic course could suggest congenital myasthenic syndrome (CMS) rather than acquired autoimmune myasthenia gravis. However, lack of ocular manifestations and diurnal variation of symptoms were against NMJ disorder. Myopathy seemed the most likely possibility given symmetric limb girdle pattern of weakness. Chronic course and early onset of symptoms suggested a genetic myopathy. Negative family history either suggested autosomal recessive inheritance or de novo mutation. Myopathies with facial weakness in children can be seen in congenital myopathies, mitochondrial myopathies, facioscapulohumeral muscular dystrophy (FSHD), myotonic dystrophy and rarely other muscular dystrophies [1].

The investigative approach in a child with myopathy includes measurement of serum CK, EMG, muscle ultrasound or muscle MRI, muscle biopsy and finally genetic testing [2, 3]. Measurement of serum CK level is an inexpensive and excellent screening tool in patients with suspected myopathies. Among the myopathic disorders with normal CK, congenital myopathies are the most common causes [2, 3]. Though high CK is commonly encountered in most of the muscular dystrophies, certain muscular dystrophies like FSHD and myotonic dystrophy can have normal CK [1, 2]. However, the pattern of weakness in this case did not suggest FSHD. SMA type 3 closely mimics myopathies due to limb girdle pattern of weakness. EMG in this case helped to rule out SMA which shows chronic neurogenic changes. Absence of myotonic discharges in EMG in this case made myotonic dystrophy less likely. EMG in CM can be myopathic or normal. Repetitive nerve stimulation was not performed, so a NMJ disorder could not be completely ruled out. A muscle biopsy was considered as the next step in this case which showed features of NM. Next generation sequencing confirmed the final diagnosis of NM due to *NEB* mutation.

Congenital myopathies are a group of clinically and genetically heterogeneous conditions characterized by muscle weakness and distinctive structural abnormalities in muscle biopsies [3, 4]. Traditionally CM is classified histologically into 4 distinct types: central core disease, multi-minicore disease, centronuclear myopathy and nemaline myopathy based on the presence of central cores, multi-minicores, central nuclei and nemaline rods respectively [5–8]. The overall prevalence of CM is not clearly known but estimated to be around 1:20,000 children [9].

NM is the commonest form of CM [10]. The hallmark feature on muscle pathology is the accumulation of Z-disk and thin filament proteins into aggregates called nemaline bodies or rods, usually accompanied by disorganization of the muscle Z-disks [11]. Nemaline rods are protein aggregates which stain red with the modified Gomori trichrome stain [4]. They can appear within the sarcoplasm as isolated or diffuse structures, compact subsarcolemmal clusters, or both [12]. On electron microscopy, nemaline rods appear as electron dense structures [13]. Another common histologic hallmark of NM is type I fiber predominance [12, 13]. Our patient's biopsy showed all those features.

NM can be classified into six clinical types based on the age of onset, severity of weakness and respiratory muscle involvement [14]. Severe neonatal form is characterized by severe hypotonia and respiratory failure at birth. Intermediate congenital NM patients fail to achieve motor milestones, or become wheelchair dependent and/or develop respiratory failure by 11 years. Typical congenital forms are characterized by delayed motor milestones, proximal limb, lower facial or bulbar weakness which is either static or progresses very slowly. The patient described in this vignette fits with this phenotype. Childhood-onset NM develop their symptoms in the late first or second decade of life and most remain ambulatory. Adult onset NM develops symptoms much later in life. NM is typically not associated with extraocular muscle weakness which differentiates it from other forms of CM like centronuclear myopathies [4]. Extramuscular manifestations are uncommon in NM [3, 4]. Patients are cognitively normal. Cardiac involvement is rare except for some patients with *ACTA1 or MYPN* mutations. Patients can develop respiratory failure, feeding difficulties or scoliosis which is usually secondary to the muscle weakness [15].

Genetics of CM is changing rapidly. To date, mutations in more than 30 different genes have been associated with CM, though it accounts for approximately 60% of the cases. There are 12 known genetic causes of NM: *ACTA1*, *NEB*, *TPM2*, *TPM3*, *TNNT1*, *CFL2*, *KBTBD13*, *KLHL40*, *KLHL41*, *LMOD3*, *MYO18B*, and *MYPN* [4]. *ACTA1* mutations are the most common dominant/de novo mutations, and *NEB* mutations are the most common recessive mutations [4]. The nebulin gene in the chromosomal region 2q23 with its 183 exons, encodes one of the biggest proteins in vertebrates (600–900 kDa) [16]. This protein plays an important role in the skeletal muscle sarcomere by determining the minimum lengths of the actin filaments and regulating actin-myosin interactions and the calcium sensitivity of force generation [17]. A repetitive region in the middle of the nebulin gene complicates analytical testing [18]. All pathogenic variants known in *NEB* have been recessive, mostly compound heterozygous. The most common types of variants are splice-site mutations (34%), followed by frameshift mutations (32%) caused by small (<20 bp) deletions or insertions, nonsense mutations (23%), missense mutations (7%); large deletions and duplications (>1 kb) are rare (4%) [18].

The clinical and histological spectrum of disorders caused by *NEB* mutations is a continuum, ranging in severity from the severe form with perinatal onset to the mild forms. The distribution of weakness can vary from generalized muscle weakness, more pronounced in proximal limb muscles, to distal-only involvement in early-onset distal myopathy without nemaline bodies, a distal form of NM, although neck flexor weakness appears to be rather consistent [3, 4, 18]. Histological patterns range from a severe, but almost invariably non-dystrophic disturbance of the myofibrillar pattern to an almost normal picture on hematoxylin-eosin staining, with or without nemaline bodies, sometimes combined with cores, core-rod myopathy with generalized muscle weakness and a childhood-onset distal myopathy with rods and cores [18].

Useful laboratory investigations include measurement of serum creatine kinase levels, which are typically normal or slightly elevated. Neurophysiological studies, such as electromyography and nerve conduction studies, are useful mainly for excluding congenital neuropathies, myotonic disorders and congenital myasthenic syndromes [3]. Muscle imaging, in particular, muscle ultrasonography as a screening test and muscle MRI for a more detailed assessment, can reveal diagnostic patterns of selective muscle involvement [19]. Assessment of muscle biopsy samples with a standard panel of histological, histochemical and immunohistochemical stains will confirm the specific congenital myopathy and exclude distinct conditions with overlapping pathological features, such as the congenital muscular dystrophies, myofibrillar myopathies and autophagic vacuolar myopathies [3]. Electron microscopy helps to clarify the pathognomonic structural abnormalities that are seen with light microscopy [3]. Analysis of multiple congenital myopathy-associated genes through next generation sequencing is rapidly becoming the preferred diagnostic approach [3].

At present, there are no specific therapies for NM, in particular those due to NEB mutations [3]. Treatment is mainly supportive with regular physical therapy and follow-up to detect and manage respiratory failure, bulbar symptoms (dysphagia and dysarthria) and orthopedic complications.

Pearls

Clinical Pearls

1. Nemaline myopathy should be considered in a child with limb girdle pattern of weakness, non-progressive course, and facial weakness.
2. CK is usually normal and EMG may not show myopathic changes.
3. NM is clinically and genetically heterogeneous; *NEB* mutations are the most common cause of autosomal recessive NM.

Pathology Pearls

1. Muscle biopsy is the gold standard in the diagnosis of NM.
2. Presence of nemaline rods within the sarcoplasm is the hallmark histologic finding in NM best visualized in modified Gomori trichrome stain.
3. Type I fibers are abundant and usually hypotrophic in NM.

References

1. Barohn RJ, Dimachkie MM, Jackson CE. A pattern recognition approach to patients with a suspected myopathy. Neurol Clin. 2014;32:569–93.
2. Al-Ghamdi F, Darras BT, Ghosh PS. Spectrum of neuromuscular disorders with HyperCKemia from a tertiary care pediatric neuromuscular center. J Child Neurol. 2018;33:389–96.
3. Jungbluth H, Treves S, Zorzato F, Sarkozy A, Ochala J, Sewry C, et al. Congenital myopathies: disorders of excitation-contraction coupling and muscle contraction. Nat Rev Neurol. 2018;14:151–67.
4. Gonorazky HD, Bönnemann CG, Dowling JJ. The genetics of congenital myopathies. Handb Clin Neurol. 2018;148:549–64.
5. Magee KR, Shy GM. A new congenital nonprogressive myopathy. Brain. 1956;79:610–21.
6. Engel AG, Gomez MR, Groover RV. Multicore disease. A recently recognized congenital myopathy associated with multifocal degeneration of muscle fibers. Mayo Clin Proc. 1971;46:666–81.

7. Spiro AJ, Shy GM, Gonatas NK. Myotubular myopathy. Persistence of fetal muscle in an adolescent boy. Arch Neurol. 1966;14:1–14.
8. Shy GH, Engel WK, Somers JE, Wanko T. Nemaline myopathy. A new congenital myopathy. Brain. 1963;86:793–810.
9. Amburgey K, McNamara N, Bennett LR, McCormick ME, Acsadi G, Dowling JJ. Prevalence of congenital myopathies in a representative pediatric United States population. Ann Neurol. 2011;70:662–5.
10. Lee JM, Lim JG, Shin JH, Park YE, Kim DS. Clinical and genetic diversity of nemaline myopathy from a single neuromuscular center in Korea. J Neurol Sci. 2017;383:61–8.
11. Wallgren-Pettersson C, Jasani B, Newman GR, Morris GE, Jones S, Singhrao S, et al. Alpha-actinin in nemaline bodies in congenital nemaline myopathy: immunological confirmation by light and electron microscopy. Neuromuscul Disord. 1995;5:93–104.
12. Gurgel-Giannetti J, Reed UC, Marie SK, Zanoteli E, Fireman MA, Oliveira AS, et al. Rod distribution and muscle fiber type modification in the progression of nemaline myopathy. J Child Neurol. 2003;18:235–40.
13. North KN, Laing NG, Wallgren-Pettersson C. Nemaline myopathy: current concepts. The ENMC international consortium and Nemaline myopathy. J Med Genet. 1997;34:705–13.
14. Wallgren-Pettersson C, Beggs AH. Laing NG. 51st ENMC international workshop: nemaline myopathy.13-15 June 1997, Naarden, the Netherlands. Neuromuscul Disord. 1998;8:53–6.
15. Colombo I, Scoto M, Manzur AY, Robb SA, Maggi L, Gowda V, et al. Congenital myopathies: natural history of a large pediatric cohort. Neurology. 2015;84:28–35.
16. Bang ML, Li X, Littlefield R, Bremner S, Thor A, Knowlton KU, et al. Nebulin-deficient mice exhibit shorter thin filament lengths and reduced contractile function in skeletal muscle. J Cell Biol. 2006;173:905–16.
17. Chandra M, Mamidi R, Ford S, Hidalgo C, Witt C, Ottenheijm C, et al. Nebulin alters cross-bridge cycling kinetics and increases thin filament activation: a novel mechanism for increasing tension and reducing tension cost. J Biol Chem. 2009;284:30889–96.
18. Lehtokari VL, Kiiski K, Sandaradura SA, Laporte J, Repo P, Frey JA, et al. Mutation update: the spectra of nebulin variants and associated myopathies. Hum Mutat. 2014;35:1418–26.
19. Jungbluth H. Myopathology in times of modern imaging. Neuropathol Appl Neurobiol. 2017;43:24–43.

Chapter 28
A 6-Week-Old Boy with Neonatal Hypotonia and Feeding and Respiratory Difficulties

Partha S. Ghosh and Hart G. W. Lidov

History

A 6-week-old boy presented to the neuromuscular clinic for evaluation of hypotonia. He was born at term gestation by induced vaginal delivery due to low biophysical profile. Fetal movements were reduced. He had low muscle tone, minimal spontaneous movements, and weak cry after birth but had normal sensorium. He received supplemental oxygen after birth and subsequently required continuous positive airway respiration (CPAP) due to desaturations. He had feeding difficulties requiring gastrostomy tube placement. There was no family history of neuromuscular disorders.

Physical Examination

On neurological examination, he was alert. There was tenting of the upper lip and high arched palate. There was no ptosis or ophthalmoparesis. He had diffuse hypotonia on pull to sit, ventral and vertical suspension. He had frog leg position of the lower limbs. He had antigravity movements at the knee extension, elbow flexion and distal joints. Knee and ankle reflexes were diminished.

P. S. Ghosh (✉)
Department of Neurology, Boston Children's Hospital,
Boston, MA, USA
e-mail: partha.ghosh@childrens.harvard.edu

H. G. W. Lidov
Department of Pathology, Boston Children's Hospital, Boston, MA, USA
e-mail: hart.lidov@childrens.harvard.edu

L. Zhou et al. (eds.), *A Case-Based Guide to Neuromuscular Pathology*,
https://doi.org/10.1007/978-3-030-25682-1_28

Investigations

He had normal serum creatine kinase (CK), lactate, carnitine, acylcarnitine, amino acids, urine organic acids and acylglycine. Genetic testing for Prader-Willi syndrome was negative. MRI brain showed a small occipital infarct and small subdural hemorrhage in the right tentorial leaflet which did not explain his clinical features. Nerve conduction study (NCS) showed normal sensory and motor responses in the upper and lower limbs. Needle electromyography (EMG) showed early recruitment of short duration, low amplitude motor unit potentials without increased insertional activity or spontaneous discharges. A left quadriceps muscle biopsy was performed.

Muscle Biopsy Findings

Muscle biopsy of the left quadriceps muscle showed excessive fiber size variation with preponderance of type I fibers which were hypotropic and abundant (Fig. 28.1). Scattered type II fibers were hypertrophic. There were no increased internal nuclei, muscle fiber necrosis or regeneration. Nemaline rods, cores were not present in the sarcoplasm. There was no increase in endomysial connective tissue. Overall features were consistent with congenital fiber type disproportion (CFTD) myopathy. Electron microscopy revealed few focal areas of disorganization of the myofibrillar apparatus.

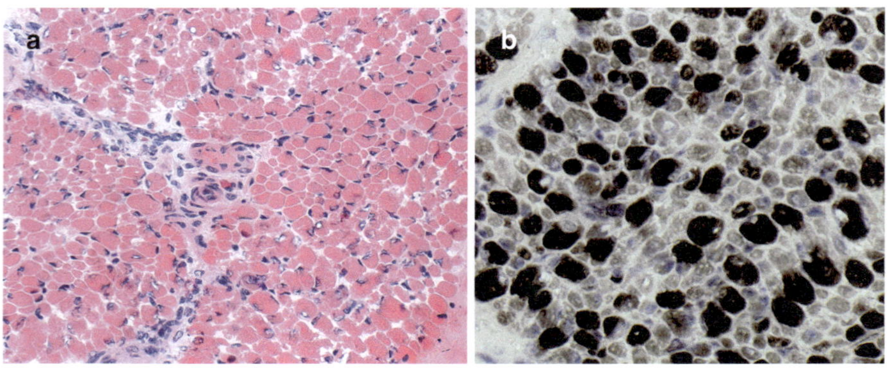

Fig. 28.1 Muscle biopsy findings of the left quadriceps muscle. (**a**), H&E shows excessive variation in fiber diameter without increased internal nuclei, muscle fiber necrosis or regeneration. Nemaline rods and cores are absent. (**b**), ATPase histochemistry (pH 9.4) demonstrates that the majority of hypotrophic fibers are Type I. Measurement of the 170 fibers in B, shows that the Type I (n = 96) has an average diameter of 7.9 microns, while the Type II fibers (n = 74) has an average diameter of 12.9 microns suggesting disproportion of both fiber diameter and fiber type population (not shown in the figure)

Additional Investigation After the Muscle Biopsy Diagnosis

Next generation sequence panel showed compound heterozygous mutations of the ryanodine receptor (*RYR1*) gene: c.3381 + 1G > A (known pathogenic mutation) and c.3235_3240dup, p.Ser1079_Tyr1080dup (predicted to be pathogenic).

Final Diagnosis

CFTD due to autosomal recessive *RYR1* myopathy (compound heterozygous)

Patient Follow-up

At the time of last follow-up, 1.5 years from the initial diagnosis, the child had significant improvements in his gross motor milestones. He could walk unassisted for few steps. He was able to feed orally and his gastrostomy tube was removed. He continued to have muscle hypotonia and diminished reflexes. He was getting regular physical therapy. Family had been counseled regarding malignant hyperthermia risk due to *RYR1* mutation.

Discussion

The child in this vignette presented with neonatal hypotonia, poor feeding, and possible respiratory muscle weakness. Pertinent negatives were absence of family history and ocular findings (ptosis and ophthalmoplegia). He most likely had peripheral hypotonia from a neuromuscular disorder rather than central hypotonia as his reflexes were diminished and he had normal sensorium. The differential diagnosis for neonatal hypotonia is broad and involves different parts of the lower motor unit [1]. Anterior horn cell disorders particularly spinal muscular atrophy (SMA) type 1 was a consideration as he had diminished tendon reflexes. Peripheral neuropathies were also possible due to depressed reflexes. He did not have ocular manifestations but had possible bulbar and respiratory muscle involvement which might suggest the possibility of a neuromuscular junction (NMJ) disorder. Lastly genetic myopathies (congenital muscular dystrophy, congenital myopathy, and congenital myotonic dystrophy) are in the differential. His mother did not have clinical features of myotonic dystrophy type 1 making congenital myotonic dystrophy less likely (frequently transmitted from the affected mother). Negative family history either suggested autosomal recessive inheritance or a de novo mutation. The genetic disorders presenting with neonatal hypotonia and feeding difficulties which frequently mimics a neuromuscular disorder is Prader-Willi syndrome [2].

The investigative approach in a child with neonatal hypotonia from a peripheral neuromuscular disorder includes measurement of serum CK and metabolic work-up (lactate, serum carnitine, acylcarnitine, urine organic acids and acylglycine) [1]. A normal CK ruled out most of the congenital muscular dystrophies, though collagen-6-related myopathies can have normal or mildly high CK [3]. Metabolic work-up and genetic testing for PWS was negative. EMG will be the next important investigation. In this case, it helped to rule out anterior horn cell disorder and peripheral neuropathy. Myopathic EMG without signs of membrane irritability suggested the possibility of congenital myopathy. It should be kept in mind that in congenital myotonic dystrophy, typical myotonic discharges may not be present in the neonatal period [4]. Repetitive nerve stimulation can show decremental response in NMJ disorders (not performed in this case).

A muscle biopsy was considered as the next step in this case which showed features of CFTD. Next generation sequencing confirmed the final diagnosis of CFTD due to *RYR1* mutation.

Congenital fiber type disproportion (CFTD) is a relatively rare subtype of congenital myopathy. In order to qualify for this diagnosis, 2 important criteria must be met: (1) type I fibers are small while type II fibers are either normal or hypertrophied in absence of other major structural abnormalities (such as cores or rods) and (2) the clinical features are consistent with congenital myopathy [5, 6]. Our patient met both these criteria. The term CFTD has been used when the mean diameter of type I fiber is at least 12% smaller than the mean type II fiber diameter irrespective of clinical features [4]. As this definition is rather nonspecific, some authors prefer to use the term fiber size disproportion (FSD) and reserve CFTD only for patients when the patients have clinical features of a congenital myopathy [7]. Two studies looking at the children's muscle biopsies found that about 7% had FSD; only 10–20% of them (approximately 1% of all children biopsied) have CFTD [6].

Using the minimum cut off of 12% FSD, 67 children were identified with CFTD which fell to 50 children when the cut off was increased to 50% FSD, the latter group had a severe phenotype [6]. Majority of the patients present with neonatal hypotonia like our patient. Patients have varying degrees of weakness ranging from mild to severe either proximal muscle or generalized weakness [8]. Reflexes are usually reduced or absent. Joint contractures can be present at birth or develop later. Spinal deformities including scoliosis, kyphoscoliosis, and lordosis are seen in 25% of the patients [8]. Facial weakness/myopathic facies (long face, high-arched palate, and tented upper lip) and ophthalmoparesis can be present [6]. Feeding difficulties and respiratory involvement can be seen in about 30% of the patients [8]. Cardiac involvement and cognitive impairment are rarely noted [8, 9]. Serum CK is usually normal or mildly elevated [6, 8]. EMG can be normal, myopathic or mixed myopathic/neuropathic [6, 8]. CFTD can be caused by mutations in several genes. The following 6 genes have been implicated in CFTD: *ACTA1* (~6% of individuals with CFTD),

MYH7 (unknown), *RYR1* (~10–20%), *SELENON* (SEPN1) (rare), *TPM2* (rare) and *TPM3* (~20–25% of individuals with CFTD) [9–15]. Patients with *RYR1* mutation may have ophthalmoparesis but our patient did not have ophthalmoparesis [8].

At present, there are no specific or effective medical therapies for different genetic types of CFTD [8]. Treatment is mainly supportive with regular physical therapy and follow-up to detect respiratory failure, bulbar symptoms and orthopedic complications.

Pearls

Clinical Pearls

1. CFTD should be considered in a child with neonatal hypotonia, facial weakness, and feeding and respiratory difficulties.
2. CK is usually normal and EMG may show myopathic changes in CFTD.
3. CFTD is clinically and genetically heterogeneous; so far 6 genes have been implicated.

Pathology Pearls

1. The characteristic muscle biopsy findings of CFTD include abundant and hypotrophic type I fibers, normal or hypertrophic type II fibers, and lacking other histologic evidence of congenital myopathies (rods or cores).

References

1. Bodensteiner JB. The evaluation of the hypotonic infant. Semin Pediatr Neurol. 2008;15:10–20.
2. Angulo MA, Butler MG, Cataletto ME. Prader-Willi syndrome: a review of clinical, genetic, and endocrine findings. J Endocrinol Investig. 2015;38:1249–63.
3. Iannaccone ST, Castro D. Congenital muscular dystrophies and congenital myopathies. Continuum. 2013;19:1509–34.
4. Streib EW. AAEE minimonograph #27: differential diagnosis of myotonic syndromes. Muscle Nerve. 1987;10(7):603–15.
5. Brooke MH. Congenital fiber type disproportion. In: Kakulas BA, editor. Clinical studies in myology. Proceedings of the 2nd International Congress on Muscle Diseases, Perth, Australia, Nov. 22–29, 1971. Amsterdam: Exerpta Medica; 1973. p. 147–59.
6. Clarke NF, North KN. Congenital fiber type disproportion-30 years on. J Neuropathol Exp Neurol. 2003;62:977–89.
7. Iannaccone ST, Bove KE, Vogler CA, Buchino JJ. Type 1 fiber size disproportion: Morphometric data from 37 children with myopathic, neuropathic, or idiopathic hypotonia. Pediatr Pathol. 1987;7:395–419.

8. DeChene ET, Kang PB, Beggs AH. Congenital fiber-type disproportion. In: Adam MP, Ardinger HH, Pagon RA, Wallace SE, LJH B, Stephens K, et al., editors. GeneReviews® [Internet]. Seattle (WA): University of Washington, Seattle; 1993–2018. 2007 Jan 12; 2013.
9. Banwell BL, Becker LE, Jay V, Taylor GP, Vajsar J. Cardiac manifestations of congenital fiber-type disproportion myopathy. J Child Neurol. 1999;14:83–7.
10. Bevilacqua JA, Monnier N, Bitoun M, Eymard B, Ferreiro A, Monges S, et al. Recessive RYR1 mutations cause unusual congenital myopathy with prominent nuclear internalization and large areas of myofibrillar disorganization. Neuropathol Appl Neurobiol. 2011;37:271–84.
11. Cagliani R, Fruguglietti ME, Berardinelli A, D'Angelo MG, Prelle A, Riva S, et al. New molecular findings in congenital myopathies due to selenoprotein N gene mutations. J Neurol Sci. 2011;300:107–13.
12. Clarke NF, Ilkovski B, Cooper S, Valova VA, Robinson PJ, Nonaka I, et al. The pathogenesis of ACTA1-related congenital fiber type disproportion. Ann Neurol. 2007;61:552–61.
13. Clarke NF, Kolski H, Dye D, Lim E, Smith RL, Patel R, et al. Mutations in TPM3 are a common cause of congenital fiber type disproportion. Ann Neurol. 2008;63:329–37.
14. Clarke NF, Waddell LB, Sie LT, van Bon BW, McLean C, Clark D, et al. Mutations in TPM2 and congenital fibre type disproportion. Neuromuscul Disord. 2012;22:955–8.
15. Ortolano S, Tarrío R, Blanco-Arias P, Teijeira S, Rodríguez-Trelles F, García-Murias M, et al. A novel MYH7 mutation links congenital fiber type disproportion and myosin storage myopathy. Neuromuscul Disord. 2011;21:254–62.

Chapter 29
A 6-Year-Old Boy with Respiratory and Feeding Difficulties at Birth, Delayed Gross Motor Milestones, and Facial and Proximal Lower Limb Weakness

Partha S. Ghosh and Chunyu Cai

History

A 6-year-old boy presented to the neuromuscular clinic for muscle weakness. He was born at 36-week via caesarian-section, fetal movements were described as normal. He developed respiratory distress after birth requiring mechanical ventilation for 2 weeks followed by continuous positive airway pressure and oxygen. He also had trouble feeding requiring nasogastric tube followed by gastrostomy tube placement. He had delayed gross motor milestones (sat at 12 months and walked at 24 months). His running was uncoordinated, needed support to stand up from sitting position and to hold railing while climbing stairs. His mouth always stayed open; there was mild droopiness of his eyelids. He fatigued quickly but there was no diurnal variation of his symptoms. His swallowing eventually improved and gastrostomy tube was removed. His language, social and cognitive skills were normal. He had two sisters and one brother who were normal. There was no family history of neuromuscular disorders.

P. S. Ghosh (✉)
Department of Neurology, Boston Children's Hospital,
Boston, MA, USA
e-mail: partha.ghosh@childrens.harvard.edu

C. Cai
Department of Pathology, University of Texas Southwestern Medical Center,
Dallas, TX, USA
e-mail: chunyu.cai@utsouthwestern.edu

L. Zhou et al. (eds.), *A Case-Based Guide to Neuromuscular Pathology*,
https://doi.org/10.1007/978-3-030-25682-1_29

Physical Examination

On neurological examination he had mild ptosis without fatigability or ophthalmoparesis, myopathic facies, and high arched palate. He had generalized hypotonia and reduced muscle bulk. He had marked neck flexor weakness (MRC grade 3−/5) and mild neck extensor weakness (4/5), proximal upper limb weakness (deltoid, triceps, biceps 4+/5), and proximal lower limb weakness (iliopsoas, gluteus medius and maximus 4/5). He had mild scapular winging. Tendon reflexes were diminished (1+) diffusely. There was no percussion or grip myotonia. He had modified Gowers sign, waddling noticed during running. There was no calf hypertrophy or joint contractures. Sensory and cerebellar examinations were normal.

Investigations

He had normal serum creatine kinase (CK), lactate, thyroid functions, total and free carnitine, and acylcarnitine. MRI brain was normal. Nerve conduction study (NCS) showed normal sensory and motor responses in the upper and lower limbs. Needle electromyography (EMG) did not show increased insertional activity or abnormal spontaneous discharges; myopathic motor unit potentials were observed in tibialis anterior muscle. Repetitive nerve stimulation of the ulnar and peroneal nerves did not show decremental response at rest and after exercise. A left quadriceps muscle biopsy was performed.

Muscle Biopsy Findings

Muscle biopsy of the left quadriceps muscle showed increased fiber size variation with preponderance of type 1 fibers. There was presence of central cores which were confirmed on electron microscopy as well-demarcated foci of disruption of sarcomeric architecture, Z-line streaming, disruption of triads, and absence of mitochondria and other organelles. Overall features were consistent with central core myopathy.

Additional Investigation After the Muscle Biopsy Diagnosis

Next generation sequencing panel showed compound heterozygous mutations of the ryanodine receptor 1 (*RYR1*) gene: c.10204 T > G, p.Cys3402Gly (known pathogenic mutation) and c.4405C > T, pArg1469Trp (potentially pathogenic mutation). Parental testing could not be performed.

Final Diagnosis

Central Core Disease from Compound Heterozygous *RYR1* Mutations

Patient Follow-up

At the time of the last follow-up 6 months from the initial presentation, there was no progression of his muscle weakness. He was getting regular physical therapy and did not require assistive devices for ambulation. Parents were counseled regarding malignant hyperthermia risk.

Discussion

The child in this vignette presented with respiratory and feeding difficulties at birth, delayed gross motor milestones, and proximal lower limb weakness. In addition to proximal limb weakness, he had neck flexor weakness, facial weakness, mild ptosis, and diminished tendon reflexes. Pertinent negatives were absence of family history, diurnal variation of symptoms, ophthalmoparesis, calf hypertrophy, joint contractures, and normal sensory examination.

The differential diagnosis for this presentation was broad and involved different parts of the lower motor unit. Anterior horn cell disorders particularly spinal muscular atrophy (SMA) type 3 was a consideration in this case due to proximal weakness and diminished tendon reflexes but facial weakness and ptosis were against that diagnosis. The non-progressive course argued against the possibility of diffuse polyradiculoneuropathy. Peripheral neuropathies seemed unlikely given lack of distal weakness and sensory findings. Presence of ptosis, facial weakness and fatigue might suggest the possibility of a neuromuscular junction (NMJ) disorder. Early onset presentation and chronic course could suggest congenital myasthenic syndrome (CMS) rather than acquired autoimmune myasthenia gravis. However, lack of diurnal variation of symptoms and fatigability of ptosis were against a NMJ disorder. Myopathy seemed the most likely possibility given symmetric limb girdle pattern of weakness. Chronic course and early onset of symptoms suggested a genetic myopathy. Negative family history either suggested autosomal recessive inheritance or de novo mutation. Myopathies with facial weakness in children include congenital myopathies, mitochondrial myopathies, facioscapulohumeral muscular dystrophy (FSHD), myotonic dystrophy and rarely other muscular dystrophies [1].

The investigative approach in a child with myopathy includes measurement of serum CK, EMG, muscle ultrasound or muscle MRI, muscle biopsy and finally genetic testing [2, 3]. Measurement of serum CK level is an inexpensive and excellent screening tool in patients with suspected myopathies. Among the myopathic disorders with normal CK, congenital myopathies (CM) are the most common causes [2, 3]. Though high CK is commonly encountered in most of the muscular dystrophies, certain muscular dystrophies like FSHD and myotonic dystrophy can have normal CK [1, 2]. However, the pattern of weakness in this case did not suggest FSHD. Absence of myotonic discharges in EMG in this case made myotonic dystrophy less likely. EMG in CM can be myopathic or normal. SMA type 3 closely mimics myopathies due to limb girdle pattern of weakness. EMG in this case helped to rule out SMA which shows chronic neurogenic changes. Repetitive nerve stimulation of the distal nerves did not show evidence of a NMJ disorder. A muscle biopsy was considered as the next step in this case which showed features of central core disease. Next generation sequencing confirmed the final diagnosis of core myopathy due to *RYR1* mutations.

Congenital myopathies are a group of clinically and genetically heterogeneous conditions characterized by muscle weakness and distinctive structural abnormalities in muscle biopsies [3, 4]. Traditionally CM is classified histologically into 4 distinct types: central core disease, multi-minicore disease, centronuclear myopathy and nemaline myopathy based on the presence of central cores, multi-minicores, central nuclei and nemaline rods respectively [3, 4]. The pathological hallmark of core myopathy is the presence of clearly demarcated areas of pale staining on light microscopy called cores which lack reactivity to the oxidative stains (NADH, succinic dehydrogenase, as well as cytochrome c oxidase), but maintained ATPase reactivity (Fig. 29.1) [4, 5]. Cores lack mitochondria and contain disorganized myofibrils on electron microscopy. Central cores span the longitudinal length of the muscle fiber whereas minicores are present in a more transverse orientation [6]. There may be more than one core per muscle fiber, either located centrally or peripherally [5]. Morphologically, the closest mimicker to central cores are target or targetoid fibers, which may have similar light microscope and ultrastructural appearances (Fig. 29.2). Unlike central cores, target or targetoid changes are usually readily visible on ATPase stains (Fig. 29.2c). Target or targetoid fibers are typically associated with denervation and reinnervation, more commonly seen in adult muscle biopsy with a background of angulated atrophic fibers, group atrophy and fiber type grouping. Central cores, on the other hand, predominantly occur in pediatric muscle biopsy with a background of type I predominance and type I hypotrophy (Fig. 29.1).

RYR1 mutations are the most common cause of congenital myopathies in general and also the most frequently encountered childhood myopathy excluding Duchenne muscular dystrophy [7]. *RYR1* gene on chromosome 19q encodes a calcium-channel of the sarcoplasmic reticulum, which, along with sarcolemmal voltage-gated calcium channels (dihydropyridine receptor), is responsible for triggering muscle contraction after sarcolemmal depolarization and subsequent calcium release (excitation-contraction coupling) [8, 9]. Myopathies due to *RYR1* mutations is thought to disrupt excitation-contraction coupling due to reduced calcium release [4].

RYR1 related myopathies (RYR1-RM) are both pathologically and phenotypically complex and diverse. Histopathological RYR1-RM subtypes include central core disease, multiminicore disease, centronuclear myopathy, core-rod myopathy, and congenital fiber-type disproportion [5, 10–15]. All these histologic types of

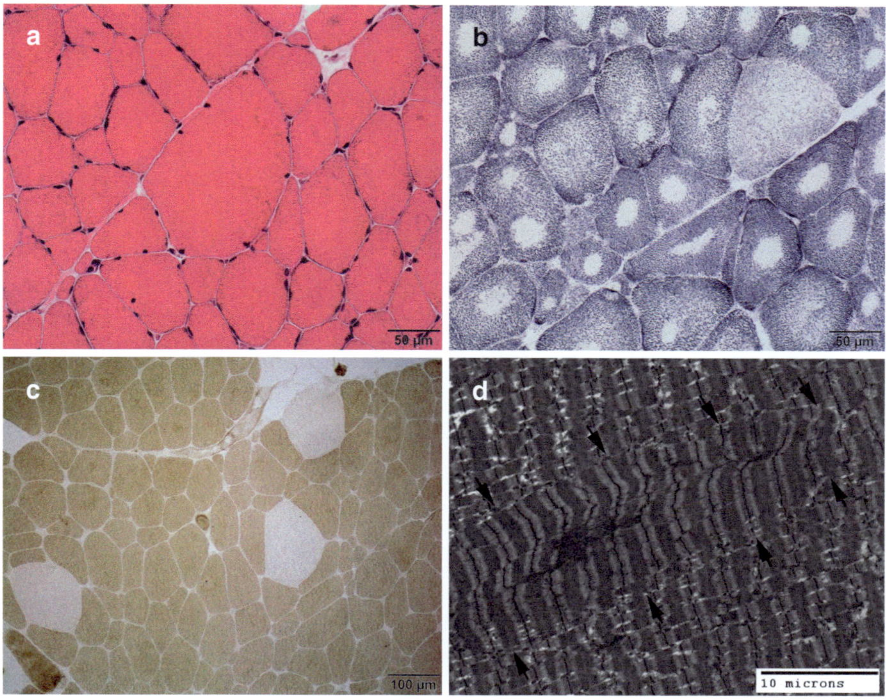

Fig. 29.1 Representative images from a separate 10-year-old boy with RYR1 mutation. (**a**) H&E stain shows marked fiber size variation. (**b**) NADH-TR stain shows well demarcated central cores in type I fibers. (**c**) ATPase at pH 4.3 shows type I (dark fibers) predominance and type I hypotrophy. Type II fibers (pale fibers) are mildly hypertrophied. (**d**) Electron microscopy shows that the central cores are composed of well demarcated mitochondria free zone (outlined by arrows) that runs parallel to the long axis of the myfiber, with or without central Z band streaming

RYR1-RM produce variable degree of muscle weakness. *RYR1* mutations can lead to other conditions including malignant hyperthermia (MH) susceptibility, exertional heat stroke, rhabdomyolysis-myalgia syndrome, King Denborough syndrome, and atypical periodic paralysis [16–19]. RYR1-RM can be inherited as autosomal dominant and recessive traits [4, 5]. Heterozygous recessive mutations have also been described due to epigenetic silencing of the wild type allele without an additional mutation in the other allele [20]. For the purpose of this vignette, we will briefly discuss central core disease due to *RYR1* mutations.

The most common phenotype encountered in patients with CCD is a nonprogressive, mild proximal limb-girdle weakness related to the dominant mutations in *RYR1*. However, some patients with CCD can have a severe infantile presentation that results in respiratory failure and impaired ambulation [4]. Such patients typically have de novo dominant mutations [21]. Patients with RYR1-related minicore myopathy usually have a severe phenotype (axial weakness more common as well musculoskeletal complications) and are usually associated with recessive *RYR1* mutations [4, 5]. Ophthalmoparesis is common in RYR1- related minicore

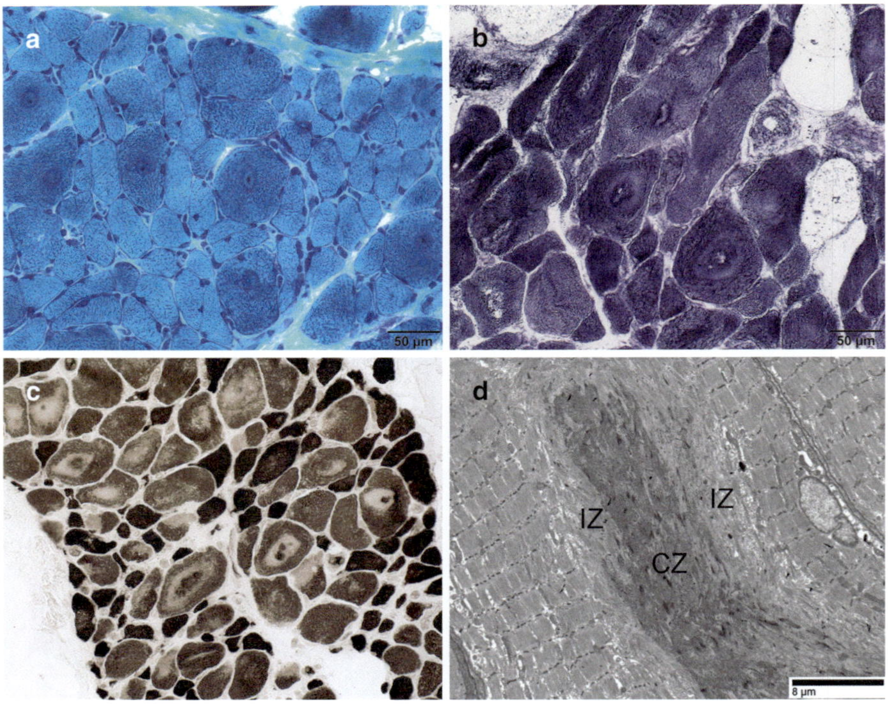

Fig. 29.2 Well-formed target fibers from a 37-year-old woman with amyotrophic lateral sclerosis (ALS). (**a**) Gomori trichrome. (**b**) NADH-TR. (**c**) ATPase at pH 9.4, dark fibers are type II, light fibers are type I. Besides target changes in type I fibers, the muscle also shows selective type II atrophy. (**d**): Electron microscopy shows a central zone (CZ) with electron dense filaments and disorganized Z band material, and an intermediate zone (IZ) with loss of normal sarcomere structure. Both CZ and IZ are devoid of mitochondria

disease and helps to clinically differentiate this from SEPN1-related minicore myopathy [22]. The patient presented in this case had a severe neonatal course with respiratory and feeding difficulty which fits with autosomal recessive inheritance and subsequently nonprogressive proximal muscle weakness which is commonly seen with CCD phenotype.

Serum creatinine kinase in CCD is usually normal or mildly elevated. EMG may show myopathic changes [5]. Muscle MRI shows selective involvement with sparing of certain muscle groups (rectus femoris, adductor longus, gracilis) in dominant RYR1-RM [23]; however, MRI findings are not consistent in recessively inherited cases. There is an overlap between CCD and MH susceptibility cases; patients with mutations at the N-terminal region have a higher probability of MH susceptibility [8]. Mutations are located in CCD hotspots including the C-terminal domain in 60% of RYR1-related CCD patients. Recessive mutations are found throughout the gene [4]. Patients with suspected RYR1-RM should have full *RYR1* gene sequencing [8, 24]. Next generation sequencing techniques are very helpful in detecting mutations in patients with suspected congenital myopathies [3].

Currently, there are no specific treatments for core myopathies but several small molecules have been tried in some patients. Dantrolene, a muscle relaxant effective against MH has been reported to be effective in a single case [25]. Salbutamol (Albuterol) had been found to be effective in a small case series [26]. N-acetylcysteine by reducing oxidative stress could be potential therapeutic agent in RYR1-RM [27]. Rycals are drugs which help to stabilize excitation-contraction coupling and thus may be helpful in this condition [28]. Gene-based therapies may be helpful in some of the RYR1-RM. Using exon-skipping strategy, researchers were able to remove a pseudo-exon formed by one of the mutations from an individual with compound heterozygous state resulting in restoration of *RYR1* expression and functional calcium release [29].

In the absence of a specific treatment, supportive management includes regular physical therapy and follow-up to detect respiratory failure, and orthopedic complications.

Pearls

Clinical Pearls

1. Core myopathy should be considered in a child with limb girdle pattern of weakness, non-progressive course, and facial weakness.
2. CK is usually normal and EMG may show myopathic changes.
3. Core myopathies are clinically and genetically heterogeneous; *RYR1* mutations are the most common cause of core myopathy.

Pathology Pearls

1. Muscle biopsy is the gold standard in the diagnosis of core myopathy.
2. Well demarcated mitochondria free zone parallel to the long axis of the myofiber on oxidative enzyme stains (e.g. NADH, SDH and COX) is the histologic hallmark of core myopathies.

References

1. Barohn RJ, Dimachkie MM, Jackson CE. A pattern recognition approach to patients with a suspected myopathy. Neurol Clin. 2014;32:569–93.
2. Al-Ghamdi F, Darras BT, Ghosh PS. Spectrum of neuromuscular disorders with HyperCKemia from a tertiary care pediatric neuromuscular center. J Child Neurol. 2018;33:389–96.
3. Jungbluth H, Treves S, Zorzato F, et al. Congenital myopathies: disorders of excitation-contraction coupling and muscle contraction. Nat Rev Neurol. 2018;14:151–67.
4. Gonorazky HD, Bönnemann CG, Dowling JJ. The genetics of congenital myopathies. Handb Clin Neurol. 2018;148:549–64.

5. Lawal TA, Todd JJ, Meilleur KG. Ryanodine receptor 1-related myopathies: diagnostic and therapeutic approaches. Neurotherapeutics. 2018;15:885–99.
6. Dubowitz V, Sewry CA, Oldfors A, et al. Muscle biopsy: a practical approach, expert consult; online and print, 4: muscle biopsy: a practical approach. Philadelphia: Elsevier - Health Sciences Division; 2013.
7. Darras BT, Royden Jones JJ, Ryan MM, et al. Neuromuscular disorders of infancy, childhood, and adolescence: a clinician's approach. London: Elsevier Science; 2014.
8. Wu S, Ibarra MC, Malicdan MC, et al. Central core disease is due to RYR1 mutations in more than 90% of patients. Brain. 2006;129:1470–80.
9. Meissner G. Regulation of mammalian ryanodine receptors. Front Biosci. 2002;7:2072–80.
10. Magee KR, Shy GM. A new congenital non-progressive myopathy. Brain. 1956;79:610–21.
11. Quane KA, Healy JM, Keating KE, et al. Mutations in the ryanodine receptor gene in central core disease and malignant hyperthermia. Nat genetics. 1993;5:51–5.
12. Ferreiro A, Monnier N, Romero NB, et al. A recessive form of central core disease, transiently presenting as multi-minicore disease, is associated with a homozygous mutation in the ryanodine receptor type 1 gene. Ann Neurol. 2002;51:750–9.
13. Fattori F, Maggi L, Bruno C, et al. Centronuclear myopathies: genotype-phenotype correlation and frequency of defined genetic forms in an Italian cohort. J Neurol. 2015;262:1728–40.
14. Scacheri PC, Hoffman EP, Fratkin JD, et al. A novel ryanodine receptor gene mutation causing both cores and rods in congenital myopathy. Neurology. 2000;55:1689–96.
15. Clarke NF, Waddell LB, Cooper ST, et al. Recessive mutations in RYR1 are a common cause of congenital fiber type disproportion. Hum Mut. 2010;31:E1544–50.
16. Dowling JJ, Lillis S, Amburgey K, et al. King-Denborough syndrome with and without mutations in the skeletal muscle ryanodine receptor (RYR1) gene. Neuromuscul Disord. 2011;21:420–7.
17. Matthews E, Neuwirth C, Jaffer F, et al. Atypical periodic paralysis and myalgia: a novel RYR1 phenotype. Neurology. 2018;90:e412–8.
18. Witting N, Werlauff U, Duno M, Vissing J. Phenotypes, genotypes, and prevalence of congenital myopathies older than 5 years in Denmark. Neurol Genet. 2017;3:e140.
19. Witting N, Werlauff U, Duno M, Vissing J. Phenotypes, genotypes, and prevalence of congenital myopathies older than 5 years in Denmark. Neurology: Genetics. 2017;3(2):e140.
20. Zhou H, Brockington M, Jungbluth H, et al. Epigenetic allele silencing unveils recessive RYR1 mutations in core myopathies. Am J Hum Genet. 2006;79:859–68.
21. Bharucha-Goebel DX, Santi M, Medne L, et al. Severe congenital RYR1-associated myopathy: the expanding clinicopathologic and genetic spectrum. Neurology. 2013;80:1584–9.
22. North KN, Wang CH, Clarke N, et al. Approach to the diagnosis of congenital myopathies. Neuromuscul Disord. 2014;24:97–116.
23. Klein A, Jungbluth H, Clement E, et al. Muscle magnetic resonance imaging in congenital myopathies due to ryanodine receptor type 1 gene mutations. Arch Neurol. 2011;68:1171–9.
24. Shepherd S, Ellis F, Halsall J, Hopkins P, Robinson R. RYR1 mutations in UK central core disease patients: more than just the C-terminal transmembrane region of the RYR1 gene. J Med Genet. 2004;41:e33.
25. Jungbluth H, Dowling JJ, Ferreiro A, et al. 182nd ENMC International Workshop: RYR1-related myopathies, 15–17th April 2011, Naarden, The Netherlands. Neuromuscul Disord. 2012;22:453–62.
26. Messina S, Hartley L, Main M, et al. Pilot trial of salbutamol in central core and multi-minicore diseases. Neuropediatrics. 2004;35:262–6.
27. Moulin M, Ferreiro A. Muscle redox disturbances and oxidative stress as pathomechanisms and therapeutic targets in early-onset myopathies. Semin Cell Dev Biol. 2017;64:213–23.
28. Marks AR. Calcium cycling proteins and heart failure: mechanisms and therapeutics. J Clin Invest. 2013;123:46–52.
29. Rendu J, Brocard J, Denarier E, et al. Exon skipping as a therapeutic strategy applied to an RYR1 mutation with pseudo-exon inclusion causing a severe core myopathy. Hum Gene Ther. 2013;24:702–13.

Chapter 30
A 12-Year-Old Girl with a 2-Year History of Progressive Limb Weakness and Difficulties with Exercise

Diana P. Castro, Chunyu Cai, and Dustin Jacob Paul

History

A 12-year-old girl with a past medical history of sensorineural hearing loss was brought to our clinic for evaluation of a 2-year history of progressive weakness and difficulties with exercise. Specifically, she reported difficulties skiing, playing basketball and physical education class. She ran slower than her classmates, had difficulties turning her feet, standing up from the floor, and going up the stairs, and had more falls than usual. During a recent travel, she had more difficulty walking on the uneven sidewalks. She also heard her hips "popping" loudly with walking. She complained of hip pain with walking for longer periods of time and her ankles also "pop". She denied any cramping pain or muscle pain though. Her birth history was remarkable for pregnancy complicated due to incompetent cervix. She was delivered vaginally at 34 weeks gestation. She required oxygen for 1 hour at birth due to respiratory distress. Her developmental history was unremarkable, in terms of gross motor, fine motor, language and social skills as well as cognition. Family history was remarkable for positive Factor V Leiden in her mother and sensorineural hearing loss in her father.

D. P. Castro (✉)
Department of Neurology and Neurotherapeutics, University of Texas Southwestern Medical Center, Children's Medical Center of Dallas, Dallas, TX, USA
e-mail: diana.castro@utsuthwestern.edu

C. Cai
Department of Pathology, University of Texas Southwestern Medical Center, Dallas, TX, USA
e-mail: chunyu.cai@utsouthwestern.edu

D. Jacob Paul
Department of Neurology and Neurotherapeutics, University of Texas Southwestern Medical Center, Dallas, TX, USA
e-mail: dustin.paul@utsouthwestern.edu

L. Zhou et al. (eds.), *A Case-Based Guide to Neuromuscular Pathology*,
https://doi.org/10.1007/978-3-030-25682-1_30

Physical Examination

On physical examination, she had long narrow face with high arched palate. Cranial nerves were normal except for eye closure weakness bilaterally and decreased hearing bilaterally. Muscle bulk and muscle tone decreased in the lower extremities. No tremors were noted. Muscle strength was decreased at the neck flexors (MRC 2/5), hip abductors (2/5), hip extensors (1/5) and ankle dorsiflexors (4+/5). Sensory exam was remarkable for decreased vibration in ankles and toes. Deep tendon reflexes were absent. Gait showed exaggerated lordosis, knee flexion and genu valgum.

Investigations

Her serum creatine kinase (CK) was elevated ranging from 1,302 to 1,506 U/L (normal 50–350). Her spine MRI was significant for a syrinx in the cervical cord. It also demonstrated a large area of fat replacement in the gluteus medius muscle. Her pelvic X-rays demonstrated subluxation of the left femoral head. Her nerve conduction study (NCS) was normal and electromyography (EMG) showed some large-amplitude and long-duration motor unit potentials in the first dorsal interosseous and vastus medialis muscles. Pulmonary function test showed evidence of the restrictive abnormality with a reduced forced vital capacity of 70%. A left quadriceps muscle biopsy was performed.

Muscle Biopsy Findings

The muscle biopsy shows striking vacuolar changes predominantly involving type 2 myofibers (Fig. 30.1a, b), many of which are atrophic. The vacuoles are variably sized, distributed throughout the myofibers, and positive on acid phosphatase stain (Fig. 30.1c) which confirms their lysosomal origin. Periodic acid Schiff (PAS) in non-aqueous solution without diastase (Fig. 30.1d) and electron microscopy (Fig. 30.1e, f) confirm abnormal glycogen storage materials within the lysosome bound vacuoles. The collective findings are those of a lysosomal glycogen storage myopathy, most consistent with acid maltase deficiency.

Additional Investigation After the Muscle Biopsy Diagnosis

The acid alpha-1,4 glucosidase (GAA) gene sequencing for Pompe disease was positive for compound heterozygous mutations described as c.-32-13 T > G and c.213 T > C.

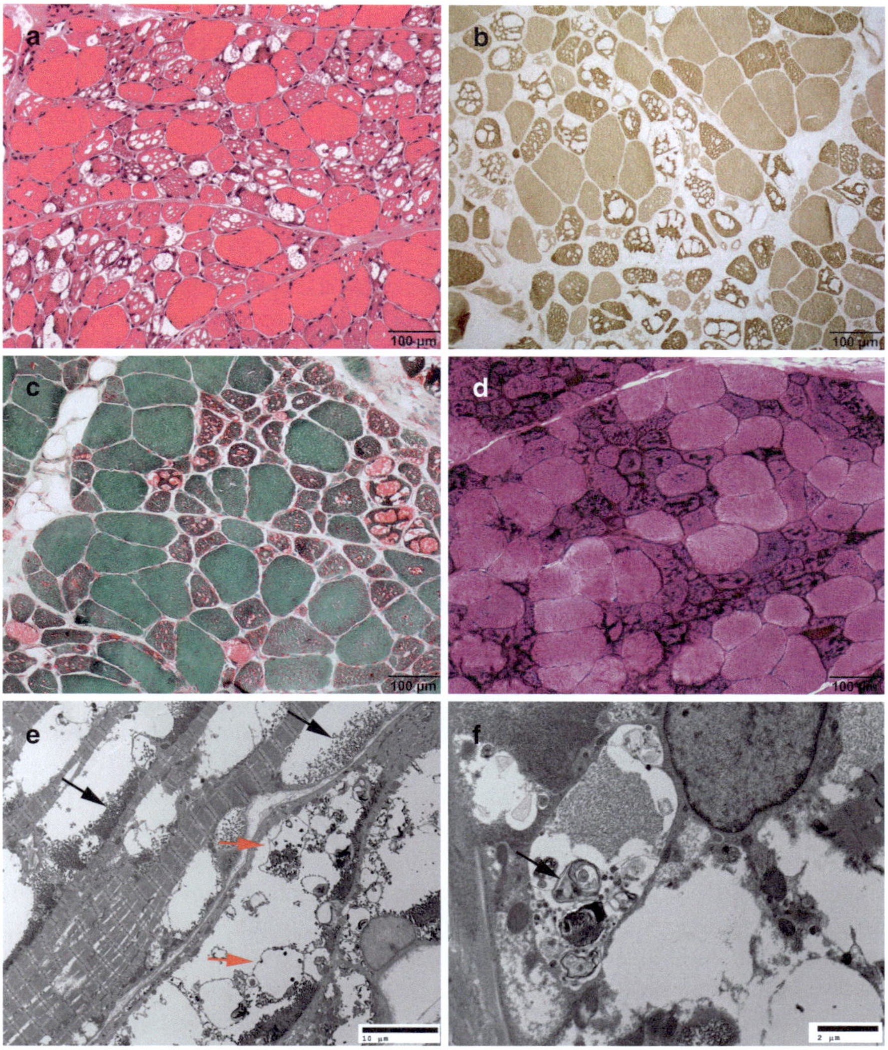

Fig. 30.1 Acid maltase deficiency. (**a**) H&E shows a vacuolar myopathy. (**b**) ATPase at pH 9.4 shows that the myofibers that contain vacuoles are predominantly type 2. There is also type 2 smallness. (**c**) Acid phosphatase stain shows that the vacuoles are stained red due to their lysosomal origin. (**d**) PAS stain without diastase confirms glycogen storage in the vacuoles. (**e**) Electron microscopy shows abundant free (black arrows) and lysosome bound (red arrows) glycogen particles in the vacuoles. (**f**) Some vacuoles also contain myeloid debris (arrow)

Final Diagnosis

Pompe Disease (Acid Maltase Deficiency)

Patient Follow-up

The patient was started on the enzyme replacement therapy (ERT) with Lumizyme every 2 weeks. Her motor function had stabilized and even improved over 5 years on the treatment. Respiratory function had also improved with better FVC. Her mild-to-moderate hearing loss was treated with a hearing aid.

Discussion

Pompe disease, also referred to as acid maltase deficiency or type II glycogen storage disease, is an autosomal recessive disease caused by mutations in the gene encoding lysosomal acid alpha-1,4 glucosidase (GAA) leading to a deficiency of the acid alpha glucosidase or acid maltase enzyme with secondary accumulation of glycogen in lysosomes [1]. The estimated incidence of GAA deficiency was 1 in 40,000 [2]. Deficiency of the enzyme leads to glycogen accumulation in lysosomes and cytoplasm, resulting in tissue destruction [3, 4]. The classic infantile form presents with hypertrophic cardiomyopathy, generalized hypotonia, and elevated CK. In the juvenile and adult forms, clinical features are widely variable. There is usually a slowly progressive myopathy with eventual respiratory muscle involvement. Children have delayed gross motor milestones with diaphragm involvement, sleep-disordered breathing and limb girdle muscle weakness. Adults also have limb girdle weakness and have diaphragm involvement relatively early. The heart is less involved with adult onset. Differential diagnosis consists of fatty oxidation disorders, mitochondrial disorders, other glycogen storage disorders, and muscular dystrophies. Initial diagnostic evaluation includes serum CK level and NCS/EMG. Patients can have neurogenic findings on EMG probably due to the co-existing motor neuron involvement, as the results from early autopsy investigations showed that spinal cord anterior horn cells, motor nuclei of the brain stem, and spinal ganglia were susceptible particularly in infantile Pompe disease [5–7]. In this clinic setting, the diagnosis of Pompe disease can be challenging, and a muscle biopsy is helpful as seen in our case. Measuring GAA enzyme activity in white blood cells or dried blood spots can be used to screen patients. Diagnostic confirmation is made through sequencing of the GAA gene. GAA gene encodes lysosomal acid alpha-1,4 glucosidase located at chromosome 17q25.2-q25.3 [1].

Pompe disease defers from all other types of glycogen storage diseases as the enzyme is located within lysosomes. Acid maltase deficiency results in glycogen accumulation within lysosomes that are positive for both acid phosphatase stain, which detects lysosomes, and PAS stain, which detects glycogen. Vacuolar changes are usually prominent in the infantile-onset form; however, they can be quite subtle or absent in selected muscle groups in patients with the late-onset disease (see Chap. 16). The most sensitive finding in a mildly affected muscle is diffusely increased sarcoplasmic punctate acid phosphatase reactivity, or in some cases, increased lipofuscin particles [8]. However, these findings are not specific. Main differential considerations include other lysosomal vacuolar myopathies associated with Danon disease, X-linked myopathy with excessive autophagy (XMEA), myotoxicities of drugs such as chloroquine, hydroxychloroquine (see Chap. 19) and colchicine, vitamin E deficiency [9] and aging. On the other hand, a muscle biopsy with normal histology does not exclude the possibility of acid maltase deficiency, especially in the late-onset cases. Mild denervation changes are relatively common in muscle biopsies from patients with acid maltase deficiency, likely due to motor neuron involvement.

Treatment of Pompe disease is ERT with alglucosidase alfa. With the advent of ERT, prognosis of Pompe disease has improved. Adverse effects of ERT include hypersensitivity reactions and development of antibodies to alglucosidase alfa [10]. Other genetic therapies are on the preclinical stages or early clinical phases [11, 12].

Pearls

Clinical Pearls

1. Infantile-onset Pompe disease presents typically very early with hypotonia and hypertrophic cardiomyopathy.
2. Pompe disease has to be considered in children with delayed motor development and problems related to limb-girdle weakness.
3. Children with Pompe disease may have myopathic face, hyporeflexia or areflexia, and scoliosis. Pulmonary function is decreased in approximately half of the patients.
4. Pompe disease should be included in the differential diagnosis in children with less familiar signs such as disproportional weakness of the neck flexors, unexplained fatigue, persistent diarrhea and unexplained high CK and liver function test.

Pathology Pearls

1. The hallmark of Pompe disease on muscle biopsy is the presence of glycogen-filled vacuoles that are positive for acid phosphatase, selectively affecting type 2 myofibers.
2. Muscle involvement is quite variable in late-onset Pompe disease. Rectus femoris, sartorius, and gracilis muscles are typically spared. A muscle biopsy with normal histology does not completely exclude late-onset Pompe disease.

3. In muscle with mild involvement, the most sensitive finding is diffusely increased, punctate sarcoplasmic acid phosphatase reactivity.
4. Neurogenic changes are common in Pompe disease, owing to motor neuron deficiency.

References

1. Martiniuk F, Mehler M, Tzall S, Meredith G, Hirschhorn R. Sequence of the cDNA and 5′-flanking region for human acid alpha-glucosidase, detection of an intron in the 5′ untranslated leader sequence, definition of 18-bp polymorphisms, and differences with previous cDNA and amino acid sequences. DNA Cell Biol. 1990;9(2):85–94.
2. Ausems MG, Verbiest J, Hermans MP, Kroos MA, Beemer FA, Wokke JH, et al. Frequency of glycogen storage disease type II in The Netherlands: implications for diagnosis and genetic counselling. Eur J Hum Genet. 1999;7(6):713–6.
3. Raben N, Plotz P, Byrne BJ. Acid alpha-glucosidase deficiency (glycogenosis type II, Pompe disease). Curr Mol Med. 2002;2(2):145–66.
4. Orth M, Mundegar RR. Effect of acid maltase deficiency on the endosomal/lysosomal system and glucose transporter 4. Neuromuscul Disord. 2003;13(1):49–54.
5. Gambetti P, DiMauro S, Baker L. Nervous system in Pompe's disease. Ultrastructure and biochemestry. J Neuropathol Exp Neurol. 1971;30(3):412–30.
6. El M, Ge A, Berry RG. Pompe's disease (Diffuse Glycogenosis) with neuronal storage. J Neuropathol Exp Neurol. 1965;24:85–96.
7. Martin JJ, De Barsy T, Van Hoof F, Palladini G. Pompe's disease: an inborn lysosomal disorder with storage of glycogen. Astudyof a brain and striated muscle. Acta Neuropathol. 1973;23(3):229–44.
8. Feeney EJ, Austin S, Chien YH, Mandel H, Schoser B, Prater S, Hwu WL, Ralston E, Kishnani PS, Raben N. The value of muscle biopsies in Pompe disease: identifying lipofuscin inclusions in juvenile and adult-onset patients. Acta Neuropathol Commun. 2014;2(2):PMC3892035. https://doi.org/10.1186/2051-5960-2-2.
9. Neville HE, Ringel SP, Guggenheim MA, Wehling CA, Starcevich JM. Ultrastructural and histochemical abnormalities of skeletal muscle in patiernts with chronic vitamin E deficiency. Neurology. 1983;33(4):483–8.
10. Nicolino M, Byrne B, Wraith JE, Leslie N, Mandel H, Freyer DR, et al. Clinical outcomes after long-term treatment with alglucosidase alfa in infants and children with advanced Pompe disease. Genet Med. 2009;11(3):210–9.
11. Falk DJ, Soustek MS, Todd AG, Mah CS, Cloutier DA, Kelley JS, et al. Comparative impact of AAV and enzyme replacement therapy on respiratory and cardiac function in adult Pompe mice. Mol Ther Methods Clin Dev. 2015;2:15007.
12. Poenaru L. Approach to gene therapy of glycogenosis type II (Pompe disease). Mol Genet Metab. 2000;70(3):163–9.

Chapter 31
A 3-Month-Old Boy with Generalized Hypotonia, Weakness, Pneumonia and Respiratory Failure

Diana P. Castro, Chunyu Cai, and Dustin Jacob Paul

History

A 3-month-old boy presented to the emergency department with a 1-day history of decreased oral intake and fever with a temperature as high as 39 degrees Celsius. His mother denied cough, congestion, vomiting, diarrhea or sick contacts. Blood, urine, and CSF cultures were obtained, and the patient was started on broad coverage antibiotics. Chest X-ray showed bilateral peri-hilar infiltrates and pneumonia, and urine analysis was concerning for urinary tract infection.

The patient was admitted to the Pediatric Intensive Care Unit. The patient was in severe respiratory distress requiring several forms of non-invasive ventilation, until he was electively intubated to place a gastrostomy tube and perform Nissen due to severe oral and pharyngeal dysphagia, as well as aspiration. He was extubated after the procedures, but his ventilation was poor, even on continuous non-invasive ventilation.

D. P. Castro (✉)
Department of Neurology and Neurotherapeutics, University of Texas Southwestern Medical Center, Children's Medical Center of Dallas, Dallas, TX, USA
e-mail: diana.castro@utsouthwestern.edu

C. Cai
Department of Pathology, University of Texas Southwestern Medical Center, Dallas, TX, USA
e-mail: Chunyu.cai@utsputhwestern.edu

D. Jacob Paul
Department of Neurology and Neurotherapeutics, University of Texas Southwestern Medical Center, Dallas, TX, USA
e-mail: dustin.paul@utsouthwestern.edu

L. Zhou et al. (eds.), *A Case-Based Guide to Neuromuscular Pathology*,
https://doi.org/10.1007/978-3-030-25682-1_31

Physical Examination

The examination upon admission showed that the patient was in respiratory distress on non-invasive ventilation. His chest wall was notable for significant pectus excavatum with a paradoxical breathing pattern. He had a weak cry and suck and would open his eyes spontaneously and look at faces. There were tongue fasciculations. He had generalized severe muscle hypotonia, minimal spontaneous movements and no antigravity movements. He was unable to hold his head with severe head lag and axillary slippage. Deep tendon reflexes were absent. Palmar and plantar reflexes were absent.

Investigations

A rectus abdominis muscle biopsy was performed.

Muscle Biopsy Findings

The rectus abdominis muscle biopsy (Fig. 31.1) showed groups of round, markedly atrophic fibers interspersed among large fibers (Fig. 31.1a). Large fibers were markedly hypertrophied and exclusively type 1; small atrophic fibers were mixed (Fig. 31.1b). The findings are consistent with spinal muscular atrophy (SMA) type 1.

Investigations After the Muscle Biopsy Diagnosis

The survival motor neuron (SMN) gene test showed a homozygous deletion of exons 7 and 8. The SMN2 copy number was not obtained.

Final Diagnosis

Spinal Muscular Atrophy Type 1

Patient Follow-up

The patient continued to deteriorate and his family decided to withdraw support at 4 months of age. At autopsy, the intercostal and psoas muscles showed marked neurogenic atrophy similar to the rectus abdominis muscle. Muscle from the diaphragm

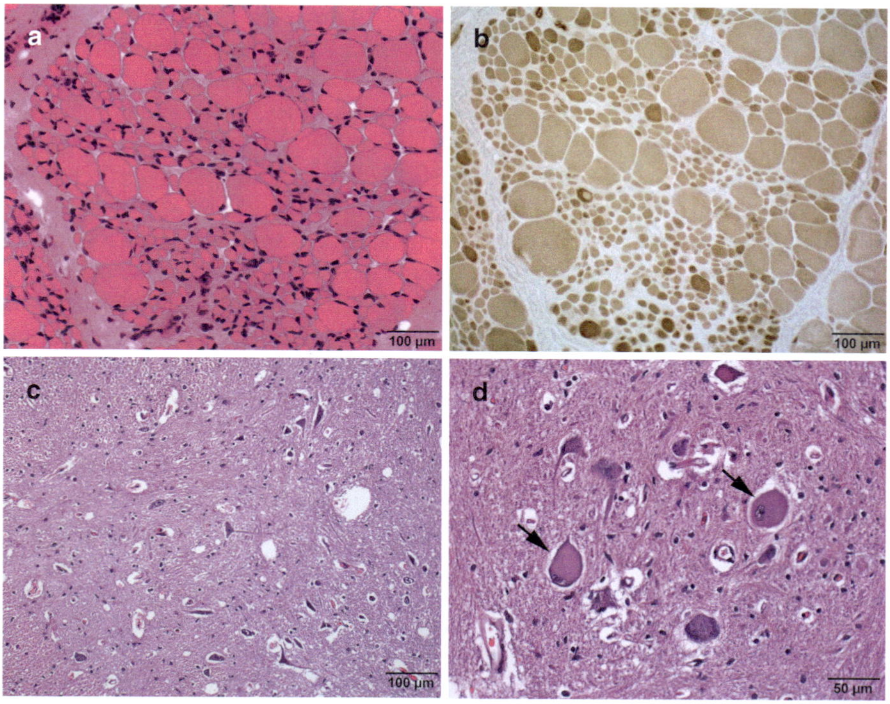

Fig. 31.1 SMA type 1. (**a**) H&E and (**b**) ATPase at pH 9.4 are images from the rectus abdominis muscle biopsy performed at age of 3 months. (**c**) H&E of spinal cord anterior horn and (**d**) thoracic cord Clark column are images from the same patient at time of autopsy, at 4 months of age. Arrows in (**d**) indicate balloon neurons

was relatively normal. The spinal cord showed moderate to severe loss of anterior horn pyramidal neurons and reactive astrocytosis (Fig. 31.1c). The thoracic cord Clarke neurons showed marked ballooning change in a background of reactive astrocytosis (Fig. 31.1d). Elsewhere, the lungs showed diffuse bilateral acute bronchopneumonia. Postmortem culture from the lungs grew multiple bacterial organisms including *Escherichia coli*, *Alpha hemolytic streptococcus*, *Staphylococcus aureus*, and *Enterobacter aerogenes*. The cause of death was determined as SMA type 1 complicated by failure to thrive, respiratory failure and pneumonia.

Discussion

Spinal muscular atrophy (SMA) is an autosomal recessive disease caused in 95% of cases by a homozygous deletion of exons 7 and 8 of the SMN1 gene [1] located on chromosome 5q. The most common mutation of SMN1 is a deletion of exon 7 [2]. The carrier frequency of SMN1 mutations ranges from 1 in 90 to 1 in 47 [3]. The number of SMN2 copies determines the clinical phenotype. It is classified into four types, depending on the age of symptom onset and maximal motor function achieved by the patient. SMA type 1 typically presents before 6 months of age with hypotonia, progressive proximal and distal weakness, fasciculations and the inability to achieve normal developmental milestones like head control or sitting without support [4, 5]. The intercostal muscles are affected, and the diaphragm is spared resulting in paradoxical breathing and a bell-shaped chest as seen in our patient. SMA type 2 presents between 6–18 months of age and are able to sit unassisted but are not able to achieve independent ambulation [6]. SMA type 3 presents weakness after 18 months and are able to achieve independent ambulation but in most cases will lose this ability with time. SMA type 4 usually has onset after 30 years of age. Sensation and cognition are usually spared. Differential diagnosis includes spinal muscular atrophy with respiratory distress type 1 (SMARD1), congenital myasthenic syndromes, congenital myopathies, congenital muscular dystrophies, glycogen storage disease type II, Prader-Willi, and Zellweger as well other conditions that can present with hypotonia. Diagnosis of SMA consists of molecular genetic testing with targeted mutation analysis of the SMN1 gene and copy number analysis of the SMN2 gene. Electrophysiological studies are rarely performed.

Muscle biopsy is becoming increasingly uncommon as the genetic test is commercially available and is the first line definitive diagnostic test when SMA is clinically suspected. The muscle pathology of SMA type 1 is characterized by a unique infantile denervation pattern. Large fibers are hypertrophied and exclusively type 1, which differs from most other types of denervation atrophy. Small fibers are mixed or predominantly type 2. The small fibers are polygonal or round rather than angular, and usually do not show strong esterase positivity. In SMA type 2, the hypertrophy of type 1 fibers are often more pronounced, giving the appearance of islands of huge type 1 fibers floating in a sea of small type 2 fibers (Fig. 31.2a, b). In SMA type 3 and 4, the muscle changes are less specific and may be difficult to differentiate from other types of denervation atrophy.

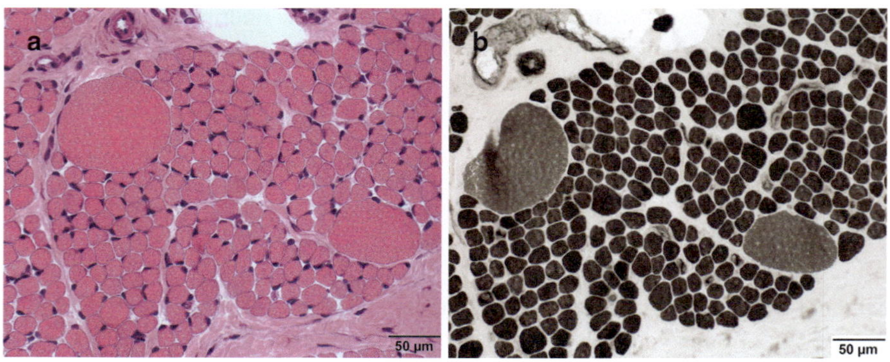

Fig. 31.2 Quadriceps muscle biopsy from a 2-year-old female with SMA type 2. (**a**) H&E. (**b**) ATPase 9.4

Differential considerations include congenital muscular dystrophy, congenital myopathies, and other types of denervation atrophy, such as Chacot-Marrie-Tooth disease. Congenital muscular dystrophies may also demonstrate marked fiber size variation and fiber hypertrophy. However, the endomysial connective tissue is usually markedly expanded, with variable presence of acute and chronic myopathic changes, which differs from SMA. Congenital myopathies may also demonstrate a bi-model fiber size variation and minimal interstitial fibrosis. However, in congenital myopathies the larger fibers are type 2 and smaller fibers type 1, opposite from SMA. Other types of denervation atrophy typically lack uniform type 1 hypertrophy.

Patient with SMA should be managed by multidisciplinary clinics that include neuromuscular specialists, therapists, and pulmonologists [7–9]. Nusinersen (Spinraza™) is the only FDA approved medication for the treatment of SMA. Nusinersen is an antisense oligonucleotide designed to increase the expression of survival motor neuron protein by enhancing the SMN2 gene and is delivered intrathecally every 4 months lifelong. This is currently changing the clinical landscape of SMA, and with other therapies in research trials it will continue to change in the years to come such as gene transfer therapy [10]. Unfortunately, when this patient presented, there were no therapies available and many families opted for withdrawing care due to the poor prognosis.

Pearls

Clinical Pearls

1. SMA should be considered in patients with generalized hypotonia, proximal and distal weakness, areflexia and tongue fasciculations.
2. Cognition and sensory examination are completely normal in patients with SMA.
3. Nusinersen (Spinraza™) is the only FDA approved medication for the treatment of patients with SMA types 1, 2 and 3. This medication has drastically changed the prognosis of this condition. According to the clinical studies, more than 50% of patients with SMA type 1 treated before 6 months of age reached milestones previously not seen in these patients, such as the capacity of holding their heads, sitting, kicking and standing [11].

Pathology Pearls

1. Islands of markedly hypertrophic type 1 fibers floating in a sea of small mixed type 1 and 2 fibers are characteristic findings in SMA type 1 and type 2.
2. The absence of myopathic changes and interstitial fibrosis distinguishes SMA from congenital muscular dystrophy and congenital myopathies.

References

1. Prior TW, Finanger E. Spinal Muscular Atrophy. In: Adam MP, Ardinger HH, Pagon RA, Wallace SE, Bean LJH, Stephens K, et al., editors. GeneReviews®. Seattle (WA): University of Washington; 1993.
2. Ogino S, Wilson RB. Genetic testing and risk assessment for spinal muscular atrophy (SMA). Hum Genet. 2002;111(6):477–500.
3. Sugarman EA, Nagan N, Zhu H, Akmaev VR, Zhou Z, Rohlfs EM, et al. Pan-ethnic carrier screening and prenatal diagnosis for spinal muscular atrophy: clinical laboratory analysis of >72,400 specimens. Eur J Hum Genet. 2012;20(1):27–32.
4. Darras BT. Spinal muscular atrophies. Pediatr Clin N Am. 2015;62(3):743–66.
5. Kolb SJ, Kissel JT. Spinal Muscular Atrophy. Neurol Clin. 2015;33(4):831–46.
6. Mercuri E, Bertini E, Iannaccone ST. Childhood spinal muscular atrophy: controversies and challenges. Lancet Neurol. 2012;11(5):443–52.
7. Arnold WD, Kassar D, Kissel JT. Spinal muscular atrophy: diagnosis and management in a new therapeutic era. Muscle Nerve. 2015;51(2):157–67.
8. Mercuri E, Finkel RS, Muntoni F, Wirth B, Montes J, Main M, et al. Diagnosis and management of spinal muscular atrophy: Part 1: Recommendations for diagnosis, rehabilitation, orthopedic and nutritional care. Neuromuscul Disord. 2018;28(2):103–15.
9. Finkel RS, Mercuri E, Meyer OH, Simonds AK, Schroth MK, Graham RJ, et al. Diagnosis and management of spinal muscular atrophy: Part 2: Pulmonary and acute care; medications, supplements and immunizations; other organ systems; and ethics. Neuromuscul Disord. 2018;28(3):197–207.
10. Mendell JR, Al-Zaidy S, Shell R, Arnold WD, Rodino-Klapac LR, Prior TW, et al. Single-dose gene-replacement therapy for spinal muscular atrophy. N Engl J Med. 2017;377(18):1713–22.
11. Finkel RS, Mercuri E, Darras BT, Connolly AM, Kuntz NL, Kirschner J. Nusinersen vs. Sham control in infantile- onset spinal muscular atrophy. N Engl J Med. 2017;377(18):1723–32.

Part III
Neuropathy Cases

Chapter 32
A 59-Year-Old Woman with Subacute Lower Limb Weakness and Painful Paresthesia

Shaida Khan and Chunyu Cai

History

A 59-year-old woman presented with a subacute onset of symmetric lower extremity weakness, painful paresthesias and gait instability. Symptom onset was 3 months prior to her presentation and symptoms were mild initially. However, there was a significant decline in neurological symptoms in the prior 3 weeks, with new painful sensory disturbances in her hands and difficulty gripping objects bilaterally. Her leg weakness progressed rapidly, and she was completely unable to ambulate upon presentation. Notably, in the past 3 months, she had a 50-pound unintentional weight loss. There was associated joint pain diffusely throughout her arms and legs. There was no associated rash, photosensitivity, fever, cough, or dryness of the eyes or mouth. Her past medical history included hypertension and diabetes mellitus type 2. There was a family history of diabetes but no neurological or rheumatologic disorders. She denied alcohol use, tobacco use, illicit drugs, or any recent travels outside the U.S. Her medications at the time of her presentation included Lasix 20 mg twice daily and Novolin 2–4 units three times daily before meals.

S. Khan (✉)
Department of Neurology and Neurotherapeutics, University of Texas Southwestern Medical Center, Dallas, TX, USA
e-mail: shaida.khan@UTSouthwestern.edu

C. Cai
Department of Pathology, University of Texas Southwestern Medical Center, Dallas, TX, USA
e-mail: Chunyu.cai@UTSouthwestern.edu

L. Zhou et al. (eds.), *A Case-Based Guide to Neuromuscular Pathology*,
https://doi.org/10.1007/978-3-030-25682-1_32

Physical Examination

She was in no acute distress and appeared well nourished. There was no malar rash, sclerodermatous changes, telangiectasias, nailfold capillary changes, palmar erythema or livedo reticularits over face or four extremities. Cardiac, lung, and abdominal examinations were normal.

Her neurological examination demonstrated severe distal > proximal upper and lower extremity weakness. Weakness was detected in the bilateral shoulder abduction (MRC 4/5), elbow flexion (4/5), elbow extension (4−/5), wrist flexion and extension (right 0/5, left 1/5), finger flexion and extension (0/5), finger abduction (right 0/5, left 1/5), hip flexion (right 2/5, left 3/5), hip abduction and adduction (4−/5), knee flexion (right 2/5, left 3/5), knee extension (4/5), and ankle and toe dorsiflexion and plantar flexion (0/5). Deep tendon reflexes were diminished at the biceps, triceps, and brachioradialis, and absent at the knees and ankles. Toes were downgoing bilaterally. Sensory impairment was noted in the upper and lower extremities, with diminished pinprick and temperature sensation in the extensor surfaces of the arms and in the hands, and absent sensation to all sensory modalities below the knees.

Investigations

Laboratory studies were notable for a positive ANA at a high titer of >1:2,560, double stranded DNA antibody >1:2,560, elevated anti-Smith antibody at 1.7, low C3 complement at 39, and low C4 complement at 6. These findings were consistent with a newly diagnosed systemic lupus erythematosus (SLE). RNP antibody was also elevated at >8 and anti-Ro (SS-A) was elevated at 1.3. Anti-La (SS-B) was <0.2. p-ANCA and c-ANCA were negative. Erythrocyte sedimentation rate (ESR) was 30 mm/hr. Hepatitis C serology, hepatitis B surface antigen, and Lyme serologies were all negative. Complete blood count (CBC) showed anemia with hemoglobin and hematocrit being 10 g/dL and 29.6%, respectively, but white blood cell (WBC) and platelet counts were normal. Comprehensive metabolic panel showed elevated AST (82 U/L) and alkaline phosphatase (295 U/L) with normal ALT (16 U/L), and normal renal function. Creatine kinase (CK) and aldolase were normal at 16 and 7.5 U/L, respectively. Cerebrospinal fluid (CSF) studies were normal. Nerve conduction studies (NCS) and electromyography (EMG) showed a severe axonal sensorimotor polyneuropathy with active denervation changes seen in all the distal upper and lower extremity muscles examined. Given the subacute onset of severe sensorimotor impairment, slight asymmetry on examination, and serologic evidence of newly diagnosed SLE, a combined right sural nerve and gastrocnemius muscle biopsy was pursued for evaluation of a potential vasculitic neuropathy.

Nerve and Muscle Biopsy Findings

The right gastrocnemius muscle showed transmural inflammation (Fig. 32.1c, d) and occasional extravascular hemosiderin deposition involving multiple small- to intermediate-sized perimysial blood vessels. The inflammation was predominantly composed of lymphocytes, plasma cells and histiocytes without granuloma formation. The background muscle fibers showed severe denervation atrophy. In the sural nerve (Fig. 32.1a, b), although no overt vasculitis was identified, one epineurial vessel with nonspecific perivascular inflammation (Fig. 32.1a) was present. The nerve fascicles showed severe depletion of myelinated axons across all fascicles. Most of the remaining myelinated axons were under monophasic Wallerian degeneration in the form of numerous myelin ovoids (Fig. 32.1b). Together these findings suggest chronic and active vasculitis involving both muscle and nerve.

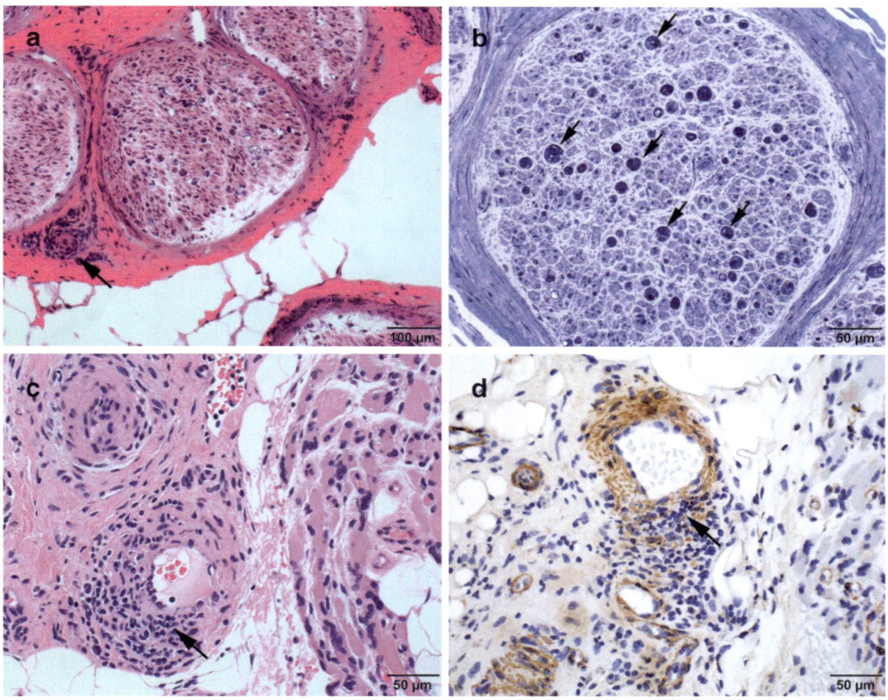

Fig. 32.1 Lupus vasculitidies. (**a**), H&E stained cryostat section of sural nerve shows one epineurial vessel with scant perivascular inflammation (arrow). (**b**), Toluidine blue stained resin embedded plastic section of the sural nerve shows severe depletion of myelinated axons. Most of the remaining axons are in the form of myelin ovoids (arrows), consistent with Wallerian degeneration. (**c**), H&E stained paraffin embedded section of the gastrocnemius muscle shows marked neurogenic atrophy. Multiple perimysial blood vessels show trans-mural inflammation (arrow). (**d**), A smooth muscle actin (SMA) immunostain shows splayed smooth muscle cells in the destructed vascular wall and intramural inflammatory cells (arrow)

Final Diagnosis

Severe active vasculitic neuropathy in a setting of newly diagnosed SLE

Patient Follow-up

The patient's clinical presentation was initially concerning for Guillain-Barre syndrome and vasculitic neuropathy. She was treated with 5 days of plasmapheresis (PLEX) without a significant improvement. She subsequently received 5 days of IV methylprednisolone 1-gram (g) daily with minor improvement. After obtaining the biopsy diagnosis of a severe active vasculitic neuropathy, which was associated with newly diagnosed SLE with no other apparent organ involvement, she was treated with oral prednisone 60 mg daily and IV cyclophosphamide 1 g monthly for 4 total infusions. She had an improvement in proximal limb muscle strength and overall functioning, but no improvement in distal limb muscle strength. She had several hospitalizations for urosepsis and cryptococcal meningitis. She was transitioned to Mycophenolate Mofetil, and Prednisone was tapered down to 10 mg daily. Several weeks later, the patient died from infectious complications related to immunosuppressive therapy.

Discussion

Vasculitic neuropathy is a debilitating neuropathy that can occur in patients with SLE as a result of immune-mediated damage to the vasa nervorum, leading to ischemic nerve damage and axonal loss [1]. Diagnosing vasculitic neuropathy can be challenging, particularly when neuropathy is isolated to the peripheral nervous system or presents as the first manifestation of systemic vasculitis with no other apparent organ involvement. Typical clinical presentation includes a distal and lower limb predominance, painful sensory disturbances, and an asymmetric or multifocal pattern of sensory or sensorimotor abnormalities [2]. While classically this type of neuropathy presents as an asymmetric painful multifocal sensorimotor process (mononeuropathy multiplex), vasculitic neuropathies can also present as a symmetric length-dependent polyneuropathy [3] in as many as 30–40% of patients [4], similar to our patient's presentation. In patients with SLE, peripheral nervous system involvement occurs more commonly as a non-vasculitic distal symmetric polyneuropathy, and is more prevalent in patients diagnosed at an older age [5, 6]. But it can also be associated with vasculitic neuropathy as seen in our case, and SLE constitutes 3% of all cases of vasculitic neuropathy [6]. The most frequently affected motor nerves in vasculitic neuropathy include peroneal nerve followed by tibial, ulnar, median, and radial nerves [6], and our patient had widespread involvement of these nerve.

Particular systemic abnormalities, laboratory findings, and electrodiagnostic testing can provide meaningful clues to expand the diagnostic workup. However, it is also noteworthy that the vasculitis can be restricted to the peripheral nerves in up to 60% of cases; these non-systemic vasculitides tend to have a better prognosis than systemic cases [4]. A positive anti-Smith antibody and low complement 3 are frequently seen in SLE polyneuropathy [7]. Laboratory findings and characteristic pathological abnormalities on biopsy proved to be very helpful in the diagnosis and management of this case.

It is considered best practice to select a nerve that is clinically and electrodiagnostically affected for biopsy [8]. Classically, the sural and superficial peroneal sensory nerves are the most commonly selected nerves in the lower extremity, given their location and low rate of post-surgical complications. The superficial radial sensory nerve is another common biopsy target [4] if it is affected. A combination of nerve and muscle biopsy has been advocated to increase the diagnostic yield for vasculitis [9]. A muscle biopsy specimen is much larger than a nerve biopsy specimen, and it contains more blood vessels for detecting vascular abnormalities. The two common combinations are sural nerve with gastrocnemius muscle, and superficial peroneal nerve with peroneal brevis muscle. With one surgical incision, both nerve and muscle biopsies can be obtained.

On biopsy, primary pathological features seen in vasculitis include transmural inflammation of the small-and medium-sized arterial vessel walls, perivascular inflammation, and significant axonal degeneration [10]. Fibrinoid necrosis and transmural inflammation are more specific for the diagnosis of vasculitis, but usually seen when large- to intermeidate-sized arteries are involved, and rarely seen in small-sized vessels that are predominantly affected in vasculitic neuropathy. In our case, the sural nerve biopsy revealed perivascular inflammation and widespread terminal complement complex (C5b-9) deposition in capillaries, which are both nonspecific findings and could also be seen in acute and chronic demyelinating neuropathies [10]. C5b-9 deposition in the endoneurial vessels is also seen in a substantial number of patients with diabetes [11]. The muscle biopsy exhibited the more specific and definitive findings of transmural vessel wall inflammation. Our case represents one of the examples that illustrates the usefulness of adding a muscle biopsy to a nerve biopsy for the evaluation of vasculitic neuropathy.

High dose corticosteroid with concomitant cyclophosphamide remains the mainstay of treatment for patients with peripheral neuropathy associated with systemic and non-systemic vasculitis [12]. Treatment with this regimen demonstrated better outcomes with significantly reduced relapse rates compared with prednisone monotherapy [1]. There are not many studies comparing different immunosuppressant treatment regimens in patients with severe ployneuropathy associated with SLE; one controlled clinical trial in this population demonstrated cyclophosphamide treatment to be more effective than pulse steroids [13]. Other maintenance immunosuppressive agents such as azathioprine, mycophenolate mofetil, IVIG, and rituximab have also been used with varying success [13]. Oral cyclophosphamide is associated with much higher toxicity and adverse side effects than intravenous (IV) dosing, thus monthly treatment with IV cyclophosphamide is preferred [4]. While several other steroids-sparing immunosuppressive agents can be used, strong evidence is lacking regarding the efficacy of these agents [12]. Many patients with significant peripheral nervous system involvement will need lifelong therapy [4], however for non-systemic cases, the treatment can be reduced if there is early response to treatment [6]. The benefits of immunosuppression must be balanced with limiting side effects; this challenge was evident in our case, where intense immunosuppressive therapy resulted in recurring and persistent infections and ultimately death. Significant systemic side effects and infectious complications should be closely monitored.

Pearls

Clinical Pearls

1. Acute or subacute onset with rapid progression of neuropathy symptoms should raise the suspicion for vasculitic neuropathy. While classically the neuropathy presents in a mononeuropathy multiplex pattern, a relatively symmetric sensorimotor polyneuropathy can also been seen.
2. Tissue diagnosis is critical for vasculitic neuropathy. A combined nerve and muscle biopsy should be pursued, as adding a muscle biopsy can increase the diagnostic yield.
3. Prompt evaluation and treatment are essential to the management of patients with vasculitic neuropathy. Better outcomes occur with earlier identification and treatment.
4. High dose corticosteroid with concomitant cyclophosphamide remains the mainstay of the treatment for vasculitic neuropathy.

Pathology Pearls

1. The most definitive evidence for active vasculitis is fibrinoid necrosis and transmural inflammation. However, these features are usually seen in large- to intermediate-sized vessels, and rarely seen in small-sized vessels that are predominantly affected in vasculitic neuropathy. The latter often shows nonspecific perivascular inflammation. Other supporting pathological features including perivascular hemosiderin deposition, epineurial microvascular proliferation, and differential fascicular axon loss should be carefully evaluated.
2. Wallerian degeneration, first described as a distal change in transected nerve [14], refers to massive monophasic axonal degeneration. Although it can be seen in association with a variety of conditions such as nerve trauma, neurotoxin exposure, and immune mediated axonal motor and sensory neuropathy (AMSAN), in peripheral nerve biopsies, Wallerian degeneration is most commonly seen in association with vasculitis.
3. Due to the patchy and asymmetric nature of vasculitis, negative findings for vasculitis on a nerve biopsy does not completely rule it out.

References

1. Mathew L, Talbot K, Love S, Puvanarajah S, Donaghy M. Treatment of vasculitic peripheral neuropathy: a retrospective analysis of outcome. QJM. 2007;100(1):41–51.
2. Collins MP, Dyck PJ, Gronseth GS, Guillevin L, Hadden RD, Léger JM, et al. Peripheral Nerve Society Guideline on the classification, diagnosis, investigation, and immunosuppressive therapy of non-systemic vasculitic neuropathy: executive summary. J Peripher Nerv Syst. 2010;15(3):176–84.
3. Lacomis D, Zivković SA. Approach to vasculitic neuropathies. J Clin Neuromuscul Dis. 2007;9(1):265–76.
4. Amato A, Russell J. Chapter 13, Vasculitis neuropathies. In: Neuromuscular disorders. Boston: The McGraw-Hill Companies; 2008. p. 261–7.
5. Toledano P, Orueta R, Rodríguez-Pintó I, Valls-Solé J, Cervera R, Espinosa G. Peripheral nervous system involvement in systemic lupus erythematosis: prevalence, clinical and immunological characteristics, treatment and outcome of a large cohort from a single centre. Autoimmun Rev. 2017;16(7):750–5.
6. Mendell JR, Cornblath DR, Kissel JT. Chapter 12, Vasculitic Neuropathy. In: Diagnosis and Management of Peripheral Nerve Disorders. Oxford: Oxford University Press; 2001. p. 202–32.
7. Xianbin W, Mingy W, Dong X, Huiying L, Yan X, Fengchun Z, et al. Peripheral neuropathies due to systemic lupus erythematosus in China. Medicine (Baltimore). 2015;94(11):e625.
8. Bennett DL, Groves M, Blake J, Holton JL, King RH, Orrell RW, et al. The use of nerve and muscle biopsy in the diagnosis of vasculitis: a 5 year retrospective study. J Neurol Neurosurg Psychiatry. 2008;79(12):1376–81.
9. Sharma A. Chapter 20, Vasculitic Neuropathy. In: Textbook of systemic Vasculitis. 1st ed. New Delhi: Jaypee Brothers Medical Publishers; 2015. p. 181.
10. Ubogu EE. Inflammatory neuropathies: pathology, molecular markers and targets for specific therapeutic intervention. Acta Neuropathol Commun. 2015;130(4):445–68.
11. Yell PC, Burns DK, Dittmar EG, White CL III, Cai C. Diffuse microvascular C5b-9 deposition is a common feature in muscle and nerve biopsies from diabetic patients. Acta Neuropathol Commun. 2018;6:11.
12. Gorson KC. Vasculitic neuropathies: an update. Neurologist. 2007;13(1):12–9.
13. Bortoluzzi A, Silvagni E, Furini F, Piga M, Govoni M. Peripheral nervous system involvement in systemic lupus erythematosus: a review of the evidence. Clin Exp Rheumatol. 2019;37(1):146–55.
14. Waller A. Experiments on the section of the glossopharyngeal and hypoglossal nerves of the frog, and observations of the alterations produced thereby in the structure of their primitive fibres. Philos Trans R Soc Lond. 1850;140:423–9.

Chapter 33
A 63-Year-Old Man with Nausea, Vomiting, Orthostatic Dizziness, and Distal Limb Paresthesia

Jeffrey L. Elliott, Lan Zhou, Chunyu Cai, and Michelle Kaku

History

A 63-year-old Caucasian man was referred to our clinic for the evaluation of neuropathy. Four years prior to the presentation, he developed tingling and numbness in the feet and fingers, which had progressed to involve the distal legs and forearms. He also developed intermittent nausea and vomiting with no obvious triggers or overall pattern. He suffered severe bowel constipation and mild lower abdominal pain. He underwent esophagogastroduodenoscopy and colonoscopy with no significant abnormalities found. Computed tomography (CT) of abdomen and pelvis only showed changes consistent with a prior cholecystectomy, which he had several years prior for gallbladder dysfunction. Gastric emptying study showed decreased gastrointestinal motility. The symptoms of nausea and vomiting worsened 1 year prior to the presentation, and he lost 30 pounds of body weight. He endorsed feeling diffusely weak and needed to use a walker occasionally. He also reported feeling

J. L. Elliott
Department of Neurology and Neurotherapeutics,
University of Texas Southwestern Medical Center, Dallas, TX, USA
e-mail: jeffrey.elliott@UTSouthwestern.edu

L. Zhou
Departments of Neurology and Pathology, Boston University Medical Center,
Boston, MA, USA
e-mail: lanzhou@bu.edu

C. Cai
Department of Pathology, University of Texas Southwestern Medical Center,
Dallas, TX, USA
e-mail: chunyu.cai@UTSouthwestern.edu

M. Kaku (✉)
Department of Neurology, Boston University Medical Center, Boston, MA, USA
e-mail: mikaku@bu.edu

L. Zhou et al. (eds.), *A Case-Based Guide to Neuromuscular Pathology*,
https://doi.org/10.1007/978-3-030-25682-1_33

dizzy when standing up from a seated position and felt that he was going to pass out. A few weeks prior to the presentation, he developed urinary retention and needed catheterization. He underwent urological evaluation, and his urinary retention was felt to be neurogenic. He denied dry mouth, dry eyes, vision changes, palpitations, abnormal sweating, skin discoloration, difficulty breathing or distal limb swelling. He admitted to erectile difficulty. He also reported mild bilateral droopy eyelids for many years, but no double vision. Besides the above conditions, he also had a past medical history of hypertension. His medications included metoclopramide as needed, furosemide, pregabalin, and multivitamins. His family history was positive for cancers involving his parents. One of his paternal cousins needed liver transplant, but he did not know the diagnosis or other details of his cousin's illness. There was no family history of neurological diseases. He was married with one daughter. He did not drink alcohol or smoke cigarettes. He was a retired office worker.

Physical Examination

General examination was notable for orthostatic hypotension. There was no evidence of cataracts, arrhythmia, abdominal tenderness, hepatosplenomegaly, distal leg or foot edema, or abnormal skin changes. Neurological examination demonstrated normal mental status and language function. Cranial nerve exam showed mild bilateral eyelid ptosis but normal extraocular movements. Motor examination showed normal muscle tone, bulk, and weakness in the bilateral hip flexors (MRC: 4+/5), finger extensors (4+/5), and interosseous hand muscles (4+/5). There was no muscle fasciculation, scapular winging, or hand grip myotonia. Pinprick sensation was reduced from the toes to the knees and from the fingers to the elbows. Vibratory sensation was reduced at the toes. Joint position sense was intact. Deep tendon reflexes were 1+ at the biceps and absent at the triceps, brachioradialis, knees, and ankles. Toes were downgoing bilaterally. His gait was unsteady due to the feeling of generalized weakness and dizziness.

Investigations

Nerve conduction study (NCS) and electromyography (EMG) showed a sensory greater than motor axonal polyneuropathy with active denervation changes in the distal and proximal muscles and no myotonic discharges. Complete blood count (CBC) showed mild anemia. Serum immunofixation showed the presence of M protein of free lambda light chain. Light chain quantification showed increased kappa light chain. Skeletal survey was negative for bony lesions. Comprehensive metabolic panel (CMP), serum creatine kinase (CK), erythrocyte sedimentation rate (ESR), anti-nuclear antibodies (ANA), rheumatoid factor (RF), vascular endothelial growth factor (VEGF), cryoglobulin, paraneoplastic antibody panel, thyroid stimulating hormone (TSH), free T4, hemoglobin A1C, vitamin B12, vitamin B6, and acetylcholine receptor antibody (AChR-Ab) were all unremarkable. Brain MRI was normal. Spine MRI showed mild degenerative joint disease at C5–6. CT of the chest, abdomen, and pelvis showed an 8 mm lung nodule in the right middle lobe and a small hiatal hernia. Transthoracic echocardiogram was normal. Myotonic dystrophy type 1 and type 2 gene tests were unrevealing. Right deltoid muscle and right superficial radial nerve biopsies were performed.

Muscle and Nerve Biopsy Findings

The right deltoid muscle and right superficial radial nerve biopsies (Fig. 33.1) showed amyloid deposits distributed around myofibers and in the interstitium, fascia, endoneurial and perineurial compartments. Transthyretin (prealbumin) immunostain showed diffuse immunoreactivity surrounding individual myofibers and in the interstitium and fascia. Kappa and lambda immunostains showed a marked immunoreactivity with the kappa immunoreactivity greater than that of lambda. These findings were suggestive of an inherited amyloidosis, possibly associated with transthyretin. In addition, the muscle biopsy showed neurogenic changes including scattered atrophic esterase-positive denervated fibers, occasional myonuclear clusters, and target/targetoid fibers. The nerve biopsy showed a significant loss of myelinated axons, particularly small-caliber axons, in all fascicles with multiple myelin ovoids and rare regenerating clusters but no selective myelin injury or onion bulb formation. There was no evidence of inflammation.

Additional Investigation After the Biopsy Diagnosis

The patient underwent genetic testing, which showed a pathological mutation c.238A > G (p.Thr80Ala) in the transthyretin (TTR) gene. This mutation has been reported in sporadic cases of hereditary amyloidosis in non-endemic areas [1–3].

Final Diagnosis

Familial Amyloid Polyneuropathy Caused by a TTR Gene Mutation

Patient Follow-up

The diagnosis of familial amyloid polyneuropathy caused by the Thr80Ala TTR mutation and the new therapies for the disease were discussed with the patient. The patient was started on Diflunisal, a TTR stabilizer, and Inotersen, a TTR silencer

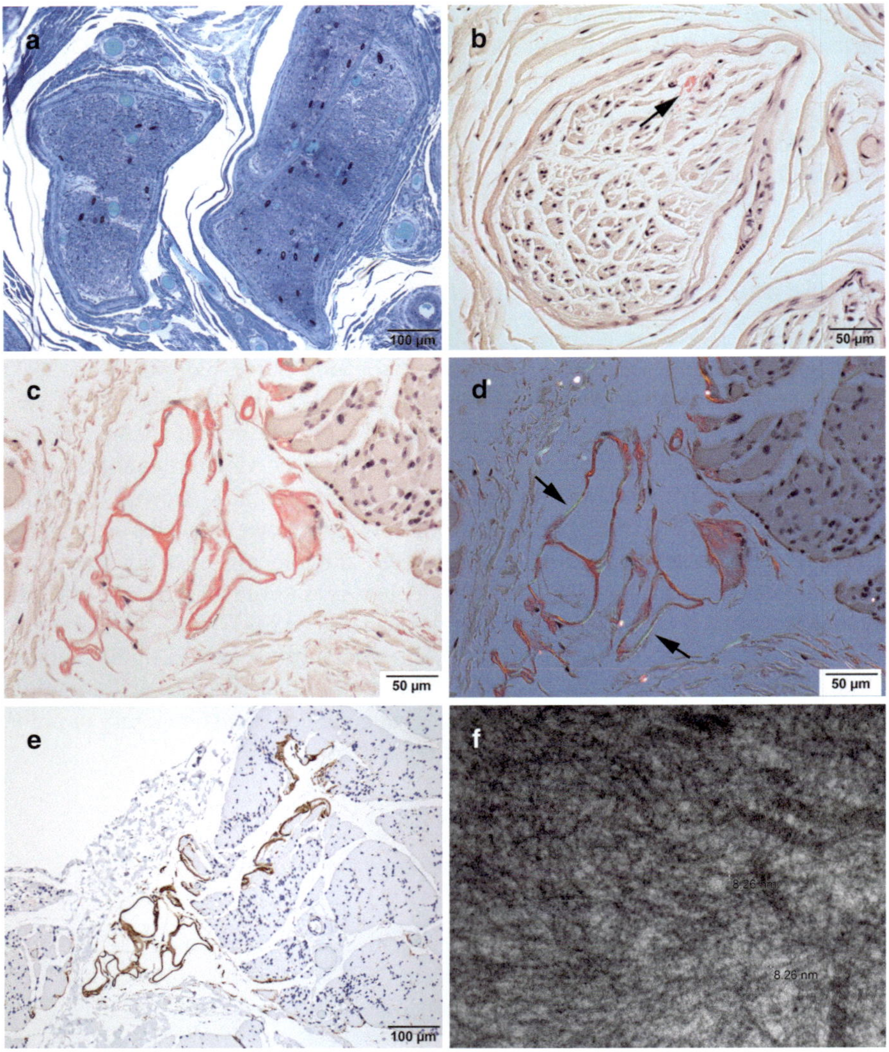

Fig. 33.1 Amyloid neuropathy. (**a**) Toluidine blue stained resin embedded plastic section of the biopsied nerve shows an end stage nerve with severe depletion of myelinated axons. (**b**) Congo red stain of the nerve shows focal perivascular amyloid deposition (arrow). (**c**) Congo red stain of the concomitant muscle biopsy shows more extensive amyloid deposition in the perimysium, fascia, and around myofibers. The background myofibers show neurogenic atrophy. (**d**) Under polarized light, the amyloid deposits show apple green birefringence (arrows). (**e**): Amyloid deposits are strongly positive for transthyretin immunostain. (**f**) On electron microscopy (EM), the amyloid deposits are composed of haphazardly arranged fibrils with diameters around 8 nm

and a transthyretin-directed antisense oligonucleotide drug. His nausea and vomiting were partially controlled by antiemetics. Orthostatic dizziness improved after taking pyridostigmine bromide. Neuropathic pain was largely controlled by maximizing the dose of pregabalin. The patient was sent for genetic counseling.

Discussion

Peripheral neuropathy commonly occurs in both hereditary and acquired amyloidosis. Immunoglobulin light chain (AL) amyloidosis is the most common form of acquired amyloidosis, whereas transthyretin (TTR) amyloidosis is the most common form of hereditary amyloidosis. When neuropathy is the primary feature of amyloidosis related to a TTR mutation, it is often referred to as neuropathic hATTR amyloidosis, or familial amyloid polyneuropathy, which is caused by one of over 140 mutations in the transthyretin gene. It is familial and transmitted in an autosomal dominant manner, although sporadic cases exist.

Transthyretin is a plasma transport protein for retinol binding protein and thyroid hormone. It is produced in the liver, with small amounts produced in the choroid plexus and retinal pigment epithelium of the eye [4–6]. When mutated, TTR misfolds and aggregates as insoluble amyloid fibrils that deposit in various organs and leads to dysfunction and even failure of affected organs. Amyloid can deposit in any part of the peripheral nervous system including nerves, nerve roots, autonomic and spinal ganglia and muscle [7, 8]. Patients often present with sensorimotor polyneuropathy, carpal tunnel syndrome and autonomic dysfunction. Small myelinated and unmyelinated axons are more affected than large myelinated axons. Depending on which organ the fibrils deposit, patients can also have cardiomyopathy, reduced gastrointestinal motility, renal insufficiency, and vitreous opacities [9].

The most common TTR mutation is a substitution of Methionine for Valine at position 30, the ATTRVal30Met mutation (or V30M mutation), whereas in the United States, the most common mutation is the substitution of isoleucine for valine at position 122, or the V122I mutation which affects 3% of African Americans [10]. The V122I mutation is commonly associated with cardiomyopathy, although neuropathy can be seen in 10–38% of patients [10, 11]. Penetrance varies by mutation type, and having a genetic mutation does not necessarily mean that patients will develop the disease [12]. Clinical presentation can vary widely worldwide. In endemic regions of Japan, northern Portugal, Sweden, and Cyprus, patients present in the third or fourth decade classically with pain and temperature abnormalities in the feet. Later, light touch and proprioception are impaired with proximal progression of symptoms up the legs and eventual weakness that can be debilitating. Autonomic dysfunction can manifest with orthostatic hypotension, dry eyes, dry mouth, gastroparesis with fluctuating constipation and diarrhea, urinary retention, and erectile dysfunction in men. Significant adrenergic, cardiovagal or sudomotor autonomic dysfunction can be detected even in patients without clinical manifestations of autonomic failure [13]. Amyloid deposits in the transverse carpal ligament can cause compression of the median nerve and manifest clinically as carpal tunnel syndrome with pain and tingling in the hands [14].

Patients living in non-endemic areas often develop symptoms later than age 50 years, and may have obscure family history, with less autonomic dysfunction. Neuropathy may involve both large and small fibers concurrently [15]. Although rare, amyloid can also deposit in muscle and cause myopathy, presenting with proximal or distal weakness. Most patients with amyloid myopathy have AL amyloidosis although amyloid myopathy has also been reported in hATTR amyloidosis. Given the rarity of this disease, it has previously been misdiagnosed as limb girdle muscular dystrophy or polymyositis [8].

The diagnosis should be considered in patients with neuropathy and a concurrent family history. In these patients, tissue diagnosis is not necessary and patients can be diagnosed by genetic testing. In patients without a known family history, the diagnosis should be considered in the presence of a progressive, length-dependent, mixed large and small fiber polyneuropathy, especially when associated with carpal tunnel syndrome, autonomic dysfunction, or other multi-systemic involvement. The most common NCS/EMG finding is a length-dependent axonal polyneuropathy. NCS/EMG may also show carpal tunnel syndrome. Conduction slowing is rare [16]. Biopsy of the affected organ, including nerve if neuropathy is present, can demonstrate the presence of amyloid deposits. Other organs that are commonly sampled include abdominal fat, salivary gland, heart, kidney, and muscle. Because of the patchy nature of amyloid deposition, a negative biopsy does not rule out amyloidosis.

In peripheral nerves, amyloid can deposit in the epi, peri or endoneurium in a patchy distribution [17]. Histologically, amyloid is an eosinophilic mass of protein fibrils that stains positive for Congo red and demonstrates yellow-green birefringence under polarized light. Teased fiber studies demonstrate various stages of axonal degeneration with nodules of amyloid indenting myelinating fibers, producing sacculations of the fiber on both sides of the point of compression [17]. When amyloid deposits in the muscle, it can be detected in the interstitium by Congo red stain viewed under polarized light or using fluorescent optics, and can also be found in intramuscular blood vessels. The transthyretin immunostain is highly sensitive and specific for transthyretin derived amyloid [18]; it thus can provide a quick diagnosis for transthyretin amyloidosis in muscle and nerve biopsies. It should be noted that besides hereditary forms, ATTR can also accumulate from wild type transthyretin protein [19], typically in patients older than 80 years. This is referred to as senile systemic amyloidosis. Wild type ATTR deposits are often weak or even negative on Congo red stain [20], but positive for transthyretin immunostain. Genetic testing is necessary to confirm hATTR, particularly in elderly patients. Electron microscopy can usually confirm the presence of amyloid fibrils but has limited utility in determining the subtype of amyloid.

Amyloidosis is a devastating disease. The mean survival is less than 10 years from the diagnosis with death typically secondary to cardiac failure, infection or malnutrition [21]. Historically, liver transplantation has been the standard of care in the treatment of hATTR amyloidosis [22]. However, new therapies have recently been approved by the United States Food and Drug Administration (FDA) for the treatment of neuropathy. These include TTR stabilizers which stabilize the TTR tetramer and suppress the TTR synthesis, and TTR silencers that inhibit hepatic production of TTR. Diflunisal, a TTR stabilizer, is a non-steroidal anti-inflammatory drug that binds to tetrameric TTR and stabilizes it, decreasing fibril formation [23]. Its use is limited largely by gastrointestinal side effects, and it is contraindicated in patients with severe congestive heart failure or renal insufficiency. Tafamidis, a thyroxine-like small ligand inhibitor, similarly stabilizes mutant tetramers. In a randomized double-blind study of patients with V30M mutation given Tafamidis or placebo, the primary outcomes in the quality of life metrics and neuropathy impairment score in the lower limbs were unfortunately not met, although the secondary end points demonstrating less neurologic deterioration were met. It is currently marketed in Europe, Japan and South America but has not been approved by US FDA [24].

TTR silencers include anti-sense oligonucleotides (ASO) and small interfering RNAs (siRNAs) which inhibit mutant and non-mutant TTR production in the liver. The ASO, Inotersen, is a string of nucleotides that prevents TTR protein expression by binding its messenger RNA and thus preventing its translation. In the NEURO-TTR study, both primary endpoints were met with significant benefit inhibiting, slowing or even improving sensorimotor polyneuropathy [25]. Patisiran is an siRNA, which is a double stranded RNA that targets a sequence of mRNA in all TTR variants, inhibiting TTR synthesis in the liver. Patisiran has been demonstrated to halt or reverse the progression of neurologic and cardiac manifestations of hATTR amyloidosis [26].

In summary, amyloidosis should be included early on in the work up of polyneuropathy, particularly with concurrent carpal tunnel syndrome, autonomic dysfunction, or other organ involvement, whether or not the patient has a family history of neuropathy or amyloidosis. With the advent of new therapies, hATTR amyloidosis has become one of the few hereditary causes of polyneuropathy that can be treated.

Pearls

Clinical Pearls

1. hATTR amyloidosis is the most common hereditary form of amyloidosis whereas AL amyloidosis is the most common acquired form of amyloidosis.
2. hATTR amyloidosis is inherited in an autosomal dominant fashion, although sporadic cases have no family history.
3. hATTR amyloidosis is a multisystem disease and can manifest clinically with cardiomyopathy, renal insufficiency, vitreous opacities, and soft tissue deposition. The common neurological presentations include a length-dependent sensorimotor polyneuropathy, carpal tunnel syndrome and autonomic dysfunction. Amyloid can also deposit in muscle causing a myopathy.
4. When large fiber neuropathy is present, NCS/EMG often shows a sensory greater than motor axonal polyneuropathy, worse in the lower extremities. When small fiber involvement is present, skin biopsy may show reduced intraepidermal nerve fiber density, but the yield of detecting amyloid

deposition in a non-lesional skin biopsy is low. Autonomic testing is useful to evaluate autonomic symptoms associated with amyloidosis.
5. Nerve biopsy can be spared in a patient with a high clinical suspicion for hATTR amyloidosis especially when a positive family history is present, as the diagnosis can be made by the TTR gene test.
6. Patients with amyloidosis are better managed by a multi-disciplinary team with experts in different fields, including neurology, cardiology, ophthalmology, nephrology, gastroenterology, and rehabilitation. Referral to a genetic counselor should also be considered.

Pathology Pearls
1. On muscle and nerve biopsies, the diagnosis of amyloidosis is established by the detection of amyloid deposits on sections stained with Congo red.
2. Transthyretin immunostain is sensitive and specific for amyloid deposits composed of TTR. Most early onset ATTR are hereditary and caused by genetic mutations, while late onset ATTR can be mutant or wild type. The latter is referred to as senile systemic amyloidosis. Genetic confirmation is necessary in differentiating senile systemic amyloidosis from late onset hATTR.
3. Amyloid deposition is patchy in amyloidosis. Concomitant nerve and muscle biopsies can increase the diagnostic yield as compared with nerve biopsy alone. Absence of amyloid on biopsy does not completely exclude amyloidosis.

References

1. Théaudin M, Lozeron P, Algalarrondo V, Lacroix C, Cauquil C, Labeyrie C, et al. Upper limb onset of hereditary transthyretin amyloidosis is common in non-endemic areas. Eur J Neurol. 2019;26(3):497–e36.
2. Dohrn MF, Röcken C, De Bleecker JL, Martin J-J, Vorgerd M, Van den Bergh PY, et al. Diagnostic hallmarks and pitfalls in late-onset progressive transthyretin-related amyloid-neuropathy. J Neurol. 2013;260(12):3093–108.
3. Brown EE, Lee YZJ, Halushka MK, Steenbergen C, Johnson NM, Almansa J, et al. Genetic testing improves identification of transthyretin amyloid (ATTR) subtype in cardiac amyloidosis. Amyloid. 2017;24(2):92–5.
4. Robbins J. Thyroxine-binding proteins. Prog Clin Biol Res. 1976;5:331–55.
5. Dickson PW, Aldred AR, Marley PD, Guo-Fen T, Howlett GJ, Schreiber G. High prealbumin and transferrin mRNA levels in the choroid plexus of rat brain. Biochem Biophys Res Commun. 1985;127(3):890–5.
6. Soprano DR, Herbert J, Soprano K, Schon E, Goodman D. Demonstration of transthyretin mRNA in the brain and other extrahepatic tissues in the rat. J Biol Chem. 1985;260(21):11793–8.

7. Takahashi K, Yi S, Kimura Y. Araki SJHp. Familial amyloidotic polyneuropathy type 1 in Kumamoto, Japan: a clinicopathologic, histochemical, immunohistochemical, and ultrastructural study. Hum Pathol. 1991;22(6):519–27.
8. Chapin JE, Kornfeld M, Harris A. Amyloid myopathy: characteristic features of a still underdiagnosed disease. Muscle Nerve. 2005;31(2):266–72.
9. Hund E, Linke R, Willig F, Grau A. Transthyretin-associated neuropathic amyloidosis pathogenesis and treatment. Neurology. 2001;56(4):431–5.
10. Maurer MS, Hanna M, Grogan M, Dispenzieri A, Witteles R, Drachman B, et al. Genotype and phenotype of transthyretin cardiac amyloidosis: THAOS (Transthyretin Amyloid Outcome Survey). J Am Coll Cardiol. 2016;68(2):161–72.
11. Connors LH, Prokaeva T, Lim A, Théberge R, Falk RH, Doros G, et al. Cardiac amyloidosis in African Americans: comparison of clinical and laboratory features of transthyretin V122I amyloidosis and immunoglobulin light chain amyloidosis. Am Heart J. 2009;158(4):607–14.
12. Hellman U, Alarcon F, Lundgren H-E, Suhr OB, Bonaïti-Pellié C, Planté-Bordeneuve V. Heterogeneity of penetrance in familial amyloid polyneuropathy, ATTR Val30Met, in the Swedish population. Amyloid. 2008;15(3):181–6.
13. Wang AK, Fealey RD, Gehrking TL, Low PA. Patterns of neuropathy and autonomic failure in patients with amyloidosis. Mayo Clinic Proceedings. 2008: Elsevier,;83:1226–30.
14. Planté-Bordeneuve V, Said G. Familial amyloid polyneuropathy. Lancet Neurol. 2011;10(12):1086–97.
15. Misu K-i, Hattori N, Nagamatsu M, Ikeda S-i, Ando Y, Nakazato M, et al. Late-onset familial amyloid polyneuropathy type I (transthyretin Met30-associated familial amyloid polyneuropathy) unrelated to endemic focus in Japan: clinicopathological and genetic features. Brain. 1999;122(10):1951–62.
16. Planté-Bordeneuve V, Ferreira A, Lalu T, Zaros C, Lacroix C, Adams D, et al. Diagnostic pitfalls in sporadic transthyretin familial amyloid polyneuropathy (TTR-FAP). Neurology. 2007;69(7):693–8.
17. Dyck PJ, Lambert EH. Dissociated sensation in amyloidosis: compound action potential, quantitative histologic and teased-fiber, and electron microscopic studies of sural nerve biopsies. Arch Neurol. 1969;20(5):490–507.
18. Schönland SO, Hegenbart U, Bochtler T, Mangatter A, Hansberg M, Ho AD, et al. Immunohistochemistry in the classification of systemic forms of amyloidosis: a systematic investigation of 117 patients. Blood. 2012;119(2):488–93.
19. Westermark P, Sletten K, Johansson B, Cornwell GG. Fibril in senile systemic amyloidosis is derived from normal transthyretin. Proc Natl Acad Sci U S A. 1990;87(7):2843–5.
20. Koike H, Misu K, Sugiura M, Iijima M, Mori K, Yamamoto M, et al. Pathology of early-vs late-onset TTR Met30 familial amyloid polyneuropathy. Neurology. 2004;63(1):129–38.
21. Coutinho P, Martins da Silva A, Lopes Lima J, Resende Barbosa A. Forty years of experience with type I amyloid neuropathy. Review of 483 cases. In: Glenner GG, Pinho e Costa P, Falcao de Freitas A, editors. Amyloid and amyloidosis. Amsterdam: Excerpta Medica; 1980. p. 88–98.
22. Yamashita T, Ando Y, Okamoto S, Misumi Y, Hirahara T, Ueda M, et al. Long-term survival after liver transplantation in patients with familial amyloid polyneuropathy. Neurology. 2012;78:637–43. https://doi.org/10.1212/WNL.0b013e318248df18.
23. Berk JL, Suhr OB, Obici L, Sekijima Y, Zeldenrust SR, Yamashita T, et al. Repurposing diflunisal for familial amyloid polyneuropathy: a randomized clinical trial. JAMA. 2013;310(24):2658–67.
24. Coelho T, Maia LF, da Silva AM, Cruz MW, Planté-Bordeneuve V, Lozeron P, et al. Tafamidis for transthyretin familial amyloid polyneuropathy A randomized, controlled trial. Neurology. 2012;79(8):785–92.
25. Benson MD, Waddington-Cruz M, Berk JL, Polydefkis M, Dyck PJ, Wang AK, et al. Inotersen treatment for patients with hereditary transthyretin amyloidosis. N Engl J Med. 2018;379(1):22–31.
26. Adams D, Gonzalez-Duarte A, O'Riordan WD, Yang C-C, Ueda M, Kristen AV, et al. Patisiran, an RNAi therapeutic, for hereditary transthyretin amyloidosis. N Engl J Med. 2018;379(1):11–21.

Chapter 34
A 47-year-old woman with progressive numbness and weakness in the limbs

Lingchao Meng, Yun Yuan, and Shan Chen

History

A 47-year-old Asian woman presented with progressive numbness and weakness in her arms and legs. Her symptoms started about one year prior to the presentation when she noticed numbness and tingling with dysesthesias in her hands followed by weakness in her legs. Gradually she developed weakness in her hands as well. The weakness became progressively worsened, and she was unable to walk without assistance eight months after the onset of the symptoms. She reported bilateral wrist drop and foot drop. She had mild weight loss. She denied any pain, muscle wasting, twitches or cramps. She denied any headaches, dizziness, visual disturbance, ptosis, dysarthria, dysphagia, or cognitive impairment. She had no urinary or bowel disturbance. She had no foreign travel prior to the onset of symptoms. She took vitamin B1 and B12 oral supplements without any symptom relief. She was otherwise healthy. There was no family history of neuromuscular disorders. She worked in a shoe factory in a rural area in China for one and a half years. She had stopped working for 2 months before presenting to our neuromuscular clinic.

L. Meng (✉) · Y. Yuan
Neuromuscular Division, Department of Neurology, Peking University First Hospital, Beijing, China

S. Chen
Peripheral Neuropathy Center, Rutgers University, Robert Wood Johnson Medical School, New Brunswick, NJ, USA
e-mail: chens5@rwjms.rutgers.edu

L. Zhou et al. (eds.), *A Case-Based Guide to Neuromuscular Pathology*,
https://doi.org/10.1007/978-3-030-25682-1_34

Physical Examination

The general examination showed that the patient was well nourished, well developed, and in no acute distress. Her vital signs were normal. She was normocephalic and atraumatic with no dysmorphic features. Her cardiac, pulmonary, and abdominal examination were unremarkable. There were no pes cavus, hammer toes, or other foot deformities. There were no skin lesions or spine tenderness. There were no hair or skin changes. Neurological examination showed normal mental status and cranial nerve functions. She was unable to walk or stand without support. There was very mild hypotonia in the limbs and very mild distal limb muscles atrophy. She had mild symmetric proximal limb weakness (Medical Research Council (MRC) grade 4/5), and moderate-to-severe symmetric distal limb weakness (MRC grade 2/5 to 3/5). She also had reduced pinprick and temperature sensation and impaired vibratory sensation and joint position sense in a stocking-glove pattern. Deep tendon reflexes were diffusely absent. Toes were down-going bilaterally.

Investigations

Laboratory evaluation revealed unremarkable CBC, basic metabolic panel, renal function, hepatic function, thyroid function, HbA1C, serum folic acid and vitamin B12 levels, antinuclear antibody (ANA), extractable nuclear antigen antibody (ENA) panel, ANCA panel, serum and urine protein electrophoresis and immunofixation, paraneoplastic antibody panel, and urine analysis. Chest x-ray was normal. Cerebral spinal fluid (CSF) study was also normal. Nerve conduction study and electromyography (NCS/EMG) showed a chronic, predominantly axonal, sensory and motor polyneuropathy. CMAP and SNAP amplitudes were all markedly reduced ranging from 5–25% of the lower limits. Mild conduction slowing was found in several nerves with conduction velocities ranging from 37–45 m/s in the upper extremities and 32–38 m/s in the lower extremities, worse in the motor nerves. There were no conduction blocks seen. A left sural nerve biopsy was performed for further evaluation.

Nerve Biopsy Findings

The left sural nerve biopsy showed a mild active neuropathy with a minimally reduced density of myelinated fibers, rare myelin ovoids, and a few giant axons with marked axonal swelling and attenuated myelin sheath (Fig. 34.1). There were no regenerating clusters or onion bulbs. Endoneurium, perineurium, epineurium, and blood vessels appeared normal. There were no inflammatory infiltrates or amyloid deposits. The findings are consistent with giant axonal neuropathy (GAN).

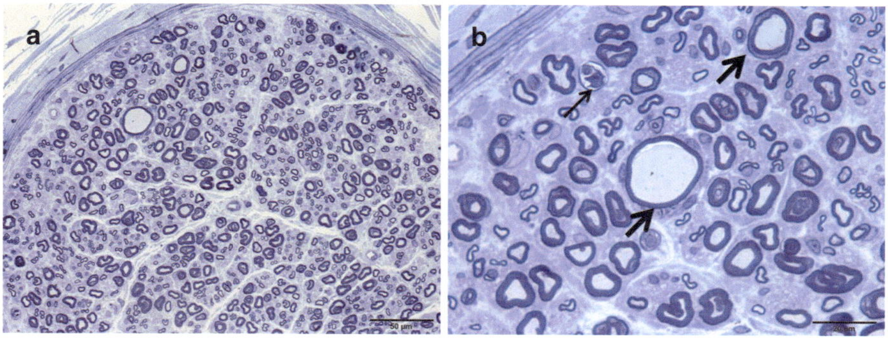

Fig. 34.1 Sural nerve biopsy. Plastic toluidine blue stained semi-thin sections at a lower magnification (**a**) and a higher magnification (**b**) show a minimally reduced density of myelinated fibers with no regenerating clusters, onion bulbs, or inflammatory infiltrates. Two axons (**b**, thick arrows) show axonal swelling and attenuated myelin sheath overlying the "giant" axons. There are rare myelin ovoids (**b**, thin arrow)

Final Diagnosis

N-hexane-induced giant axonal neuropathy

Patient Follow-up

The patient was advised to avoid any route of exposure to leather cements at her work. She underwent physical and occupational therapy with her symptoms improved gradually. In a follow-up visit one and a half years later, she was able to walk on her own with mild residual numbness and tingling sensation. Examination showed mild residual distal limb weakness and sensory impairment as well as absent ankle jerks.

Discussion

N-hexane used as solvents in shoe, furniture, automotive, and printing industries as well as recreational glue/gasoline sniffing is neurotoxic [1–3]. Chronic n-hexane intoxication can result in sensory and motor axonal polyneuropathy with secondary demyelination [4, 5]. Rarely conduction blocks can be seen on the nerve conduction studies [6]. The neuropathy symptoms are often slowly progressive, but the disease onset can be insidious or subacute. Sensory symptoms are usually the initial complaints followed by muscle weakness with a pattern of distal predominance [5]. Paresthesias and dysesthesias are common, but pain is usually minimal. The development of neuropathy seems to have no direct relationship to the duration of exposure; hence, factors such as individual susceptibility may be important. Optic neuropathy and central nervous system (CNS) involvement are uncommon, and autonomic neuropathy is rarely encountered [2, 5]. The hallmark of the nerve pathology is segmental swelling of axons with thinning of the overlying myelin sheath without marked active nerve fiber degeneration or regeneration as seen in our case [1–6]. Electron microscopic (EM) examination of nerve biopsies often shows accumulation of packed intermediate neurofilaments [1–6], which is suggestive of disorganized network of cytoskeleton [1]. This may affect axonal transportation and other cellular functions, resulting in primary axonopathy. Aggregation of intermediate neurofilaments has been shown to impair mitochondrial motility with resultant metabolic and oxidative stress [7]. Ultrastructural studies of n-hexane neuropathy in the animal models showed that there was a retrograde, temporal spread of axonal swelling from distal paranodal sites and up along the affected nerve trunks, but the axonal degeneration did not begin in the nerve terminal or spread centripetally along individual nerve fibers; it was rather in a multifocal pattern [8, 9]. The exact pathogenic mechanism of n-hexane-induced GAN remains unknown. Nevertheless, n-hexane neuropathy shares these above-mentioned neuropathological features with the hereditary form of GAN [10–12].

Hereditary GAN is a rare, autosomal recessive, and progressive neurodegenerative disease seen in pediatric population. It is characterized by progressive motor and sensory peripheral neuropathy, CNS involvement with pyramidal and cerebellar signs, and characteristic kinky hair [10, 11]. In the hereditary form of GAN, the GAN gene mutations cause reduced or dysfunctional gigaxonin which is crucial for ubiquitin-proteasomal degradation of neuronal intermediate neurofilaments, resulting in accumulation of intermediate neurofilaments [12, 13]. In n-hexane-induced GAN, it has been postulated that n-hexane is converted to toxic gamma-diketone metabolite 2,5-hexanedione (2,5-HD), which can cause covalent crosslinking of neurofilaments, resulting in intermediate neurofilaments aggregation [14].

Acquired GAN induced by n-hexane can be differentiated from hereditary GAN by a late age at onset, a history of industrial or recreational exposure, a lack of kinky hair or CNS involvement, and improvement after removing the exposure as seen in our patient. Thorough history taking, especially the occupational and recreational history, is important to raise the suspicion. Nerve biopsy is diagnostic as seen in our case, which may otherwise be misdiagnosed with and wrongly managed for chronic inflammatory demyelinating polyneuropathy or other forms of polyneuropathy.

The clinical course of polyneuropathy induced by n-hexane exposure tends to be biphasic with “coasting” phenomenon (continued symptoms after removal of insulting agent, as seen in some chemotherapy-induced polyneuropathy) for 2–3 months, followed by a slow improvement or recovery in about 1–2 years after the cessation of the n-hexane exposure [1–3, 5, 15]. Prognosis is usually favorable, but some patients may have a protracted recovery course or permanent disability if initial axonal damage is severe.

N-hexane exposure at workplace needs to be investigated and recreational exposure needs to be considered in a patient with acquired GAN. Using safer solvents with adequate ventilation system in factories of shoe furniture, automotive, and printing industries is critical to prevent the disease. This case has profound implications for occupational health.

Pearls

Clinical pearls

1. Workers in shoe, furniture, automotive, and printing industries and glue sniffers are at risk for developing n-hexane-induced toxic polyneuropathy.
2. Chronic n-hexane-induced toxic polyneuropathy often manifests insidious or subacute onset, progressive, sensorimotor deficits affecting all four extremities with distal predominance.
3. NCS/EMG usually shows a predominantly axonal polyneuropathy with mild secondary demyelination changes.
4. Unlike hereditary GAN, optic neuropathies, kinky hair, CNS involvement, and autonomic neuropathy are uncommon in n-hexane-induced GAN.
5. N-hexane exposure needs to be investigated in a patient with acquired GAN.
6. N-hexane-induced toxic polyneuropathy is preventable and treatable by avoiding the exposure. It is often reversible after the exposure is removed.

Pathology pearls

1. N-hexane intoxication can cause aquired GAN. Nerve biopsy often shows giant axons caused by segmental swelling of axons, thinning of myelin sheath, widened nodal gaps and loss of some large myelinated nerve fibers.
2. Active nerve fiber degeneration and regeneration in nerve biopsy of n-hexane-induced GAN are often very mild, which is relatively distinct from the dying back pattern of axonal degeneration caused by other toxic and metabolic etiologies such as diabetes mellitus.
3. EM usually shows accumulation of packed neurofilaments as seen in the hereditary form of GAN.

References

1. Rizzuto N, Terzian H, Galiazzo-Rizzuto S. Toxic polyneuropathies in Italy due to leather cement poisoning in shoe industries. A light- and electron-microscopic study. J Neurol Sci. 1977;31(3):343–54.

2. Chang CM, Yu CW, Fong KY, Leung SY, Tsin TW, Yu YL, Cheung TF, Chan SY. N-hexane neuropathy in offset printers. J Neurol Neurosurg Psychiatry. 1993;56(5):538–42.
3. Smith AG, Albers JW. n-Hexane neuropathy due to rubber cement sniffing. Muscle Nerve. 1997;20(11):1445–50.
4. Neghab M, Soleimani E, Khamoushian K. Electrophysiological studies of shoemakers exposed to sub-TLV levels of n-hexane. J Occup Health. 2012;54(5):376–82.
5. Misirli H, Domaç FM, Somay G, Araal O, Ozer B, Adigüzel T. N-hexane induced polyneuropathy: a clinical and electrophysiological follow up. Electromyogr Clin Neurophysiol. 2008;48(2):103–8.
6. Chang AP, England JD, Garcia CA, Sumner AJ. Focal conduction block in n-hexane polyneuropathy. Muscle Nerve. 1998;21(7):964–9.
7. Israeli E, Dryanovski DI, Schumacker PT, Chandel NS, Singer JD, Julien JP, et al. Intermediate filament aggregates cause mitochondrial dysmotility and increase energy demands in giant axonal neuropathy. Hum Mol Genet. 2016;25(11):2143–57.
8. LoPachin RM, Lehning EJ. The relevance of axonal swellings and atrophy to gamma-diketone neurotoxicity: a forum position paper. Neurotoxicology. 1997;18(1):7–22.
9. Spencer PS, Schaumburg HH. Ultrastructural studies of the dying-back process. III. The evolution of experimental peripheral giant axonal degeneration. J Neuropathol Exp Neurol. 1977;36(2):276–99.
10. Wang L, Zhao D, Wang Z, Zhang W, Lv H, Liu X, et al. Heterogeneity of axonal pathology in Chinese patients with giant axonal neuropathy. Muscle Nerve. 2014;50(2):200–5.
11. Hentati F, Hentati E, Amouri R. Giant axonal neuropathy. Handb Clin Neurol. 2013;115:933–8. Review
12. Johnson-Kerner BL, Roth L, Greene JP, Wichterle H, Sproule DM. Giant axonal neuropathy: An updated perspective on its pathology and pathogenesis. Muscle Nerve. 2014;50(4):467–76.
13. Bomont P. Degradation of the intermediate filament family by gigaxonin. Methods Enzymol. 2016;569:215–31.
14. Graham DG, Anthony DC, Szakál-Quin G, Gottfried MR, Boekelheide K. Covalent cross-linking of neurofilaments in the pathogenesis of n-hexane neuropathy. Neurotoxicology. 1985;6(4):55–63.
15. Huang CC. Polyneuropathy induced by n-hexane intoxication in Taiwan. Acta Neurol Taiwan. 2008;17(1):3–10.

Chapter 35
A 65-Year-Old Woman with Acute Limb Weakness and Worsening of Paresthesia

Susan C. Shin, Michelle Kaku, and Lan Zhou

History

A 65-year-old Hispanic woman presented to the emergency room with worsening pain and weakness of the distal lower extremities. Two months prior to the presentation, she developed a deep aching, cramping pain throughout both legs and the lower lumbar region. There was no shooting pain. Shortly after, she also developed tingling and numbness in the feet. She was evaluated by a neurologist. Nerve conduction study (NCS) showed normal motor and sensory conduction responses in the upper and lower limbs, but needle electromyography (EMG) showed a few fibrillation potentials and positive sharp waves in the bilateral L5-S1-innervated distal limb muscles and paraspinal muscles, which was interpreted to be consistent with a lumbosacral radiculopathy. A lumbosacral spine MRI, however, was unremarkable. Two weeks prior to the presentation, she developed acute onset of cold sensation in the bilateral lower extremities and mild proximal leg weakness. One week prior to the presentation, she developed acute onset of bilateral foot drop followed by mild hand weakness. She could no longer walk. She denied saddle anesthesia or change in bowel or bladder function. She denied fevers, weight loss, cough, diarrhea, or skin rashes. She denied preceding vaccinations or travels. There was no toxin

S. C. Shin
Department of Neurology, Icahn School of Medicine at Mount Sinai, New York, NY, USA
e-mail: Susan.shin@mssm.edu

M. Kaku
Department of Neurology, Boston University Medical Center, Boston, MA, USA
e-mail: Michelle.Kaku@bmc.org

L. Zhou (✉)
Departments of Neurology and Pathology, Boston University Medical Center, Boston, MA, USA
e-mail: lanzhou@bu.edu

L. Zhou et al. (eds.), *A Case-Based Guide to Neuromuscular Pathology*,
https://doi.org/10.1007/978-3-030-25682-1_35

exposure. She had a past medical history of breast cancer treated with mastectomy and chemotherapy 6 years prior, and a remote history of cutaneous sarcoidosis at age 20s that was treated with a course of oral prednisone for a few months. The diagnosis of cutaneous sarcoidosis was made based on a biopsy of a skin lesion. She also had a history of hypertension, hypothyroidism, and asthma. Her medications included levothyroxine 75 μg daily, aspirin 81 mg daily, losartan/hydrochlorothiazide 100/12.5 mg daily, gabapentin 600 mg three times daily, calcium, vitamin D, alendronate, and albuterol inhaler as needed. Family history was negative for neuropathy. She did not smoke cigarettes or drink alcohol.

Physical Examination

General examination was unremarkable including pulmonary and skin examination. Neurological examination showed normal mental status and cranial nerve functions. Motor examination was notable for mildly reduced tone in both lower extremities along with weakness in both proximal and distal lower limb muscles as well as distal upper limb muscles. Strength was MRC 4/5 in the bilateral hip flexors, 4+/5 in the knee flexors, 2/5 in the foot and toe dorsiflexors, 3/5 in the foot and toe plantar flexors, and 4+/5 in the finger extensors and interossei hand muscles. Deep tendon reflexes were 2+ at the biceps, triceps, and brachioradialis, 1+ at the knees, and absent at the ankles. Sensory examination showed intact vibratory sensation and joint position sense. Pinprick sensation was reduced in a stocking distribution. Coordination testing was normal. Toes were downgoing bilaterally. She was unable to walk.

Investigations

The patient was admitted to our neurology inpatient service. A repeat NCS/EMG was performed. NCS revealed reduced bilateral peroneal and tibial compound muscle action potential (CMAP) amplitudes with normal conduction velocities and distal motor latencies. Sensory conduction responses were normal. H-reflexes were absent. Needle EMG revealed abundant fibrillation potentials and positive sharp waves in the majority of the muscles tested both proximally and distally in the bilateral lower extremities, including the lumbar paraspinal muscles but to a much lesser degree compared to the limb muscles. Motor unit recruitment was markedly reduced; motor unit morphology appeared relatively normal except for a few polyphasic units. Cerebrospinal fluid (CSF) study revealed mildly elevated protein 68 mg/dL (normal: 15–45 mg/dL), normal cells, glucose, and IgG index and synthesis, and absent oligoclonal bands. Blood tests showed a mildly elevated serum angiotensin converting enzyme (ACE) level at 74.6 (normal: 12–68 U/L). GM1 antibodies were negative. Complete blood count (CBC), comprehensive metabolic panel, HbA1C, serum immunofixation, ANA, ENA, ANCAs, cryoglobulins, TSH, B12, Lyme serology, and paraneoplastic antibody panel were all unremarkable. She was treated with intravenous immunoglobulin (IVIg) 0.4 gm/kg/day for 5 days for a presumed diagnosis of the axonal variant of Guillian Barré syndrome (GBS). Her weakness and pain minimally improved after the first course of IVIg, and she was discharged to the inpatient rehabilitation unit. Her sensorimotor deficits did not show further improvement even after two more courses of IVIG (2 gm/kg per course), 2 weeks apart. NCS/EMG was repeated again 2 months after the second one. NCS revealed absent motor and sensory nerve conduction responses in the lower extremities. EMG showed ongoing denervation changes in the proximal and distal lower extremity muscles. The findings are consistent with a severe, progressive, sensorimotor, axonal polyneuropathy. A combined right sural nerve and gastrocnemius muscle biopsy was performed.

Nerve and Muscle Biopsy Findings

The right sural nerve biopsy (Fig. 35.1) revealed a mildly-to-moderately severe, active, axonal neuropathy with striking perineuritis but no granulomas or acid fast bacilli. Several fascicles showed focal or irregular inflammation and thickening of perineurium. Chronic mononuclear inflammatory cells were seen infiltrating perineurium and surrounding epineurial and endoneurial blood vessels. Vasculitis was absent. The degree of perineurial inflammation was variable among different fascicles. In one fascicle, the perineurial inflammation extended into endoneurium. Many of the inflammatory cells were CD68+ macrophages. Fite stain was negative for acid fast bacilli. The semithin plastic sections also showed prominent perineurial inflammation and scattered perivascular inflammation. Many foamy macrophages were noted in perineurium; a few were also seen in endoneurium. The majority of the fascicles showed focal inflammation and thickening of perineurium. Subperineurial edema was absent. The myelinated fiber density was mildly-to-moderately reduced with no significant interfascicular or intrafascicular variations. Some myelin ovoids were present, indicating active axonal degeneration. There was no regenerating cluster. There was no large thinly-myelinated fiber or onion bulb to suggest demyelination and remyelination. The right gastrocnemius muscle biopsy (Fig. 35.1) showed prominent chronic active neurogenic changes, including abundant target and targetoid fibers, mild fiber type grouping, and grouped atrophy. It also showed mild-to-moderate type 2 myofiber atrophy. There were two tiny endomysial collections of chronic mononuclear inflammatory cells, but no necrotic or regenerating fibers.

Additional Investigations After the Nerve and Muscle Biopsy Diagnoses

Given the sterile perineuritis revealed by the nerve biopsy and the remote history of cutaneous sarcoidosis, the patient underwent high resolution chest computed tomography (CT). It showed trace bibasilar atelectasis but no lymphadenopathy. CT of abdomen and pelvis was also unremarkable. There was no evidence of systemic sarcoidosis.

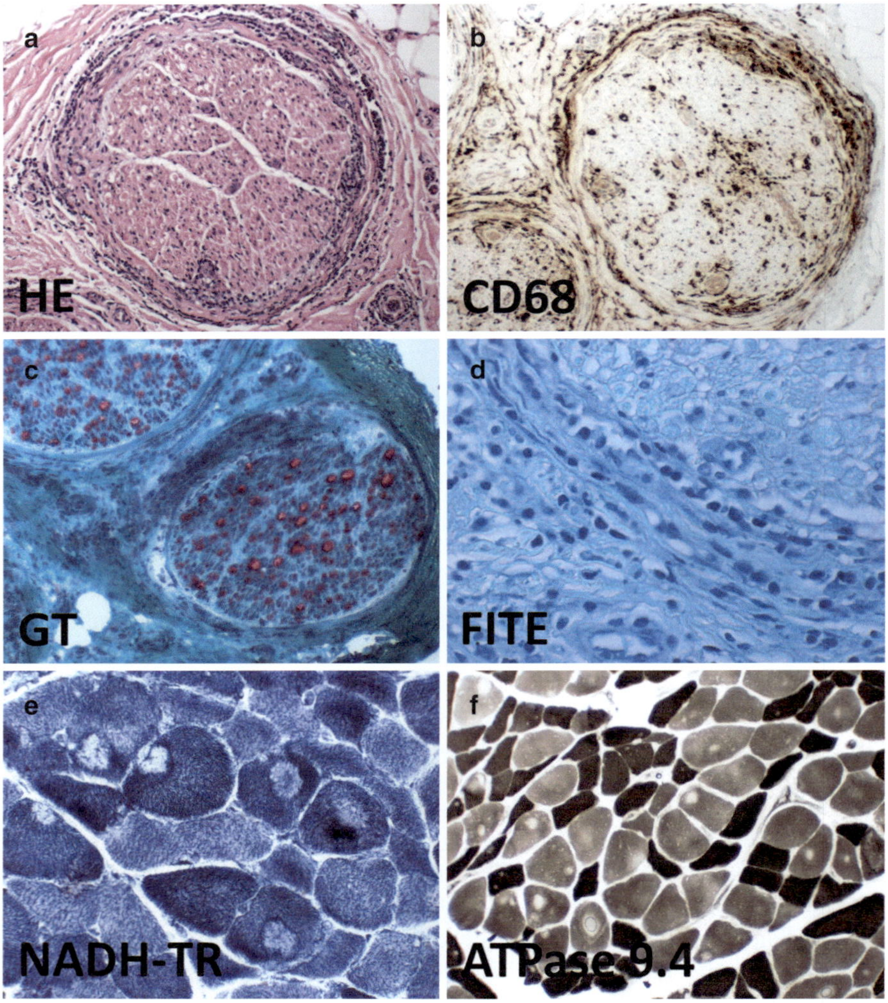

Fig. 35.1 Hematoxylin and eosin stain (HE) of the sural nerve biopsy section shows chronic mononuclear inflammatory cells infiltrating perineurium and surrounding epineurial and endoneurial blood vessels. There is irregular thickening of perineurium. CD68 immunostain (CD68) shows many of the inflammatory cells in perineurium are macrophages. The number of endoneurial macrophages also appears mildly increased. Gomori trichrome stain (GT) shows mildly-to-moderately reduced myelinated axons. FITE stain (FITE) shows no acid fast bacilli. NADH-TR stain (NADH-TR) of the gastrocnemius muscle biopsy section shows several target fibers. ATPase pH 9.4 stain (ATPase 9.4) shows grouped atrophy and type 2 myofiber atrophy

Final Diagnosis

Perineuritis with Active Axonal Polyradiculoneuropathy.

Patient Follow-up

After the diagnosis of active perineuritis was made based on the biopsy, the patient received intravenous infusions of methylprednisolone 1 gram daily for 5 consecutive days, followed by oral prednisone 60 mg daily. The patient's pain markedly reduced. Strength also improved. She was able to ambulate with a walker within a few weeks. Mycophenolate mofetil 1 gram twice daily was added. The patient had a near complete recovery of her motor function within a year. She only had mild residual weakness in the foot and toe dorsiflexors. Immunosuppressant medications were gradually tapered and discontinued after 3 years with close monitoring.

Discussion

Perineuritis is a rare clinicopathological entity. Patients with perineuritis may present with sensory polyneuropathy [1, 2], sensorimotor axonal polyneuropathy [3], chronic polyneuropathy with mixed demyelinating and axonal features [4], or mononeuropathy multiplex [5]. Perineuritis that manifests acute, progressive, sensorimotor, axonal polyneuropathy mimicking Guillian Barre syndrome (GBS) as seen in our case has also been described [6]. Painful paresthesia is a prominent symptom. Perineuritis can be idiopathic but is more often seen in association with a systemic disease such as sarcoidosis, leprosy, cryoglobulinemia, ulcerative colitis, intoxication with adulterated rapeseed oil, or systemic malignancy [5–8]. Our case appears to represent idiopathic perineuritis. Although the patient had a remote history of cutaneous sarcoidosis and breast cancer, there was no evidence of systemic sarcoidosis or malignancies at the time of neuropathy evaluation. The combined sural nerve and gastrocnemius muscle biopsy did not show granulomas or micro-organisms. The link between the perineuritis and prior cutaneous sarcoidosis is uncertain.

The differential diagnosis of an acute, painful, rapidly progressive, polyneuropathy includes GBS, vasculitic neuropathy, other inflammatory neuropathies such as sarcoid granulomatous neuritis and perineuritis, infectious neuropathies, and toxic neuropathies. GBS mimics should be considered when the disease course is atypical and the treatment response is poor. Our patient presented with acute worsening of paresthesia and rapid progression of limb weakness with reduced peroneal and tibial CMAP amplitudes and normal sensory NCS, which made the initial consideration of GBS reasonable. However, the onset of mild sensory symptoms 2 months prior to the acute worsening, and the lack of any improvement over the course of 3 months despite the repeated courses of IVIg treatment made the GBS diagnosis questionable.

It raised a strong suspicion for an active inflammatory myopathy other than GBS such as vasculitic neuropathy. Given the past medical history of breast cancer and sarcoidosis, paraneoplastic neuropathy and sarcoid neuritis were also of concern. The patient did not have signs of infection or a history of neurotoxin exposure. A nerve biopsy was needed in this clinical setting to address the GBS mimics.

The sural nerve biopsy in our patient showed striking active perineuritis. Perineuritis is a rare but distinct pathological diagnosis. The nerve pathology of perineuritis is characterized by prominent perineural inflammation, damage, and thickening along with axonal degeneration as seen in our case [6]. Endoneurial and epineurial perivascular inflammation is commonly seen. The inflammation and thickening of perineurium are often focal or irregular with fascicle-to-fascicle variations. Electron microscopy (EM) typically reveals foamy histiocytes and lymphocytes infiltrating and splitting perineurial lamellae, perineurial cell necrosis, and thickening of perineurium with excessive collagen deposition [3, 5, 6]. When associated with sarcoidosis, granulomas may be present in the endoneurium or epineurium (see Fig. 2.6 in Chap. 2) [6]. When associated with leprosy neuritis, additional features such as granulomas, acid fast bacilli, more severe epineurial and endoneurial inflammation, and neural architectural damage are often present [9] (see the chapter of "Leprous Neuropathy"). The nerve biopsy finding of perineuritis should prompt a careful search for sarcoidosis and leprosy. In our case, although the patient had a remote history of cutaneous sarcoidosis, the high resolution chest CT and the abdomen and pelvis CT did not reveal any evidence of systemic sarcoidosis. The nerve biopsy did not show granulomas. The nerve inflammation was relatively confined to perineurium, and the FITE stain did not show acid fast bacilli to suggest leprosy neuritis.

A sural nerve biopsy can differentiate GBS from other inflammatory neuropathies which can clinically mimic GBS. A nerve biopsy in GBS typically shows prominent endoneurial inflammation rather than perineurial inflammation, along with active demyelination and/or axonal degeneration. A nerve biopsy in acute vasculitic neuropathy often shows acute vasculitis changes and axonal degeneration with interfascicular and/or intrafascicular variations (see Figs. 2.2, 2.3, and 2.13 in Chap. 2 and the chapter of "Vaculitic Neuropathy").

As perineuritis is rare, the natural history and the treatment response to immunosuppressive or immune modulating therapies have not been studied. According to the limited number of case reports, steroids appears effective.

Pearls

Clinical Pearls

1. Perineuritis is a rare clinicopathological entity that may manifest sensory neuropathy, sensorimotor axonal polyneuropathy, chronic polyneuropathy with mixed demyelinating and axonal features, or mononeuropathy multiplex. It can also mimic the axonal variant of GBS.

2. Perineuritis can be idiopathic but is more often seen in association with a systemic disease such as sarcoidosis, leprosy, cryoglobulinemia, ulcerative colitis, intoxication with adulterated rapeseed oil, or systemic malignancy. Adequate workup is needed for appropriate patient management.
3. The differential diagnosis of an acute, painful, rapidly progressive, axonal polyneuropathy includes GBS, vasculitic neuropathy, other inflammatory neuropathies such as sarcoid granulomatous neuritis and perineuritis, infectious neuropathies, and toxic neuropathies.
4. GBS mimics should be considered when the disease course is atypical and the treatment response is poor. A nerve biopsy is essential to address the GBS mimics.
5. A prompt diagnosis of GBS mimics is critical, as it changes clinical management. While the therapy for GBS is IVIg or plasmapheresis, the treatment of vasculitic neuropathy, sarcoid granulomatous neuritis, and sterile perineuritis usually requires steroids and other immunosuppressive agents. Infectious neuritis such as leprosy neuritis needs antibiotics treatment.

Pathology Pearls

1. Perineuritis is characterized by predominant inflammation, damage, and thickening of perineurium along with axonal degeneration. The inflammation and thickening of perineurium are often focal or irregular with fascicle-to-fascicle variations. EM typically shows foamy histiocytes and lymphocytes infiltrating and splitting perineurial lamellae, perineurial cell necrosis, and thickening of perineurium with excessive collagen deposition.

References

1. Asbury AK, Picard EH, Baringer JR. Sensory perineuritis. Arch Neurol. 1972;26(4):302–12.
2. Matthews WB, Squier MV. Sensory perineuritis. J Neurol Neurosurg Psychiatry. 1988;51(4):473–5.
3. Bourque CN, Anderson BA, Martin del Campo C, Sima AA. Sensorimotor perineuritis—an autoimmune disease? Can J Neurol Sci. 1985;12(2):129–33.
4. Chad DA, Smith TW, DeGirolami U, Hammer K. Perineuritis and ulcerative colitis. Neurology. 1986;36(10):1377–9.
5. Simmons Z, Albers JW, Sima AA. Case-of-the-month: perineuritis presenting as mononeuritis multiplex. Muscle Nerve. 1992;15(5):630–5.
6. Midroni G, Bilbao JM. Idiopathic inflammatory neuropathies: sarcoidosis and perineuritis. In: Midroni G, Bilbao JM, editors. Biopsy diagnosis of peripheral neuropathy. Boston: Butterworth-Heinemann; 1995. p. 197–207.
7. Konishi T, Saida K, Ohnishi A, Nishitani H. Perineuritis in mononeuritis multiplex with cryoglobulinemia. Muscle Nerve. 1982;5(2):173–7.
8. Ricoy JR, Cabello A, Rodriguez J, Tellez I. Neuropathological studies on the toxic syndrome related to adulterated rapeseed oil in Spain. Brain. 1983;106(Pt 4):817–35.
9. Midroni G, Bilbao JM. Leprous neuropathy. In: Mildroni G, Bilbao JM, editors. Biopsy diagnosis of peripheral neuropathy. Boston: Butterworth-Heinemann; 1995. p. 223–40.

Chapter 36
A 34-Year-Old Man with Right Hand and Left Foot Numbness

Sharon P. Nations and Dennis K. Burns

History

A 34-year-old Indian man presented for evaluation of right hand and left foot numbness. Eighteen months earlier, he noted right index finger numbness that spread over months to involve entire hand up to mid-forearm. He had burned his fingers without feeling it. He also noted the skin of the right hand was dry. About 6 months after onset, he noted a small patch of numbness, slowly enlarging, on the lateral left foot. He denied pain, rashes or skin discoloration, nasal congestion or nose bleeds, or weight loss. He had no history of diabetes, hepatitis or renal disease. He did not smoke or drink alcohol and worked in a clerical position, without exposure to toxins.

Physical Examination

His examination revealed no rash or skin hypopigmentation. His mental status and cranial nerve functions were normal. He had normal strength, coordination, deep tendon reflexes, and gait. He had decreased light touch, pinprick and temperature sensation in the right hand and left lateral foot. Vibratory sensation was decreased in his right index finger. Proprioception was normal.

S. P. Nations (✉)
Department of Neurology & Neurotherapeutics,
University of Texas Southwestern Medical Center, Dallas, TX, USA
e-mail: sharon.nations@utsouthwestern.edu

D. K. Burns
Department of Pathology, Neuropathology Section,
University of Texas Southwestern Medical Center, Dallas, TX, USA

L. Zhou et al. (eds.), *A Case-Based Guide to Neuromuscular Pathology*,
https://doi.org/10.1007/978-3-030-25682-1_36

Investigations

The following tests were negative or normal: serum glucose, erythrocyte sedimentation rate, antinuclear antibody, anti-neutrophil cytoplasmic antibodies, and serum protein electrophoresis. Nerve conduction studies (NCS) revealed slightly prolonged right ulnar distal latency, mildly reduced right ulnar motor amplitude and normal conduction velocity across the forearm. Across the elbow, conduction velocity was mildly slowed by 21% and amplitude decrease by 21%. Right median motor response was normal. Right median and ulnar sensory responses were absent. Right radial sensory response had mildly prolonged peak latency and moderately reduced amplitude. Left peroneal and tibial motor responses were normal. Left sural sensory response had normal peak latency and severely reduced amplitude. Overall findings were of a predominantly sensory axonal multifocal neuropathy with superimposed right ulnar neuropathy at the elbow.

Skin biopsy of the right hand was performed and showed mild nonspecific inflammation without abnormal stains for acid fast bacilli (AFB). Since the biopsy was non-diagnostic, the patient was referred for biopsy of the right superficial radial nerve. Biopsy of overlying skin was performed at the same time.

Nerve and Skin Biopsy Findings

Cryostat and paraffin sections of the right superficial radial nerve biopsy revealed a striking endoneurial mononuclear inflammatory infiltrate, particularly pronounced in the subperineurial region of the largest fascicle and extending more diffusely through the remainder of the endoneurial compartment. Granulomas were present in some areas (Fig. 36.1a). Myelinated axons were decreased in number in an irregular distribution in all fascicles. Fite modified acid fast stain highlighted scattered acid fast bacilli dispersed singularly and in small clusters throughout the endoneurial compartment, some within the cytoplasm of inflammatory cells and some within myelin sheaths (Fig. 36.1b). Toluidine blue-stained semithin Epon sections revealed a generalized decrease in myelinated fiber numbers, with a substantial number of the remaining myelinated axons invested by disproportionately thin myelin sheaths (Fig. 36.1c). Electron microscopy revealed endoneurial mononuclear infiltration and additional evidence of axonal loss in the form of numerous collections of Schwann cell cytoplasmic processes devoid of axoplasm, as well numerous thinly myelinated axons and an occasional myelin ovoid. In some instances, myelin sheaths were disrupted by intramyelinic vesicular profiles, consistent with active demyelination. Electron dense bacilli were identified in the cytoplasm of some Schwann cells and occasional endoneurial mononuclear cells (Fig. 36.1d). No definite intra-axonal bacilli were identified. Simultaneous skin biopsy showed a patchy mononuclear inflammatory infiltrate around dermal appendages and nerve twigs, the latter most conspicuous at the dermal-subcutaneous junction. No granulomas were identified. Fite-stained sections revealed scattered AFB adjacent to adnexal structures and within the deeper dermal nerve twigs. Slit skin scrapings for tissue

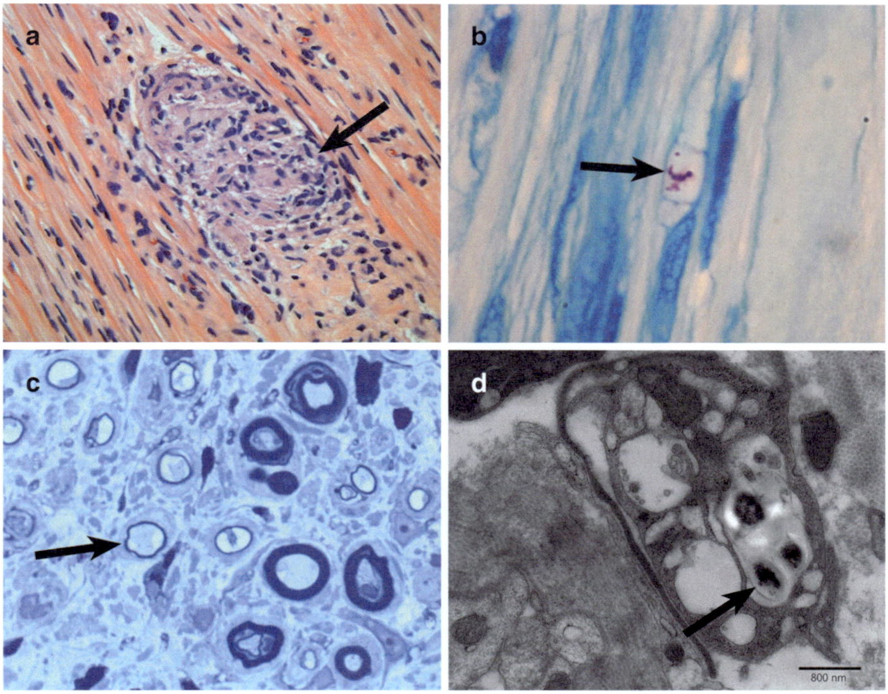

Fig. 36.1 Nerve biopsy, leprous neuropathy. (**a**), An H&E-stained paraffin section of the superficial radial nerve biopsy, demonstrating a well-formed granuloma (arrow). (**b**), Fite stained longitudinally oriented paraffin section, demonstrating clusters of acid fast bacilli intimately associated with a myelin sheath (arrow). (**c**), Epon-embedded 1.5 mm transverse section, demonstrating numerous axons invested by disproportionately thin myelin sheaths, compatible with demyelination (arrow). (**d**), Transmission electron micrograph, demonstrating irregular, electron dense bacilli within an endoneurial mononuclear cell. A prominent mycolic acid coat (arrow), typical of *M. tuberculosis*, surrounds the degenerating bacilli

fluid of bilateral ear lobes, elbows and knees, tested by modified Fite stain, demonstrated AFB at the right elbow.

Final Diagnosis

Multibacillary Hansen's disease

Patient Follow-up

The patient was treated with dapsone, rifampin and clofazimine for 2 years per the National Hansen's disease program guidelines [1]. His sensory exam improved dramatically in the right hand and normalized in the left foot.

Four years after completing therapy, he returned for evaluation of worsening right-hand numbness, new weakness of the right hand, and new numbness and weakness of the right foot. He had partial recurrence of numbness in left lateral foot. His hemoglobin A1c was normal. Skin biopsy of the numb area of the right foot showed chronic perivascular and perineurial inflammatory infiltrates in the mid and deep dermis. One focus clearly involved a cutaneous nerve. No AFB could be identified by Fite stain. The patient was treated with prednisone, gradually tapering over several months. He was also treated with dapsone, rifampin and clofazimine for a year for possible recurrent infection. However, in retrospect, this episode most likely represented a reversal reaction [2], an increase in the body's immune response to bacteria, which can be seen before, during or even years after completion of antibiotic treatment [3]. Nonviable bacteria are cleared from the body very slowly over years and may provoke an inflammatory response, producing new neuropathies, with or without pain. Reversal reactions can be successfully treated with steroids or other immune suppressants. The patient's right hand weakness improved but did not return to baseline. His right foot numbness was unchanged.

Discussion

Leprosy, or Hansen's disease, is a common cause of neuropathy in the developing world, but may be seen in immigrants to developed countries or in endemic regions of the United States. It is an infection caused by *Mycobacterium leprae*, affecting skin and nerves. Its neurotropism can be explained, at least in part, by its affinity for Schwann cells. The cell wall of *M. leprae* contains phenolic glycolipid-1 (PGL-1), which is not found in other mycobacteria [4]. PGL-1 binds to the laminin alpha-2 chain of the Schwann cell basal lamina, an interaction sufficient to induce the uptake of *M. leprae* into the Schwann cell [5]. Manifestations of the disease range on a spectrum from tuberculoid to lepromatous. Tuberculoid patients have a well-developed cell-mediated immune response, with disease limited to a few hypoesthetic skin lesions and at most a mononeuropathy. Lepromatous patients present with widespread rash and a symmetric polyneuropathy. Interestingly, deep tendon reflexes are typically preserved in leprous neuropathy. Patients may have loss of eyelashes and eyebrows, and inflammatory infiltration of ear lobes, nose and forehead, leading to the so-called "leonine facies". In between these polar extremes are patients with more asymmetric presentations, called borderline leprosy [6]. For treatment purposes, patients are classified as either paucibacillary (5 or fewer skin lesions) or multibacillary (more than 5 skin lesions) and treated according to World Health Organization protocols. Paucibacillary patients are treated with dapsone and rifampin for 6 months. Multibacillary patients are treated with dapsone, rifampin and clofazimine for 1 year [7]. In the United States, treatment is continued for 1 year for paucibacillary and 2 years for multibacillary disease per the National Hansen's Disease Program recommendations [1].

One of the challenges of treating this disease is its propensity for causing autoimmune reactions, which can occur as long as the bacterial antigens are present in the body. These are of two types: type 1 or reversal reaction and type 2 or erythema nodosum leprosum (ENL). In reversal reaction, there is an increase in cell-mediated immune response, leading to increased erythema and swelling of skin lesions and new numbness or weakness, with or without pain. ENL is caused by deposition of antigen-antibody complexes in various tissues, leading to fever, painful skin nodules, hepatosplenomegaly, neuritis, nephritis, orchitis, and iridocyclitis [2]. Both reversal reaction and ENL are treated with prednisone, particularly when there is nerve involvement. In addition, thalidomide is used to treat ENL in non-pregnant patients. It is not helpful in treating neuropathy. Both male and female patients treated with thalidomide must use adequate contraception due to the well-known teratogenic effects of the medication.

Leprosy is typically diagnosed by biopsy of skin rash. In tuberculoid cases, well-formed epithelioid granulomas, sometimes caseating, may be seen with bacteria absent or only demonstrable by polymerase chain reaction (PCR) for *M. leprae*. In lepromatous cases, skin biopsy reveals disorganized inflammatory cells, including lipid-laden ("foamy") macrophages containing many bacilli in clumps ("globi"). Destruction of sweat glands and hair follicles results in dry skin and loss of hair, respectively [2].

As illustrated in this case, "neuritic leprosy" may occur, without associated skin hypopigmentation or rash. A high index of suspicion in patients from endemic areas (which include Texas and Louisiana in the United States) should prompt referral for biopsy. Skin biopsy in a symptomatic area may reveal inflammation involving dermal nerves, which is highly suggestive of leprosy by itself without AFB. If skin biopsy is not definitive, biopsy of an affected nerve may confirm the diagnosis.

Nerve biopsy shows variable degrees of inflammatory changes, involving some fascicles, sparing others. Perineurial inflammation is common, and its presence in any nerve biopsy should always prompt a search for acid fast bacilli. Animal studies have demonstrated that the mycobacteria collect in epineurial lymphatics, thus spreading to endoneurial blood vessels [8]. *M. leprae* may be seen in endothelial cells of human patients, suggesting a vascular entry through the perineurial sheath [9]. In tuberculoid disease, granuloma formation is prominent and destroys nerve. Staining with S-100 may be necessary to verify presence of nerve tissue. In lepromatous cases, the nerve structure may be relatively preserved and well-formed granulomas are absent. Myelin injury is best demonstrated in toluidine blue stained semithin resin-embedded semithin sections and in teased fiber preparations. The perineurium may be split into layers by sheets of foamy cells or edema, giving an "onion bulb" appearance [2].

Prognosis depends on the duration of symptoms and is good to excellent if the disease is diagnosed in early stages before significant nerve damage occurs. Close monitoring of patients is required during treatment and periodically after treatment is completed, in order to promptly detect and treat reactions that can lead to further nerve damage.

Pearls

Clinical Pearls

1. Leprous neuropathy should be a diagnostic consideration in any patient with neuropathy, with or without rash, from an endemic region.
2. Nerve biopsy is not usually necessary but helpful for diagnosis.
3. The disease is curable with recommended antibiotic therapy but prolonged treatment is necessary.
4. Patients must be monitored for worsening or new neuropathy symptoms, which may signal an immune mediated reaction, requiring treatment with immune suppressants. Thalidomide may be used to treat ENL reactions but does not treat neuropathy.

Pathology Pearls

1. Nerve biopsy in leprous neuropathy may reveal characteristic inflammation and AFB as well as demyelination of axons. Acid fast bacilli may be exceedingly rare in some cases of the tuberculoid form of the disease, but are typically abundant in the lepromatous variants.

References

1. Health Resources and Services Administration. National Hansen's Disease (Leprosy) Program Caring and Curing Since 1894. www.hrsa.gov/hansens-disease. Accessed 4 Mar 2019.
2. Sabin TD, Swift TR, Jacobson RR. Leprosy. In: Dyck PJ, Thomas PK, Griffin JW, Low PA, Poduslo JF, editors. Peripheral neuropathy, vol. 2. 3rd ed. Philadelphia: WB Saunders; 1993. p. 1354–79.
3. Naafs B. Current views on reactions in leprosy. Indian J Lepr. 2000;72:99–124.
4. Sang-Nae C, Yanagihara DL, et al. Serological specificity of phenolic glycolipid 1 from Mycobacterium leprae and use in diagnosis of leprosy. Infect Immun. 1983;41:1077–83.
5. Rambukkana A. Molecular basis for the peripheral nerve predilection of *Mycobacterium leprae*. Curr Opin Microbiol. 2001;4:21–7.
6. Ridley DS, Jopling WH. Classification of leprosy according to immunity—a five-group system. Int J Lepr Other Mycobat Dis. 1966;34:235–74.
7. World Health Organization. WHO recommended MDT regimens. www.who.int/lep/mdt/regimens/en. Accessed 4 Mar 2019.
8. Scollard DM, McCormick G, Allen J. Localization of *Mycobacterium leprae* to endothelial cells of epineural and perineural blood vessels and lymphatics. Am J Pathol. 1999;154:1611–20.
9. Scollard DM, Truman RW, Ebenezer GJ. Mechanisms of nerve injury in leprosy. Clin Dermatol. 2015;33:46–54.

Chapter 37
A 64-Year-Old Woman with Progressive Pain, Numbness and Weakness in the Right Lower Limb

Lan Zhou, Susan Morgello, Rajeev Motiwala, and Susan C. Shin

History

A 64-year-old woman presented to the emergency room with progressive pain, weakness, and numbness in the right lower extremity. She developed a relatively acute onset of pain in the right gluteal area shooting towards the right posterior thigh, calf, and lateral foot 2 months prior to the presentation. This was followed by progressive weakness and numbness in the right leg and foot, which affected her gait. She also developed focal swelling in the lateral aspect of the right distal leg. She denied other limb involvement. She denied bowel or urinary incontinence. There had been no fever, weight loss, night sweats, or skin rash. Her past medical history was significant for uterine fibroids status-post hysterectomy. Her family history, social history, and review of systems were unremarkable.

L. Zhou (✉)
Departments of Neurology and Pathology, Boston University Medical Center, Boston, MA, USA
e-mail: lanzhou@bu.edu

S. Morgello
Departments of Neurology, Neuroscience, and Pathology, Icahn School of Medicine at Mount Sinai, New York, NY, USA
e-mail: Susan.morgello@mssm.edu

R. Motiwala
Department of Neurology, New York University, New York, NY, USA
e-mail: Rajeev.Motiwala@nyulangone.org

S. C. Shin
Department of Neurology, Icahn School of Medicine at Mount Sinai, New York, NY, USA
e-mail: Susan.shin@mssm.edu

L. Zhou et al. (eds.), *A Case-Based Guide to Neuromuscular Pathology*,
https://doi.org/10.1007/978-3-030-25682-1_37

Physical Examination

Her general examination was unremarkable except for mild focal edema with tenderness involving the lateral aspect of the right distal leg. There was no spine tenderness. Her neurological examination showed normal mental status and cranial nerve functions. Sensorimotor deficits were only detected in the right lower limb with weakness in the knee flexors (MRC 4−/5), foot dorsiflexors (4/5) and plantar flexors (4−/5), foot evertors and invertors (4−/5), and toe dorsiflexors (3/5) and plantar flexors (4−/5). Pinprick sensation was reduced in the right posterior thigh, posterior and lateral distal leg, and the dorsal and lateral aspects of the foot. Vibratory sensation was reduced at the right toes and ankle. Joint position sense was intact. Deep tendon reflexes were 2+ except for the absent right ankle jerk. Plantar responses were flexor bilaterally. Her gait was antalgic, and she dragged her right foot.

Investigations

Nerve conduction study (NCS) and electromyogram (EMG) showed severely reduced right peroneal compound muscle action potential (CMAP) amplitude recording the extensor digitorum brevis muscle (0.1 mV). The right peroneal CMAP amplitude recording the tibialis anterior muscle was also reduced (1.4 mV) with a partial (42%) conduction block and conduction slowing (28 m/s) across the fibular head. Right tibial CMAP amplitude was also markedly reduced (0.8 mV) with normal distal latency and conduction velocity. Right tibial H-reflex was absent. Right sural sensory nerve action potential (SNAP) amplitude was more than 50% reduced as compared to the left (right 9 μV and left 19 μV). Right superficial peroneal sensory response was absent. Right femoral motor conduction study was normal and similar to the left. NCS of the left lower extremity was normal. Concentric needle EMG revealed 1+ to 3+ fibrillation potentials and positive sharp waves with reduced motor unit recruitment and slightly large motor unit potentials in the right tibialis anterior, peroneal longus, gastrocnemius, extensor hallucis longus, biceps femoris, and gluteus medius muscles. Fibrillation potentials and positive sharp waves were also noted in the right L5 and S1 paraspinal muscles. Needle EMG of the right vastus lateralis muscle and the left lower extremity and paraspinal muscles was normal. The complex electrodiagnostic findings were consistent with a right lumbosacral radiculoplexus neuropathy with associated acute right peroneal neuropathy at the fibular head. Magnetic resonance imaging (MRI) of the lumbar and sacral spine showed no significant degenerative changes of the spine but thickening and contrast enhancement of cauda equine nerve roots, most prominently the right S1 nerve root. MRI of the right leg showed a 4.9 cm × 1.2 cm × 1.0 cm lobular enlargement with contrast enhancement of the right superficial peroneal nerve adjacent to the distal fibular shaft. There was also thickening and enhancement of the distal sciatic, tibial, or common peroneal nerve. MRIs of brain and cervical and thoracic spine were unrevealing. Rheumatological markers, ACE level, and HIV, EBV, CMV, HSV, and Lyme serology were all unremarkable. A cerebrospinal fluid (CSF) study demonstrated an elevated protein level (112 mg/dL), normal otherwise. CSF cytology displayed rare atypical lymphocytes, and flow cytometry was suspicious for a B-cell lymphoproliferative disorder. Computed tomography (CT) scan of chest, abdomen and pelvis with contrast was unremarkable. Whole body fludeoxyglucose-positron emission tomography (FDG-PET) scan showed intense radiotracer activity along the course of the right S1 nerve root, discrete focus of increased tracer uptake in the posterior compartment of the lower right thigh and popliteal fossa, and intensely hypermetabolic tubular mass in the anterior compartment of the right distal leg. There were no other hypermetabolic lesions in the rest of the body. A right superficial peroneal nerve lesion biopsy was performed.

Nerve Lesion Biopsy Findings

The right superficial peroneal nerve lesion biopsy (Fig. 37.1) showed diffuse large B-cell lymphoma (DLBCL) involving the nerve and surrounding soft tissue; the lymphoma cells were immunoreactive to CD20 and Bcl-2 but not CD10.

Final Diagnosis

Primary Neurolymphomatosis

Patient Follow-up

The patient underwent chemotherapy with the R-MPV regimen (rituximab, methotrexate, procarbazine, and vincristine) developed for primary CNS lymphoma [1]. She also received radiation therapy to her right distal leg. She presented to our neurology clinic for follow up 15 months after the symptom onset, when she had received 7 cycles of chemotherapy and 17 radiation treatments. She showed remarkable interval improvement with the right leg pain completely resolved. Only mild weakness was detected in the right foot dorsiflexors (4+/5) and toe dorsiflexors (4/5). Pinprick sensation was slightly reduced at the lateral aspect of her right distal leg and the lateral, dorsum, and bottom of her right foot. She was able to walk without dragging her right foot. The repeat FDG-PET showed no evidence of residual lymphoma.

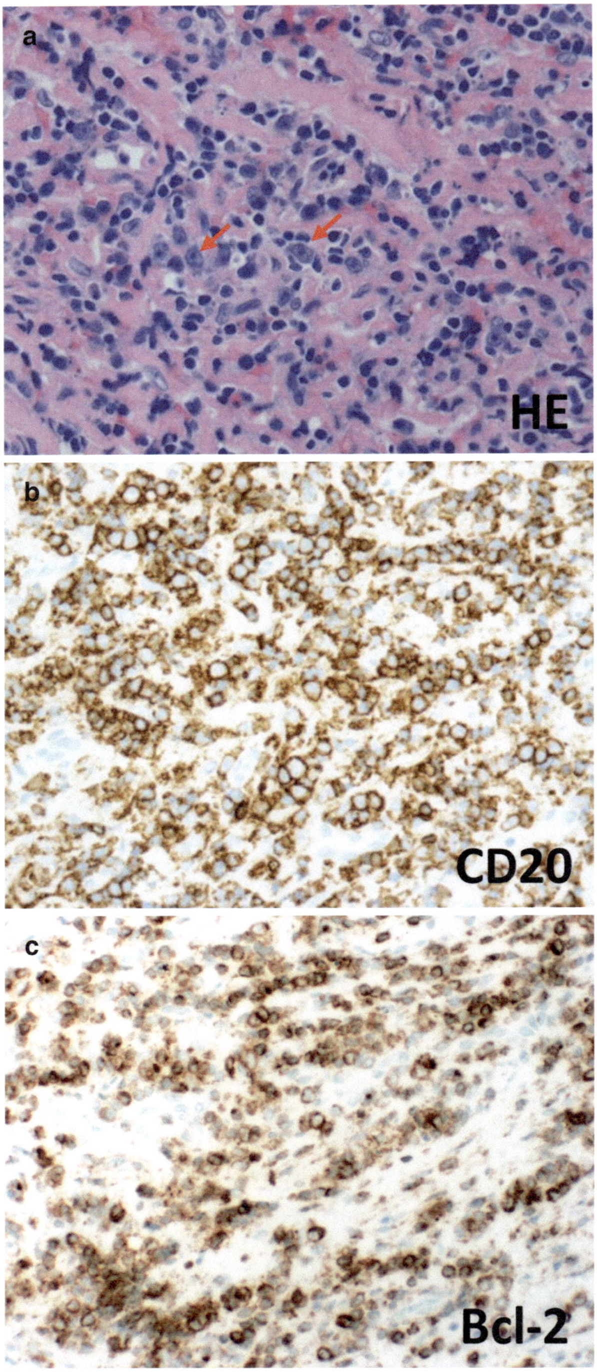

Fig. 37.1 H&E stain (**a**) shows nerve infiltration by abundant tumor cells (arrows). The tumor cells have large nuclei and prominent nucleoli; these features are typical of a large cell B-cell lymphoma. Immunostains show that these cells expressed CD20 (**b**) and Bcl-2 (**c**)

Discussion

Neurolymphomatosis (NL), defined as lymphoma infiltrating the nerve, occurs both in isolation as primary neurolymphomatosis (PNL), or secondary to systemic or central nervous system (CNS) disease [2–4]. As a secondary phenomenon, it can present at initial lymphoma diagnosis, during the course of disease, or during relapse; as a primary condition, it is exceedingly rare [5]. It is typically due to non-Hodgkin's lymphoma, most commonly diffuse large B-cell lymphoma (DLBCL), but T-cell lymphomas are also reported [6, 7].

NL is a rare disease which can affect cranial nerves, spinal nerve roots, brachial and lumbosacral plexus, and peripheral nerves. The median age at onset is about 50 years, and the disease has male predominance [3, 8, 9]. A few cases of PNL have been reported affecting focal individual peripheral nerves, nerve roots, or both [4, 6, 9–12], with the sciatic nerve involvement being the most common [10–12]. Our case represents PNL with painful unilateral lower limb involvement caused by polyradiculoneuropathy, which is very rare. The patient had unilateral multiple lesions involving the right S1 root, sciatic nerve, common peroneal nerve, superficial peroneal nerve, and tibial nerve.

Due to the lack of systemic and CNS involvement, early diagnosis of PNL can be quite challenging, which requires a high clinical suspicion and adequate evaluation to avoid delay [4]. Comprehensive evaluation of patients is essential to achieve early diagnosis of PNL as seen in our patient. NCS/EMG is helpful to localize the lesion(s) [3, 13]. Neuroimaging study with MRI is useful to further localize and evaluate the lesion(s) and to target a lesion for biopsy. Whole body PET scan is more sensitive than MRI for staging the disease [3, 5, 9, 13–15]. MRI in PLN usually shows enhancing lesions in the affected nerves and nerve roots. But MRI enhancing nerve and root lesion(s) can also be seen in other malignancies such as nerve sheath tumors, inflammatory diseases such as inflammatory demyelinating polyradiculoneuropathy or sarcoid radiculoneuropathy, and infectious neuritis and radiculitis [16]. Blood tests and CSF study are important in the initial evaluation to address the differential diagnosis. CSF cytology may show lymphoma cells but the sensitivity is low [2, 9]. Therefore, successful nerve or nerve root lesion biopsy is often needed and is the gold standard for the diagnosis of PNL. In the present case, the definitive diagnosis was made by the superficial peroneal nerve lesion biopsy.

Histologically, tumor cells can infiltrate in an annular fashion just beneath the perineurium, can extend from the sub-perineurium into the endoneurial space, or can diffusely, confluently infiltrate the endoneurium [7]. Foci of demyelination devoid of macrophage infiltrates can occur in the region of NL, but without direct apposition of tumor cells to the demyelinated axons [7]. Distal to tumor, Wallerian degeneration of axons with macrophage infiltrates can be seen. As NL often has a proximal distribution, it is important to recognize that "false negative" biopsies with degenerative features may occur, thus, radiographic localization of lesions prior to biopsy is recommended [17]. In one recent review, histology with immunohistochemistry for lymphocyte markers was sufficient to make the diagnosis of NL on nerve biopsy in only 40% of cases; with the use of multiplex PCR to detect lymphoma gene rearrangements in the nerve tissue, close to 90% could be ascertained [18].

The pathogenesis of PNL is currently unclear. There is a high rate of extranodal primary presentations in a variety of organ systems in DLBCL. Gene expression profiling has identified two distinct forms of DLBCL, germinal centre B-like DLBCL and activated B-like DLBCL. Germinal centre B-like DLBCL cells resemble germinal centre cells in the lymph node and express CD10 and Bcl-6, while activated B-like DLBCL cells look like activated peripheral blood cells and express Bcl-2 [19]. Since the DLBCL cells in the NL lesion of our patient expressed Bcl-2 but not CD10, they appeared originated from peripheral blood. But the primary site of the extranodal generation of the lymphoma and how the activated circulating B cells preferentially home to and infiltrate the local peripheral nerves and nerve roots remain unclear. It may involve systemic tumor cells crossing the blood-nerve barrier mediated through aberrant NCAM expression on lymphocytes homing to CD56 in the nerve [4].

There is no standard treatment for NL. It is usually treated with chemotherapy alone or in combination with radiotherapy. Systemic chemotherapy is critical if multiple sites are involved. Radiotherapy is added if a focal lesion is prominent. High-dose intravenous methotrexate (MTX)-based poly-chemotherapy is the preferred treatment with encouraging results [3, 4]. Adding rituximab appears beneficial [10, 20]. The prognosis of NL is generally poor [2, 3, 9], but PNL appears to have a more favorable prognosis [9] with a median survival of 24 months in a small series treated with high-dose MTX-based poly-chemotherapy [3]. Our patient underwent chemotherapy with the R-MPV regimen (rituximab, methotrexate, procarbazine, and vincristine). She also received radiation therapy to her right distal leg for the lymphoma mass lesion in the right superficial peroneal nerve. She responded very well to the treatment with complete resolution of the PET scan lesions and marked improvement of her sensorimotor deficits.

Pearls

Clinical Pearls

1. NL is a rare disease which can affect cranial nerves, spinal nerve roots, brachial or lumbosacral plexus, and peripheral nerves.
2. Early diagnosis of PNL can be challenging due to a broad spectrum of clinical presentation and the lack of CNS or systemic involvement at the time of evaluation.
3. Comprehensive evaluation including NCS/EMG, MRI with contrast, whole body PET scan, and nerve lesion biopsy is essential to achieve the early diagnosis of PNL.
4. In PNL, MRI usually shows enhancing lesion(s), CSF study may show lymphoma cells but it is insensitive, and nerve lesion biopsy is often needed for the diagnosis.

5. The current preferred treatment of PNL includes systemic chemotherapy using high-dose intravenous MTX-based poly-chemotherapy and radiotherapy for focal lesions. Adding rituximab can be beneficial.
6. A good treatment response can be obtained by aggressive chemotherapy using the R-MPV (rituximab, methotrexate, procarbazine, and vincristine) regimen coupled with radiation treatments starting at a relatively early stage.

Pathology Pearls

1. Nerve lesion biopsy is the gold standard for the diagnosis of PNL.
2. PNL is typically due to non-Hodgkin's lymphoma, most commonly diffuse large B-cell lymphoma (DLBCL). The diagnostic finding of nerve lesion biopsy is the invasion by CD20+ lymphoma cells.

References

1. Morris PG, Correa DD, Yahalom J, Raizer JJ, Schiff D, Grant B, et al. Rituximab, methotrexate, procarbazine, and vincristine followed by consolidation reduced-dose whole-brain radiotherapy and cytarabine in newly diagnosed primary CNS lymphoma: final results and long-term outcome. J Clin Oncol. 2013;31(31):3971–9.
2. Baehring JM, Batchelor TT. Diagnosis and management of neurolymphomatosis. Cancer J. 2012;18(5):463–8.
3. Kamiya-Matsuoka C, Shroff S, Gildersleeve K, Hormozdi B, Manning JT, Woodman KH. Neurolymphomatosis: a case series of clinical manifestations, treatments, and outcomes. J Neurol Sci. 2014;343(1–2):144–8.
4. Lagarde S, Tabouret E, Matta M, Franques J, Attarian S, Pouget J, et al. Primary neurolymphomatosis diagnosis and treatment: a retrospective study. J Neurol Sci. 2014;342(1–2):178–81.
5. Gan HK, Azad A, Cher L, Mitchell PL. Neurolymphomatosis: diagnosis, management, and outcomes in patients treated with rituximab. Neuro-Oncology. 2010;12(2):212–5.
6. Kim J, Kim YS, Lee EJ, Kang CS, Shim SI. Primary CD56-positive NK/T-cell lymphoma of median nerve: a case report. J Korean Med Sci. 1998;13(3):331–3.
7. Tomita M, Koike H, Kawagashira Y, Iijima M, Adachi H, Taguchi J, et al. Clinicopathological features of neuropathy associated with lymphoma. Brain. 2013;136.(Pt 8:2563–78.
8. Baehring JM, Damek D, Martin EC, Betensky RA, Hochberg FH. Neurolymphomatosis. Neuro-Oncology. 2003;5(2):104–15.
9. Grisariu S, Avni B, Batchelor TT, van den Bent MJ, Bokstein F, Schiff D, et al. Neurolymphomatosis: an international primary CNS lymphoma collaborative group report. Blood. 2010;115(24):5005–11.
10. Descamps MJ, Barrett L, Groves M, Yung L, Birch R, Murray NM, et al. Primary sciatic nerve lymphoma: a case report and review of the literature. J Neurol Neurosurg Psychiatry. 2006;77(9):1087–9.
11. Pillay PK, Hardy RW Jr, Wilbourn AJ, Tubbs RR, Lederman RJ. Solitary primary lymphoma of the sciatic nerve: case report. Neurosurgery. 1988;23(3):370–1.
12. Purohit DP, Dick DJ, Perry RH, Lyons PR, Schofield IS, Foster JB. Solitary extranodal lymphoma of sciatic nerve. J Neurol Sci. 1986;74(1):23–34.

13. Ye BS, Sunwoo IN, Suh BC, Park JP, Shim DS, Kim SM. Diffuse large B-cell lymphoma presenting as piriformis syndrome. Muscle Nerve. 2010;41(3):419–22.
14. Salm LP, Van der Hiel B, Stokkel MP. Increasing importance of 18F-FDG PET in the diagnosis of neurolymphomatosis. Nucl Med Commun. 2012;33(9):907–16.
15. Toledano M, Siddiqui MA, Thompson CA, Garza I, Pittock SJ. Teaching NeuroImages: diagnostic utility of FDG-PET in neurolymphomatosis. Neurology. 2013;81(1):e3.
16. Kelly JJ, Karcher DS. Lymphoma and peripheral neuropathy: a clinical review. Muscle Nerve. 2005;31(3):301–13.
17. van den Bent MJ, de Bruin HG, Bos GM, Brutel de la Riviere G, Sillevis Smitt PA. Negative sural nerve biopsy in neurolymphomatosis. J Neurol. 1999;246(12):1159–63.
18. Duchesne M, Roussellet O, Maisonobe T, Gachard N, Rizzo D, Armand M, et al. Pathology of nerve biopsy and diagnostic yield of PCR-based Clonality testing in neurolymphomatosis. J Neuropathol Exp Neurol. 2018;77(9):769–81.
19. Alizadeh AA, Eisen MB, Davis RE, Ma C, Lossos IS, Rosenwald A, et al. Distinct types of diffuse large B-cell lymphoma identified by gene expression profiling. Nature. 2000;403(6769):503–11.
20. Brandstadter R, Brody J, Morgello S, Motiwala R, Shin S, Lublin F, et al. Primary neurolymphomatosis presenting with polyradiculoneuropathy affecting one lower limb. J Clin Neuromuscul Dis. 2015;17(1):6–12.

Chapter 38
A 68-Year-Old Man with Progressive Lower Limb Numbness and Weakness and Urinary Incontinence

Lan Zhou, Susan Morgello, and Susan C. Shin

History

A 68-year-old Asian American man developed numbness in the left leg, mostly involving the left toes, and intermittent low back pain 6 months prior to the presentation. The symptoms worsened in the last 3–4 weeks with slowly progressive numbness and weakness of both lower extremities which caused difficulty with ambulation requiring a cane. He also had had urinary incontinence and bowel constipation for 2–3 weeks. Initial workup by his primary care physician with lumbar spine and hip X-rays was unremarkable. His symptoms did not improve with physical therapy, acupuncture, Gabapentin, or epidural injections. He acutely lost the ability to walk when he was trying to go for spine magnetic resonance imaging (MRI), and he was brought to the emergency room. He had a past medical history of pre-diabetes, asthma, and gout. His medications included Gabapentin, Allopurinol, and Monteleukast. Family history was non-contributory. He denied any smoking or alcohol drinking history. He denied any fevers, malaise or skin rashes but did note unintentional 20-pound weight loss.

L. Zhou (✉)
Departments of Neurology and Pathology, Boston University Medical Center, Boston, MA, USA
e-mail: lanzhou@bu.edu

S. Morgello
Departments of Neurology, Neuroscience, and Pathology, Icahn School of Medicine at Mount Sinai, New York, NY, USA
e-mail: Susan.morgello@mssm.edu

S. C. Shin
Department of Neurology, Icahn School of Medicine at Mount Sinai, New York, NY, USA
e-mail: Susan.shin@mssm.edu

L. Zhou et al. (eds.), *A Case-Based Guide to Neuromuscular Pathology*,
https://doi.org/10.1007/978-3-030-25682-1_38

Physical Examination

General examination was unremarkable. Neurological examination showed normal mental status and cranial nerve functions. Motor examination showed normal tone and bulk, but weakness was detected in the right hip flexors and bilateral knee flexors (MRC 4/5). There were patchy reduction of pinprick sensation in the distal lower extremities, reduced vibratory sensation in the toes and ankles, and impaired proprioception of the right toes and foot. Pinprick sensation was intact in the perineum, and anal sphincter tone was normal. Deep tendon reflexes were absent at the ankles, and 2+ elsewhere. Toes were equivocal. Gait was broad based and ataxic.

Investigations

The patient was admitted to the neurology service. His brain MRI with and without contrast showed an incidental small, chronic appearing, right subdural hematoma. Whole spine MRI without contrast was unrevealing. Extensive laboratory workup including CBC, comprehensive metabolic panel, B12, serum immunofixation, paraneoplastic antibody panel, copper level, rapid plasma reagin (RPR), Lyme serology, and HIV serology were all unremarkable. Comprehensive rheumatologic markers did not yield any positive values other than a weakly positive ANA 1:160 and elevated sedimentation rate 62 mm/hr. Cerebrospinal fluid (CSF) studies revealed mild lymphocytic pleocytosis with white blood cells 12/UL (normal: 0–5/UL) and elevated protein 173 mg/dL (normal:15.0–45.0) but normal glucose 80 mg/dL. CSF Gram stain, cryptococcal antigen, and Lyme, EBV, CMV, and VZV antibodies were all negative. CSF cytology was negative. Computed tomography (CT) of chest, abdomen, and pelvis revealed a few bilateral subcentimeter pulmonary nodules, several small renal cysts, and a mildly enhancing focal soft tissue density lesion in the spleen measuring 2.5 × 2.4 cm that showed a higher density than simple fluid but not hypervascular. The etiology of the lesion was indeterminate without a known history of malignancy. Nerve conduction studies (NCS) and electromyography (EMG) revealed a polyradiculopathy affecting the right L3-S1 myotomes and the left L5-S1 myotomes, sparing the thoracic and cervical spinal segments. NCS/EMG also showed a mild, distal, sensorimotor axonal polyneuropathy.

The patient's leg weakness and numbness continued to progress after the admission. A repeat lumbosacral spine MRI with gadolinium revealed diffuse enhancement of the cauda equina. An autoimmune or neoplastic etiology was considered, given the negative infection workup. He was empirically treated with IV steroids with transient improvement. His symptoms then progressively worsened despite oral Prednisone and intravenous immunoglobulin (IVIG) treatment. Over the course of 6 weeks, he became flaccid paraplegic. He also developed anasarca, pleural effusion, hypoxia, hyponatremia, leukocytopenia, anemia, mildly impaired liver function, metabolic encephalopathy, and left distal leg deep venous thrombosis. Bone marrow biopsy was non-diagnostic. A combine left superficial peroneal nerve and peroneus brevis muscle biopsy was performed.

Nerve and Muscle Biopsy Findings

Both nerve and muscle biopsy specimens (Fig. 38.1) showed scattered blood vessels containing markedly atypical cells in their lumens with large nuclei and prominent nucleoli. Immunohistochemical stains showed that these cells were reactive for CD79a, CD20, CD5, and Bcl-2, but not CD10, CD30, CD3, BCL-1, CD4, CD8, or CD68. In situ hybridization for EBV EBER RNA was negative. The findings are consistent with intravascular large B-cell lymphoma. The nerve biopsy also showed

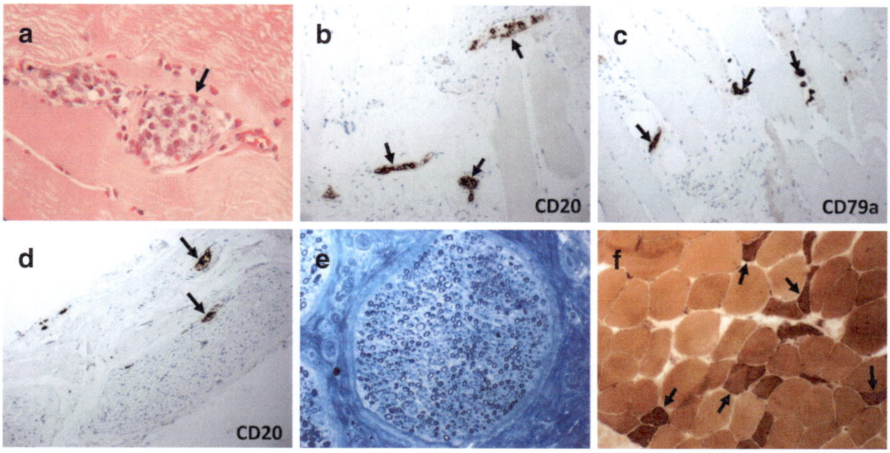

Fig. 38.1 (**a**), Intravascular lymphoma in an endomyseal blood vessel (arrow). Tumor cells distend the vascular lumen, have large nuclei and prominent nucleoli; these features are typical of a large cell B-cell lymphoma (high power photomicrograph of hematoxylin and eosin stain). (**b** and **c**), Lymphoma cells in endomyseal blood vessels expressing pan-B cell markers CD20 (**b,** arrows) and CD79a (**c,** arrows) (high power photomicrographs of immunohistochemical stains with diaminobenzidene chromogen and hematoxylin counterstain). (**d**), Lymphoma cells in perineurial and epineurial medium- and small-caliber blood vessels (arrows), expressing pan-B cell marker CD20 (low power photomicrograph of immunohistochemical stain with diaminobenzidene chromogen and hematoxylin counterstain). (**e**), There is no evidence of neuritis or vasculitis in the peripheral nerve; this fascicle displays mild depopulation of myelinated axons (one micron-thick, toluidene blue-stained section of plastic-embedded peripheral nerve). (**f**), In the skeletal muscle, acute denervation of myofibers is demonstrated by diffuse, dark reactivity for esterase (arrows). Many of these fibers are atrophic and angulated (frozen section histochemistry for non-specific esterase)

mild depopulation of myelinated axons and occasional degenerating nerve fibers. The muscle biopsy also showed numerous esterase-positive denervated fibers, rare necrotic fibers undergoing myophagocytosis, and scattered regenerating fibers.

Final Diagnosis

Intravascular Large B-cell Lymphoma

Patient Follow-up

The patient underwent chemotherapy for the lymphoma. He received R-CHOP (rituximab, cyclophosphamide, doxorubicin, vincristine, and prednisone) and methotrexate (MTX) with marked improvement. He was discharged to subacute rehab after 3 months of hospitalization. After another 3 months, he was discharged home. He was disease-free with negative whole body fludeoxyglucose-positron emission tomography (FDG-PET) scan. He had mild residual bilateral hip flexor and knee extensor weakness. He still had sensory ataxia and needed a walker for ambulation.

Discussion

Intravascular large B-cell lymphoma (IVLBCL) is a rare form of lymphoma with an incidence of 0.095 cases/1,000,000 according to a population-based study in the United States [1]. It is characterized by almost exclusive growth of lymphoma cells within the lumens of blood vessels [2]. Almost all blood vessels can be involved [3]. The most commonly affected sites include central nervous system, skin, and hematopoietic system [4–6]. There are three variants according to the clinical features: classical variant, cutaneous variant, and hemophagocytic syndrome-associated variant [2, 7]. The classical variant has a wide spectrum of clinical presentation depending on the organ involvement. The median age is 70 years with no sex prevalence. Patients may present with systemic symptoms and organ-specific symptoms. The most common systemic symptom is fever of unknown origin. Weight loss without fever is present in 10% of patients. The cutaneous variant predominantly manifests skin lesions, and it is more frequently seen in Western Countries. The hemophagocytic syndrome-associated variant predominantly manifests bone marrow abnormalities and hepatosplenomegaly with rapid onset and progression; it is mostly seen in Asians.

Neurological symptoms are present in 35% of IVLBCL patients, which include encephalopathy, aphasia, visual loss, vertigo, sensorimotor deficits, seizures, and others. Central nervous system (CNS) is much more frequently affected than peripheral nervous system (PNS). CNS involvement is present in about 25% of patients with IVLBCL at the time of diagnosis [8]. Neurologically, our patient had PNS involvement and presented with progressive cauda equina syndrome with gadolinium enhancement of cauda equine nerve roots but no MRI abnormalities in the spinal cord or brain, which is very rare [9, 10].

Tissue biopsy is essential for the diagnosis of IVLBCL, as no discrete tumor masses can be appreciated on radiographic studies, blood and CSF usually do not show malignant lymphocytes, symptoms are non-specific, and cutaneous lesions, when present, display a variety of gross morphologies [7]. As IVLBCL is aggressive, rare, and lacks a characteristic clinical presentation, it has been stated that diagnosis is often made at autopsy; however, recent studies reveal antemortem ascertainment in up to 80% of patients [11]. Muscle, skin and nerve biopsies constitute important diagnostic modalities; even in the absence of macroscopic lesions, skin biopsies may achieve upwards of 75% sensitivity for definitive diagnosis [12]. The peripheral tissue biopsy is less invasive than brain or internal organ biopsy.

Histologically, tumor cells reflect the morphology of large B-cell lymphoma, with large nuclei, prominent nucleoli, and scant cytoplasm. The cells often crowd and distend the lumens of small caliber blood vessels; importantly, they do not invade the vascular wall, and there is no evidence of an angiodestructive process (as might be seen with lymphomatoid granulomatosis, infection, or vasculitis) [7]. The aggregation of tumor cells within vascular lumens is thought to reflect expression of cell surface molecules promoting endothelial adhesion; the lack of tumor cell infiltration into parenchymal structures is thought to reflect an absence of cell surface molecules enabling vascular extravasation, such as the b1 integrin CD29 [11]. When vascular lumens are distended by monomorphous tumor cells, IVLBCL can be easily recognized on routine light microscopy, but when admixed with other blood elements, care must be taken to distinguish atypical tumor morphology from benign but immature circulating blood elements. Immunohistochemical analysis of lymphocyte markers is therefore a critical part of the diagnostic work-up. The vast majority of IVLBCL express pan B cell markers such as CD79a and CD20; MUM1/IRF4, Bcl-2, and CD19 are also extremely frequent; but there is known variation in immunophenotypes, with some tumors displaying germinal center (20%) and others non-germinal center (80%) surface marker patterns [7]. Through immunohistochemical analysis, rare T cell intravascular lymphomas have been recognized [11].

Due to the rarity of IVLBCL, there have been no prospective therapy trials for the disease. Since IVLBCL is a rapidly progressive disseminated disease except for the cutaneous variant, it requires aggressive treatment. The R-CHOP regimen has been shown to achieve an 88% complete remission rate, a 91% overall response rate, and a 60% two year survival rate [13–15]. Our patient also responded very well to this regimen. MTX is recommended to use for CNS prophylaxis and treatment in IVLBCL patients given its better CNS bioavailability [3]. The outcomes depend largely on the early diagnosis and treatment of the disease.

Pearls

Clinical Pearls

1. Intravascular large B-cell lymphoma is a rare and mostly systemic disease which frequently involves CNS.
2. PNS involvement is uncommon and can present with rapidly progressive cauda equine syndrome.
3. MRI with contrast is useful to evaluate the nervous system involvement; CSF study usually shows lymphocytic pleocytosis, elevated protein level, and negative cytology.
4. Intravascular large B-cell lymphoma is difficult to diagnose based solely on the clinical presentation, routine laboratory tests, and imagine studies. Tissue biopsy is essential for the diagnosis.
5. R-CHOP regimen is used for treating intravascular large B-cell lymphoma. MTX may be added for CNS prophylaxis and treatment.
6. Clinical outcomes depend largely on the early diagnosis and treatment.

Pathology Pearls

1. Nerve and muscle biopsies can play an important role in diagnosing intravascular large B-cell lymphoma.
2. The diagnostic finding is the aggregation of lymphoma cells within vascular lumens. These cells have large nuclei, prominent nucleoli, and scant cytoplasm, express pan B cell markers such as CD20 and CD79a, and frequently express MUM1/IRF4, Bcl-2, and CD19.

References

1. Rajyaguru DJ, Bhaskar C, Borgert AJ, Smith A, Parsons B. Intravascular large B-cell lymphoma in the United States (US): a population-based study using Surveillance, Epidemiology, and End Results program and National Cancer Database. Leuk Lymphoma. 2017;58(9):1–9.
2. Nakamura S, Ponzoni M, Campo E. Intravascular large B-cell lymphoma. In: Swerdlow SH, Campo E, Harris NL, editors. WHO classification of tumours of haematopoietic and lymphoid tissues. 4th ed. Lyon: International Agency for Research of Cancer; 2017. p. 317–8.
3. Ponzoni M, Ferreri AJ, Campo E, Facchetti F, Mazzucchelli L, Yoshino T, et al. Definition, diagnosis, and management of intravascular large B-cell lymphoma: proposals and perspectives from an international consensus meeting. J Clin Oncol. 2007;25(21):3168–73.
4. Chapin JE, Davis LE, Kornfeld M, Mandler RN. Neurologic manifestations of intravascular lymphomatosis. Acta Neurol Scand. 1995;91(6):494–9.
5. Ferreri AJ, Campo E, Seymour JF, Willemze R, Ilariucci F, Ambrosetti A, et al. Intravascular lymphoma: clinical presentation, natural history, management and prognostic factors in a series of 38 cases, with special emphasis on the 'cutaneous variant'. Br J Haematol. 2004;127(2):173–83.

6. Glass J, Hochberg FH, Miller DC. Intravascular lymphomatosis. A systemic disease with neurologic manifestations. Cancer. 1993;71(10):3156–64.
7. Ponzoni M, Campo E, Nakamura S. Intravascular large B-cell lymphoma: a chameleon with multiple faces and many masks. Blood. 2018;132(15):1561–7.
8. Shimada K, Murase T, Matsue K, Okamoto M, Ichikawa N, Tsukamoto N, et al. Central nervous system involvement in intravascular large B-cell lymphoma: a retrospective analysis of 109 patients. Cancer Sci. 2010;101(6):1480–6.
9. Nakahara T, Saito T, Muroi A, Sugiura Y, Ogata M, Sugiyama Y, et al. Intravascular lymphomatosis presenting as an ascending cauda equina: conus medullaris syndrome: remission after biweekly CHOP therapy. J Neurol Neurosurg Psychiatry. 1999;67(3):403–6.
10. Yu Y, Govindarajan R. Intravascular large B-cell lymphoma presenting as an isolated cauda equina-conus medullaris syndrome – a case report. J Spinal Cord Med. 2018:1–4.
11. Orwat DE, Batalis NI. Intravascular large B-cell lymphoma. Arch Pathol Lab Med. 2012;136(3):333–8.
12. Yamada E, Ishikawa E, Watanabe R, Matsumura H, Sakamoto N, Ishii A, et al. Random skin biopsies before brain biopsy for intravascular large B-cell lymphoma. World Neurosurg. 2018; pii: S1878-8750(18)32156-9.
13. Ferreri AJ, Dognini GP, Bairey O, Szomor A, Montalban C, Horvath B, et al. The addition of rituximab to anthracycline-based chemotherapy significantly improves outcome in 'Western' patients with intravascular large B-cell lymphoma. Br J Haematol. 2008;143(2):253–7.
14. Ferreri AJ, Dognini GP, Govi S, Crocchiolo R, Bouzani M, Bollinger CR, et al. Can rituximab change the usually dismal prognosis of patients with intravascular large B-cell lymphoma? J Clin Oncology. 2008;26(31):5134–6; author reply 6–7
15. Shimada K, Matsue K, Yamamoto K, Murase T, Ichikawa N, Okamoto M, et al. Retrospective analysis of intravascular large B-cell lymphoma treated with rituximab-containing chemotherapy as reported by the IVL study group in Japan. J Clin Oncol. 2008;26(19):3189–95.

Chapter 39
A 53-Year-Old Woman with Pain, Burning, Tingling, and Numbness in the Distal Limbs

Lan Zhou

History

A 53-year-old African American woman presented to our clinic with pain, burning, tingling, and numbness in the distal limbs. She first noticed burning pain and tingling (pins and needles) sensation in the feet about 5 years prior to the presentation. She then developed numbness in the toes, which gradually progressed to involve the entire feet and distal legs. The burning and tingling sensation also progressed to involve the distal legs and fingers. The symptoms were initially intermittent and then became constant, worse with prolonged standing or walking and also worse at night, which affected her sleep. She also reported intermittent sharp pain in the feet and distal legs, and coldness in the feet. She denied weakness. She did have mild chronic low back pain which was non-radiating. She denied dry mouth, dry eyes, palpitations, orthostatic dizziness, bowel constipation, urinary retention, or sweating abnormalities. She saw a neurologist 2 years prior, who did nerve conduction study (NCS) and electromyography (EMG) which was unrevealing. She had been taking Gabapentin with an initial dose of 300 mg three times a day and then increased to 600 mg three times a day with limited benefit. She had type 2 diabetes mellitus diagnosed 6 years prior. Her glycemic control was suboptimal. She also had a past medical history of hypertension and hypothyroidism. She took Glucophage, Lisinopril, and levothyroxine in addition to Gabapentin. Her family history was positive for diabetes mellitus and hypertension. She did not drink alcohol, smoke cigarettes, or abuse illicit drugs.

L. Zhou (✉)
Departments of Neurology and Pathology, Boston University Medical Center, Boston, MA, USA
e-mail: lanzhou@bu.edu

L. Zhou et al. (eds.), *A Case-Based Guide to Neuromuscular Pathology*,
https://doi.org/10.1007/978-3-030-25682-1_39

Physical Examination

Her general examination was significant for skin dark-red discoloration and coldness in the feet and distal legs. Neurological examination showed normal mental status, cranial nerve functions, motor strength, coordination, and gait. Pinprick sensation was reduced from toes to knees and from fingers to mid-forearms with a distal-to-proximal gradient. Vibratory sensation and joint position sense were normal. Romberg sign was absent. Deep tendon reflexes were normal except for reduced ankle jerks. Toes were downgoing bilaterally.

Investigations

NCS/EMG was repeated, which was normal. Blood tests revealed a high level of HbA1C at 8.6%. ANA, ENA, TSH, free T4, B12, folate, serum and urine immunofixation, and lipid panel were all unremarkable. Skin biopsy of the left lower limb with intraepidermal nerve fiber density (IENFD) evaluation was performed for diagnostic evaluation.

Skin Biopsy Findings

3-mm punch skin punch biopsy showed absent intraepidermal nerve fibers (IENF) at the distal leg and distal thigh, and a reduced IENFD at the proximal thigh (4.3 fibers/mm; normal: ≥8) (Fig. 39.1). The findings are consistent with a severe, length-dependent, small fiber sensory neuropathy.

Final Diagnosis

Severe length-dependent small fiber sensory neuropathy associated with diabetes mellitus

Patient Follow-up

The patient had been followed in our clinic for 2 years. Her diabetes treatment regimen was adjusted by her endocrinologist with a significant improvement of the glycemic control. Her last HbA1C level was 6.9%. She also underwent diet control, weight control, and regular exercise. The dose of Gabapentin was gradually

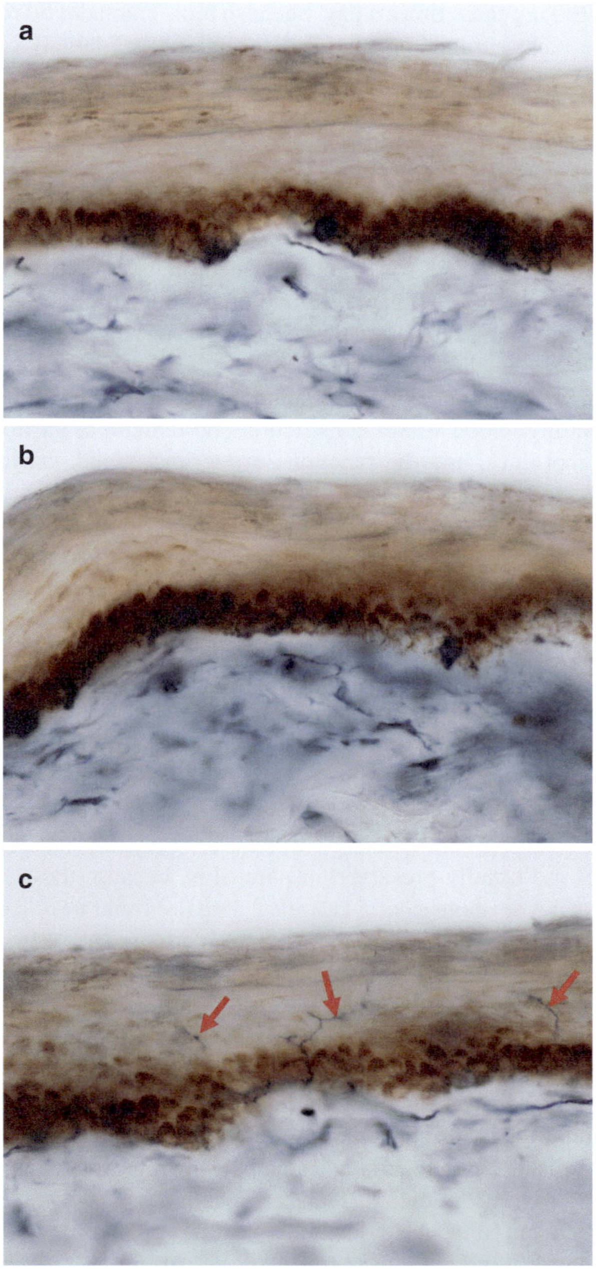

Fig. 39.1 PGP9.5 immunostaining of skin biopsy sections show absent intraepidermal nerve fibers at the left distal leg (**a**) and distal thigh (**b**). A few intraepidermal nerve fibers are seen at the left proximal thigh (**c**, arrows)

increased to 1200 mg three times a day. She also took Tramadol 50 mg twice a day as needed. Her pain, burning, and tingling sensation were largely controlled. Her numbness was stabilized with no further progression.

Discussion

Small fiber neuropathy (SFN) is a common neuromuscular disorder which predominantly affects small myelinated Aδ and unmyelinated C fibers. According to a Dutch study, the minimum prevalence of SFN is 52.95 per 100,000 population [1]. SFN can affect small somatic sensory fibers which control the perception of pinprick and thermal stimuli, or small autonomic C fibers which control cardiac muscle contractility, blood vessel constriction and dilatation, gastrointestinal and genitourinary motilities, and the functions of lacrimal gland, salivary gland and sweat gland, among others [2].

Patients with small somatic sensory fiber involvement commonly present with pain, burning, tingling, and/or numbness [3] as seen in our patient. They may also report squeeze sensation, coldness, or itchy skin in the affected areas [4, 5]. The symptoms are usually worse at night. The paresthesias frequently cause intolerance to bed sheet or socks. Unlike the pain caused by musculoskeletal or joint diseases, which is mostly dull ache, the pain caused by SFN is typically sharp and described as burning, pins and needles, stabbing, lancinating, and electric shock-like sensation. Examination often shows allodynia (non-painful stimuli perceived as painful), hyperalgesias (painful stimuli perceived as more painful than expected), and/or reduced pinprick and thermal sensation in the affected areas. Examination can also be unrevealing. Motor strength, proprioception, and deep tendon reflexes are usually preserved in pure SFN, because these modalities are the functions of large nerve fibers. However, impaired vibratory sensation at the toes and reduced ankle jerks may be detected in elderly patients with SFN, as these findings are not uncommon in elderly people without neuropathy. SFN is mostly length-dependent, with the most distal sites affected the first and the most. All the small sensory nerve fibers derive from dorsal root ganglions along the spine. So, the most distal sites are the toes and feet. The common initial symptoms in patients with a length-dependent small fiber neuropathy (LD-SFN) are burning feet and numb toes as reported by our patient. The sensory symptoms then gradually progress to involve distal legs, fingers, and hands, showing a stocking-glove pattern with a distal-to-proximal gradient [2]. Our patient had typical symptoms and signs of a length-dependent SFN.

When autonomic fibers are affected, patients may develop autonomic symptoms including dry eyes, dry mouth, palpitations, orthostatic dizziness, bowel constipation, urinary retention, sexual dysfunction, sweating abnormalities, and skin discoloration. Patients may develop reduced sweating in the feet (distal anhidrosis) due to the impaired sudomotor autonomic function, and increased sweating in the trunk or face (compensatory proximal hyperhidrosis) to maintain thermoregulation.

Examination may detect coldness and skin white, red or purple discoloration in the feet and distal legs due to dysregulation of vasomotor autonomic functions [2, 3, 6] as seen in our patient. So, our patient also had autonomic involvement. Autonomic symptoms are present in nearly half of the patients with SFN in one study population [1]. The involvement of autonomic fibers is frequently seen in SFN associated with amyloidosis, diabetes mellitus, sarcoidosis, and Sjogren syndrome. In rare occasions, patients with SFN may present with prominent dysautonomia with limited or no somatic sensory fiber involvement [6].

Skin biopsy with IENDF evaluation is the gold standard diagnostic test for SFN, as routine NCS/EMG, a valuable test for evaluating large fiber neuropathy, is typically normal in SFN and cannot confirm or exclude SFN. However, NCS/EMG should be done first when evaluating SFN to rule out a large fiber polyneuropathy and bilateral S1 radiculopathies which can also cause paresthesia in the feet, although these patients often have low back pain shooting towards the feet. The diagnosis of distal SFN is based on the clinical symptoms, examination findings, and diagnostic test findings. The graded diagnostic criteria developed by the NeuroDiab expert panel [7] can be used for all forms of SFN regardless of etiology [7–9]. The possible SFN is define as the presence of length-dependent symptoms and/or signs of small fiber damage. The probable SFN is defined as the presence of length-dependent symptoms and signs of small fiber damage, and normal sural nerve conduction study. The definitive SFN is defined as the presence of length-dependent symptoms and signs of small fiber damage, normal sural nerve conduction study, and reduced intraepidermal nerve fiber density (IENFD) at the ankle and/or abnormal quantitative sensory testing (QST) thermal thresholds in the foot [7]. Based on the diagnostic criteria, our patient had definitive distal SFN. It was quite severe as all three biopsy sites showed small fiber depopulation with a distal-to-proximal gradient. It is worth noting that quantitative sudomotor axon reflex test (QSART) and cardiovascular autonomic testing may also be ordered to evaluate autonomic functions in SFN patients if autonomic symptoms are present. Adding QSART has been shown to increase the diagnostic sensitivity for SFN [10, 11].

SFN can be associated with many medical conditions, including diabetes mellitus, prediabetes, metabolic syndrome, connective tissue diseases, sarcoidosis, B12 deficiency, monoclonal gammopathy, thyroid dysfunction, HIV and hepatitis C infections, sodium channelopathy, and paraneoplastic syndrome, among others [2, 8, 12–15]. The associated conditions can be identified in about half of the cases [12, 13, 16]. The frequencies of the individual associated conditions vary depending on the geographic location, ethnicity, and environmental factors. Overall, glucose dysmetabolism, including diabetes and prediabetes, is the most common. The most sensitive test for detecting diabetes and prediabetes is 2-hour oral glucose tolerance test [17]. In our study of patients with skin biopsy-confirmed pure SFN, including 175 patients with LD-SFN and 63 patients with non-length-dependent small fiber neuropathy (NLD-SFN), glucose dysmetabolism was present in 37.7% of the LD-SFN cases and 15.9% of the NLD-SFN cases [13]. Our case represents diabetic LD-SFN. It has been shown that a rapid improvement of glycemic control in diabetic patients by insulin or oral hypoglycemic medications can also induce painful

SFN which is acute [18, 19]. It usually occurs when HbA1C level is reduced by 2 or more percentage points over a 3-month period of time. The pain is severe and refractory to treatment, but it spontaneously improves after 12–24 months [18, 19].

When evaluating a patient with SFN, a battery of blood and urine tests should be ordered to search for the associated conditions even a known associated condition is present. A recent study showed that additional associated conditions were identified in 26.7% of SFN patients who had known associated conditions prior to the neuropathy etiology evaluation [12]. The tests may include CBC, comprehensive metabolic panel, 2-hour oral glucose tolerance test (OGTT), lipid panel, ESR, TSH, free T4, ANA, ENA, serum and urine immunofixation, and B12 level. If there is a history of gastrointestinal symptoms or gluten intolerance, gliadin antibody, tissue transglutaminase antibodies, and small bowel biopsy may be pursued to evaluate for celiac sprue. HIV or HCV serology should be ordered if the risk factors are present. If there is a significant family history, further genetic testing should be considered. Lip biopsy or bone marrow biopsy should be considered if clinical suspicion for Sjögren's syndrome, seronegative sicca syndrome or amyloidosis is high. Because of the low sensitivity and specificity of a serum ACE level, if sarcoidosis is suspected clinically, additional confirmatory testing, such as a chest CT, should be ordered [20].

Management of SFN consists of identifying and treating underlying causes, controlling neuropathic pain, and modifying lifestyle. Etiology-specific treatment is the key to prevent or slow down SFN progression. As glucose dysmetabolism is the most common associated condition of SFN and individual components of the metabolic syndrome are potential risk factors for SFN [21–23], a tight glycemic control and lifestyle modification with diet control, weight control, and regular exercise are of paramount importance in patients with these conditions. Impaired glucose tolerance (IGT) neuropathy may represent the earliest stage of diabetic neuropathy, and the neuropathy at this stage may be potentially reversible with lifestyle intervention and IGT improvement [24]. Lifestyle modification has also been shown to improve painful neuropathy symptoms in overweight patients with diabetes [25]. The SFN progression was also halted in our patient after improving glycemic control and modifying lifestyle.

SFN is often painful, especially when associated with amyloidosis, diabetes mellitus, HIV infection, sarcoidosis, and sodium channelopathy [6, 26]. Although SFN is mostly non-debilitating as motor strength and proprioception are preserved, it often negatively impacts the quality of life both physically and mentally due to the annoying neuropathic pain and autonomic symptoms [27]. Diabetic peripheral neuropathy has become a significant economic burden to the healthcare in the United States [28]. Pain control is crucial in the treatment of SFN. The recommended first-line medications include tricyclic antidepressants, serotonin norepinephrine reuptake inhibitors (SNRIs), anticonvulsants Pregabalin and Gabapentin, and topical anesthetics if the pain is localized [29–34]. Tramadol, a semisynthetic opioid analgesic, is a second-line choice. These medications can be used as monotherapy or polytherapy. Combining medications with different mechanisms, such as Gabapentin with Nortriptyline, can be more effective than monotherapy [35].

Combining Pregabalin or Gabapentin with Tramadol can also improve pain control if Pregabalin or Gabapentin alone is inadequate. Chronic use of opioids for noncancer-related neuropathy is not recommended due to the high rates of addiction and overdose and the worse functional outcomes [36]. Non-pharmacological management includes transcutaneous electrical nerve stimulation (TENS), heat, ice, and massage of painful areas. The efficacy of alternative therapies, including meditation, yoga, and acupuncture, needs to be studied.

The overall clinical progression of idiopathic SFN or diabetic SFN with a good glycemic control is usually slow as seen in our patient. However, most SFN patients require chronic pain management. In one study that followed 124 SNF patients, only 13% showed evidence of large fiber involvement over a period of 2 years [16]. None went on to develop Charcot joints, foot ulcers, weakness, or sensory ataxia as often seen in patients with longstanding or severe large fiber neuropathy. Another longitudinal study of patients with idiopathic SNF and SFN associated diabetes and prediabetes showed that after a mean follow up for 2–3 years, there was no change in Neuropathy Impairment Score of the Lower Limb (NIS-LL), but the IENFD at all three biopsy sites, including the distal leg, distal thigh, and proximal thigh, were reduced [37]. A longitudinal study with a follow up duration longer than 2–3 years is needed to further address the long-term prognosis of SFN.

Pearls

Clinical Pearls

1. Common SFN symptoms include pain, burning, tingling, and numbness. The initial symptoms are often burning feet and numb toes.
2. Common SFN signs include allodynia, hyperesthesia, reduced pinprick sensation, and skin white, red, or purple discoloration in the affected area.
3. SFN is mostly length-dependent with symptoms and signs in a stocking-glove pattern with a distal-to-proximal gradient.
4. SFN can affect autonomic C fibers, causing dry mouth, dry eyes, orthostatic intolerance, bowel constipation, urinary retention, sexual dysfunction, sweating abnormalities, and skin discoloration.
5. SFN can be associated with many medical conditions, with glucose dysmetabolism being the most common. The associated conditions can be identified in about half of the SFN cases, and glucose dysmetabolism in over 1/3 of LD-SFN cases.
6. Skin biopsy with IENFD evaluation is the gold standard diagnostic test for SFN. QSART and cardiovascular autonomic testing are valuable in evaluating autonomic symptoms.
7. The management of SFN consists of identifying and treating underlying associated conditions, controlling pain, and modifying lifestyle.

Pathology Pearls

1. Skin biopsy in LD-SFN typically shows reduced IENFD at the biopsy sites with a distal-to-proximal gradient. While mild cases show reduced IENFD only at the distal leg, severe cases often show additional involvement of the proximal biopsy sites.

References

1. Peters MJ, Bakkers M, Merkies IS, Hoeijmakers JG, van Raak EP, Faber CG. Incidence and prevalence of small-fiber neuropathy: a survey in the Netherlands. Neurology. 2013;81(15):1356–60.
2. Tavee J, Zhou L. Small fiber neuropathy: a burning problem. Cleve Clin J Med. 2009;76(5):297–305.
3. Lacomis D. Small-fiber neuropathy. Muscle Nerve. 2002;26(2):173–88.
4. Gemignani F, Giovanelli M, Vitetta F, Santilli D, Bellanova MF, Brindani F, et al. Non-length dependent small fiber neuropathy. A prospective case series. J Peripher Nerv Syst. 2010;15(1):57–62.
5. Misery L, Brenaut E, Le Garrec R, Abasq C, Genestet S, Marcorelles P, et al. Neuropathic pruritus. Nat Rev Neurol. 2014;10(7):408–16.
6. Gibbons CH. Small fiber neuropathies. Continuum (Minneap Minn). 2014;20(5 Peripheral Nervous System Disorders):1398–412.
7. Tesfaye S, Boulton AJ, Dyck PJ, Freeman R, Horowitz M, Kempler P, et al. Diabetic neuropathies: update on definitions, diagnostic criteria, estimation of severity, and treatments. Diabetes Care. 2010;33(10):2285–3.
8. Cazzato D, Lauria G. Small fibre neuropathy. Curr Opin Neurol. 2017;30(5):490–9.
9. Terkelsen AJ, Karlsson P, Lauria G, Freeman R, Finnerup NB, Jensen TS. The diagnostic challenge of small fibre neuropathy: clinical presentations, evaluations, and causes. Lancet Neurol. 2017;16(11):934–44.
10. Tavee JO, Karwa K, Ahmed Z, Thompson N, Parambil J, Culver DA. Sarcoidosis-associated small fiber neuropathy in a large cohort: clinical aspects and response to IVIG and anti-TNF alpha treatment. Respir Med. 2017;126:135–8.
11. Thaisetthawatkul P, Fernandes Filho JA, Herrmann DN. Contribution of QSART to the diagnosis of small fiber neuropathy. Muscle Nerve. 2013;48(6):883–8.
12. de Greef BTA, Hoeijmakers JGJ, Gorissen-Brouwers CML, Geerts M, Faber CG, Merkies ISJ. Associated conditions in small fiber neuropathy - a large cohort study and review of the literature. Eur J Neurol. 2018;25(2):348–55.
13. Khan S, Zhou L. Characterization of non-length-dependent small-fiber sensory neuropathy. Muscle Nerve. 2012;45(1):86–91.
14. Chan AC, Wilder-Smith EP. Small fiber neuropathy: Getting bigger! Muscle Nerve. 2016;53(5):671–82.
15. The Diabetes Control and Complications Trial Research Group. The effect of intensive treatment of diabetes on the development and progression of long-term complications in insulin-dependent diabetes mellitus. N Engl J Med. 1993;329(14):977–86.
16. Devigili G, Tugnoli V, Penza P, Camozzi F, Lombardi R, Melli G, et al. The diagnostic criteria for small fibre neuropathy: from symptoms to neuropathology. Brain. 2008;131.(Pt 7:1912–25.
17. Sumner CJ, Sheth S, Griffin JW, Cornblath DR, Polydefkis M. The spectrum of neuropathy in diabetes and impaired glucose tolerance. Neurology. 2003;60(1):108–11.

18. Gibbons CH, Freeman R. Treatment-induced diabetic neuropathy: a reversible painful autonomic neuropathy. Ann Neurol. 2010;67(4):534–41.
19. Gibbons CH, Freeman R. Treatment-induced neuropathy of diabetes: an acute, iatrogenic complication of diabetes. Brain. 2015;138.(Pt 1:43–52.
20. Tavee JO. Office approach to small fiber neuropathy. Cleve Clin J Med. 2018;85(10):801–12.
21. Smith AG, Rose K, Singleton JR. Idiopathic neuropathy patients are at high risk for metabolic syndrome. J Neurol Sci. 2008;273(1–2):25–8.
22. Tesfaye S, Chaturvedi N, Eaton SE, Ward JD, Manes C, Ionescu-Tirgoviste C, et al. Vascular risk factors and diabetic neuropathy. N Engl J Med. 2005;352(4):341–50.
23. Zhou LLJ, Ontaneda D, Sperling J. Metabolic syndrome in small fiber sensory neuropathy. J Clin Neuromuscul Dis. 2011;12(4):235–43.
24. Smith AG, Russell J, Feldman EL, Goldstein J, Peltier A, Smith S, et al. Lifestyle intervention for pre-diabetic neuropathy. Diabetes Care. 2006;29(6):1294–9.
25. Look ARG. Effects of a long-term lifestyle modification programme on peripheral neuropathy in overweight or obese adults with type 2 diabetes: the Look AHEAD study. Diabetologia. 2017;60(6):980–8.
26. Lauria G, Hsieh ST, Johansson O, Kennedy WR, Leger JM, Mellgren SI, et al. European Federation of Neurological Societies/Peripheral Nerve Society Guideline on the use of skin biopsy in the diagnosis of small fiber neuropathy. Report of a joint task force of the European Federation of Neurological Societies and the Peripheral Nerve Society. Eur J Neurol. 2010;17(7):903–12, e44–9.
27. Bakkers M, Faber CG, Hoeijmakers JG, Lauria G, Merkies IS. Small fibers, large impact: quality of life in small-fiber neuropathy. Muscle Nerve. 2014;49(3):329–36.
28. Gordois A, Scuffham P, Shearer A, Oglesby A, Tobian JA. The health care costs of diabetic peripheral neuropathy in the US. Diabetes Care. 2003;26(6):1790–5.
29. Acevedo JC, Amaya A, Casasola Ode L, Chinchilla N, De Giorgis M, Florez S, et al. Guidelines for the diagnosis and management of neuropathic pain: consensus of a group of Latin American experts. J Pain Palliat Care Pharmacother. 2009;23(3):261–81.
30. Bohlega S, Alsaadi T, Amir A, Hosny H, Karawagh AM, Moulin D, et al. Guidelines for the pharmacological treatment of peripheral neuropathic pain: expert panel recommendations for the middle East region. J Int Med Res. 2010;38(2):295–317.
31. Bril V, England J, Franklin GM, Backonja M, Cohen J, Del Toro D, et al. Evidence-based guideline: treatment of painful diabetic neuropathy: report of the American Academy of Neurology, the American Association of Neuromuscular and Electrodiagnostic Medicine, and the American Academy of Physical Medicine and Rehabilitation. Neurology. 2011;76(20):1758–65.
32. Dworkin RH, O'Connor AB, Audette J, Baron R, Gourlay GK, Haanpaa ML, et al. Recommendations for the pharmacological management of neuropathic pain: an overview and literature update. Mayo Clin Proc. 2010;85(3. Suppl):S3–14.
33. Hovaguimian A, Gibbons CH. Diagnosis and treatment of pain in small-fiber neuropathy. Curr Pain Headache Rep. 2011;15(3):193–200.
34. Moulin D, Boulanger A, Clark AJ, Clarke H, Dao T, Finley GA, et al. Pharmacological management of chronic neuropathic pain: revised consensus statement from the Canadian Pain Society. Pain Res Manag. 2014;19(6):328–35.
35. Gilron I, Bailey JM, Tu D, Holden RR, Jackson AC, Houlden RL. Nortriptyline and gabapentin, alone and in combination for neuropathic pain: a double-blind, randomised controlled crossover trial. Lancet. 2009;374(9697):1252–61.
36. Hoffman EM, Watson JC, St Sauver J, Staff NP, Klein CJ. Association of long-term opioid therapy with functional status, adverse outcomes, and mortality among patients with polyneuropathy. JAMA Neurol. 2017;74(7):773–9.
37. Khoshnoodi MA, Truelove S, Burakgazi A, Hoke A, Mammen AL, Polydefkis M. Longitudinal assessment of small fiber neuropathy: evidence of a non-length-dependent distal axonopathy. JAMA Neurol. 2016;73(6):684–90.

Chapter 40
A 40-Year-Old Woman with Patchy Painful Paresthesia

Lan Zhou

History

A 40-year-old Caucasian woman presented to our clinic with painful paresthesias. She first developed sharp pain over her chest about 1 year prior to her presentation, and the symptom was severe and intermittent with no obvious triggers. She underwent a thorough cardiac evaluation which was unrevealing. She then developed intermittent burning and tingling sensation in the limbs which were patchy and migrating. Sometimes, these symptoms involved her face. She also reported mild numbness in the feet and legs. She reported episodes of orthostatic dizziness and palpitations. She admitted to difficulty sweating in her feet even in the hot summer but no excessive sweating. She did not notice skin discoloration. She admitted to dry mouth and bowel constipation but no dry eyes or urinary disturbance. She went to a neurologist several months prior, who did nerve conduction study (NCS) and electromyography (EMG) which was reportedly normal. She had been taking Gabapentin 1200 mg three times a day and Tramadol 50 mg two to four times a day for pain control with a partial response. She had sarcoidosis diagnosed 15 months prior by a mediastinal lymph node biopsy which showed non-necrotizing granulomatous lymphadenitis. At that time, she also had diffuse joint pain and blurry vision. She was treated with oral Prednisone initially 60 mg daily which gradually tapered to 20 mg daily. She also took Methotrexate 10 mg weekly. Her respiratory symptoms, joint pain, and blurry vision significantly improved but not the painful paresthesias or orthostatic intolerance. Her family history was positive for diabetes mellitus and hyperlipidemia. She did not drink alcohol, smoke cigarettes, or abuse illicit drugs.

L. Zhou (✉)
Departments of Neurology and Pathology, Boston University Medical Center, Boston, MA, USA
e-mail: lanzhou@bu.edu

L. Zhou et al. (eds.), *A Case-Based Guide to Neuromuscular Pathology*,
https://doi.org/10.1007/978-3-030-25682-1_40

Physical Examination

Her general examination was significant for orthostatic intolerance with tachycardia. Neurological examination showed normal mental status, cranial nerve functions, motor strength, coordination, and gait. There was patchy reduction of pinprick sensation in her limbs and trunk. Vibratory sensation and joint position sense were intact. Deep tendon reflexes were normal. Toes were downgoing bilaterally.

Investigations

ANA, ENA, 2-hour oral glucose tolerance test, TSH, free T4, B12, folate, serum and urine immunofixation, and lipid panel were all unremarkable. Quantitative sudomotor axon reflex test (QSART) showed reduced sweat production in the foot and forearm. Cardiovasular autonomic testing showed diffuse autonomic impairment. PET scan of the heart did not show evidence of cardiac sarcoidosis. Brain and spine MRIs were unremarkable. Skin biopsy of the left lower limb with intraepidermal nerve fiber density (IENFD) evaluation was performed.

Skin Biopsy Findings

3-mm punch skin punch biopsy showed reduced intraepidermal nerve fiber densities (IENFD) at the distal leg (3.8 fibers/mm; normal: ≥5.7), distal thigh (4.3 fibers/mm; normal: ≥7), and proximal thigh (3.1 fibers/mm; normal: ≥8) with no distal-to-proximal gradient (Fig. 40.1). The findings are consistent with a non-length-dependent small fiber neuropathy.

Final Diagnosis

Non-length-dependent small fiber neuropathy associated with systemic sarcoidosis

Patient Follow-up

The patient was started on intravenous immunoglobulin (IVIG) infusion 2 grams/kg followed by 1 gram/kg every 1 month. The painful paresthesias and orthostatic intolerance markedly improved within 2 months, and she could function better. Prednisone was tapered off in 6 months. She continued to take Gabapentin 900 mg three times a day and Tramadol 50 mg twice a day as needed.

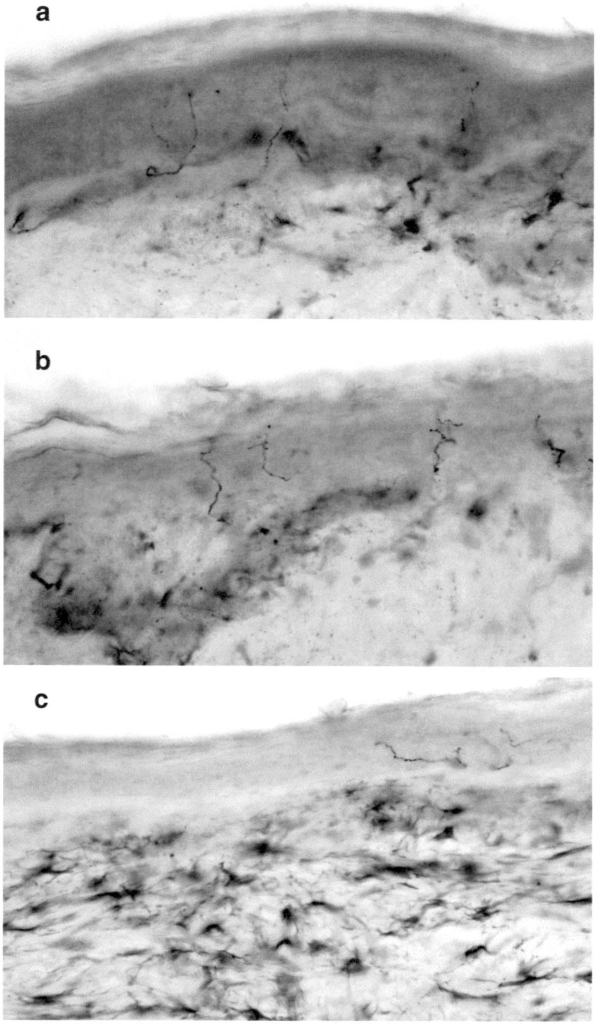

Fig. 40.1 PGP9.5 immunostaining of skin biopsy sections shows reduced intraepidermal nerve fiber densities at the left distal leg (**a**), distal thigh (**b**) and proximal thigh (**c**) with no distal-to-proximal gradient

Discussion

Small fiber neuropathy (SFN) is a common neuromuscular disorder which predominantly affects small myelinated Aδ and unmyelinated C fibers. Small fibers mediate sensory and autonomic functions [1]. Patients with small somatic sensory fiber involvement commonly present with pain, burning, tingling, and/or numbness. When autonomic fibers are affected, patients may develop autonomic symptoms including dry eyes, dry mouth, palpitations, orthostatic dizziness, bowel constipation, urinary retention, sexual dysfunction, sweating abnormalities, and skin discoloration [1–3]. Autonomic symptoms are present in nearly half of the patients with SFN in one study population [4]. Our patient also has SFN with both somatic and autonomic involvement, which is frequently seen in association with amyloidosis, diabetes mellitus, sarcoidosis, and Sjogren's syndrome. The SFN in our patient is associated with sarcoidosis.

SFN is mostly length-dependent (LD-SFN) with symptoms and signs in a stocking-glove pattern with a distal-to-proximal gradient [1]. Non-length-dependent SFN (NLD-SFN) is relatively rare, accounting for 20–25% of cases of pure SFN [5, 6]. The sensory symptoms and signs in NLD-SFN are usually patchy, asymmetrical, migrating or diffuse, which often involve trunk and face in addition to limbs [6]. There is no distal-to-proximal gradient of the sensory symptoms or signs in the affected limbs. The sensory symptoms and signs in our patient are typical for NLD-SFN. Chest pain is relatively common in SFN associated with sarcoidosis as seen in our patient. Many of these patients undergo cardiac evaluation due to the concern of cardiac ischemia, and the cardiac work-up is usually unrevealing as the symptom is caused by SFN. The symptoms of NLD-SFN are frequently suspected to be psychogenic as NLD-SFN is less well recognized than LD-SFN. By comparing 63 patients who had pure NLD-SFN with 175 patients who had pure LD-SFN, we found that the age at onset (Mean ± SD years) was younger in NLD-SFN (45.5 ± 13.1) than in LD-SFN (55.1 ± 11.4; $p < 0.001$), more women were affected in NLD-SFN (73.0%) than in LD-SFN (48.0%; $p < 0.001$), and the neuropathy was more likely to be association with immune-mediated conditions in NLD-SFN (14.3%) than in LD-SFN (3.4%; $p = 0.012$) [6]. The increased association of NLD-SFN with immune-mediated conditions such as sarcoidosis and Sjogren's syndrome has also been reported by other studies [7–10].

Skin biopsy with IENDF evaluation is the gold standard diagnostic test for SFN, as routine NCS/EMG, a valuable test for evaluating large fiber neuropathy, is typically normal in SFN and cannot confirm or exclude SFN. Skin biopsy in NLD-SFN typically shows reduced IENFD with no distal-to-proximal gradient and with a high distal leg:proximal thigh IENFD ratio as compared with that in LD-SFN [6, 11]. The skin biopsy findings in our patient are typical for NLD-SFN. QSART and cardiovascular autonomic testing are valuable in evaluating autonomic symptoms when present. Combining these tests can increase the diagnostic yield [9, 12].

Our patient had systemic sarcoidosis before developing the SFN symptoms. We still ordered a battery of blood tests to search for other possible associated conditions. It has been shown that additional conditions can be identified in over 25% of SFN patients with known underlying associated conditions prior to the neuropathy etiology evaluation [13]. Therefore, a thorough evaluation of associated conditions should be done in every patient with SFN. Treating the underlying associated conditions is the key to prevent or slow down SFN progression. It can also improve SFN symptoms [3, 9, 10]. Our patient did not have an associated condition other than sarcoidosis. She had sarcoidosis-associated NLD-SFN.

SFN symptoms have been reported in up to 40% of patients with sarcoidosis [14]. A retrospective study of 115 patients with sarcoidosis-associated SFN without other causes showed that 63% were women and mean age at onset was 46 years. Over 50% of these patients presented with NLD-SFN affecting both somatic sensory and autonomic small fibers. Combining skin biopsy and QSART increased the diagnostic yield. The development of SFN in sarcoidosis is felt to be mediated by inflammatory cytokines rather than granulomatous inflammation [15]. The non-lesion skin biopsy for diagnosing SFN usually shows reduced IENFD in a non-length-dependent pattern but not granulomas.

Unlike other forms of neurosarcoidosis, sarcoidosis-associated SFN symptoms respond poorly to steroids or immunosuppressants such as methotrexate, but they may respond very well to IVIG and/or anti-TNF therapy infliximab [9, 10, 16, 17]. In a large cohort of sarcoidosis-associated SFN [9], 75.8% of patients responded to IVIG, 66.7% responded to infliximab, and 71.4% responded to IVIG and infliximab. The mechanism underlying this is not entirely clear. Large prospective controlled studies are needed to further determine the therapeutic effects of IVIG and infliximab to direct the long-term management.

Pearls

Clinical Pearls

1. NLD-SFN accounts for 20–25% of cases of pure SFN.
2. NLD-SFN is more common in women, presents at a younger age, and is more likely to be associated with immune-mediated conditions than LD-SFN.
3. NLD-SFN usually manifests diffuse, patchy, or migrating painful paresthesias and autonomic symptoms. Examination often shows reduced pinprick or temperature sensation with no distal-to-proximal gradient.
4. The important diagnostic tests for NLD-SFN include skin biopsy with IENFD evaluation, QSART, and cardiovascular autonomic testing.
5. NLD-SFN warrants diligent search for immune-mediated associated conditions such as sarcoidosis and Sjogren's syndrome, as treating these underlying conditions may improve the neuropathy symptoms and halt the disease progression.
6. Sarcoidosis-associated SFN symptoms usually do not respond to steroids or immunosuppressants such as methotrexate, but may respond very well to IVIG and/or infliximab.

Pathology Pearls

1. Skin biopsy in NLD-SFN typically shows reduced IENFD at the biopsy sites with no distal-to-proximal gradient.
2. Over 50% sarcoidosis-associated SFN are NLD-SFN. The development of sarcoidosis-associated SFN is most likely mediated by inflammatory cytokines not granulomatous inflammation. Non-lesion skin biopsy for diagnosing SFN in this setting shows reduced IENFD but not granulomas.

References

1. Tavee J, Zhou L. Small fiber neuropathy: a burning problem. Cleve Clin J Med. 2009;76(5):297–305.
2. Lacomis D. Small-fiber neuropathy. Muscle Nerve. 2002;26(2):173–88.
3. Gibbons CH. Small fiber neuropathies. Continuum (Minneap Minn). 2014;20(5 Peripheral Nervous System Disorders):1398–412.
4. Peters MJ, Bakkers M, Merkies IS, Hoeijmakers JG, van Raak EP, Faber CG. Incidence and prevalence of small-fiber neuropathy: a survey in the Netherlands. Neurology. 2013;81(15):1356–60.
5. Gemignani F, Giovanelli M, Vitetta F, Santilli D, Bellanova MF, Brindani F, et al. Non-length dependent small fiber neuropathy. A prospective case series. J Peripher Nerv Syst. 2010;15(1):57–62.
6. Khan S, Zhou L. Characterization of non-length-dependent small-fiber sensory neuropathy. Muscle Nerve. 2012;45(1):86–91.
7. Chai J, Herrmann DN, Stanton M, Barbano RL, Logigian EL. Painful small-fiber neuropathy in Sjogren syndrome. Neurology. 2005;65(6):925–7.
8. Gorson KC, Herrmann DN, Thiagarajan R, Brannagan TH, Chin RL, Kinsella LJ, et al. Non-length dependent small fibre neuropathy/ganglionopathy. J Neurol Neurosurg Psychiatry. 2008;79(2):163–9.
9. Tavee JO, Karwa K, Ahmed Z, Thompson N, Parambil J, Culver DA. Sarcoidosis-associated small fiber neuropathy in a large cohort: clinical aspects and response to IVIG and anti-TNF alpha treatment. Respir Med. 2017;126:135–8.
10. Parambil JG, Tavee JO, Zhou L, Pearson KS, Culver DA. Efficacy of intravenous immunoglobulin for small fiber neuropathy associated with sarcoidosis. Respir Med. 2011;105(1):101–5.
11. Provitera V, Gibbons CH, Wendelschafer-Crabb G, Donadio V, Vitale DF, Loavenbruck A, et al. The role of skin biopsy in differentiating small-fiber neuropathy from ganglionopathy. Eur J Neurol. 2018;25(6):848–53.
12. Thaisetthawatkul P, Fernandes Filho JA, Herrmann DN. Contribution of QSART to the diagnosis of small fiber neuropathy. Muscle Nerve. 2013;48(6):883–8.
13. de Greef BTA, Hoeijmakers JGJ, Gorissen-Brouwers CML, Geerts M, Faber CG, Merkies ISJ. Associated conditions in small fiber neuropathy - a large cohort study and review of the literature. Eur J Neurol. 2018;25(2):348–55.
14. Hoitsma E, Marziniak M, Faber CG, Reulen JP, Sommer C, De Baets M, et al. Small fibre neuropathy in sarcoidosis. Lancet. 2002;359(9323):2085–6.
15. Tavee JO, Stern BJ. Neurosarcoidosis. Continuum (Minneap Minn). 2014;20(3 Neurology of Systemic Disease):545–59.
16. Hoitsma E, Faber CG, van Santen-Hoeufft M, De Vries J, Reulen JP, Drent M. Improvement of small fiber neuropathy in a sarcoidosis patient after treatment with infliximab. Sarcoidosis Vasc Diffuse Lung Dis. 2006;23(1):73–7.
17. Hoitsma E, Faber CG, Drent M, Sharma OP. Neurosarcoidosis: a clinical dilemma. Lancet Neurol. 2004;3(7):397–407.

Chapter 41
A 39-Year-Old Woman with Intermittent Bilateral Foot and Leg Pain since Childhood

Ryan Castoro, Jun Li, and Lan Zhou

History

A 39-year-old woman presented for evaluation of intermittent bilateral foot and leg pain since childhood. She described the pain as deep aching and it was rated at 6–7/10. In childhood she would have pain daily, but lately had pain approximately two times per week. The pain usually lasted between 15–30 minutes with a rapid onset. Exacerbating factors included weather changes and physical exertion. Relieving factors were rest and non-steroidal anti-inflammatory drugs (NSAIDs). There was no radiation of the pain, associated erythema or weakness. She denied dry eyes, dry mouth, orthostatic dizziness, bowel constipation, and difficulty sweating. Prior to this visit the patient had been followed by rheumatology for possible fibromyalgia. Her past medical history was unremarkable except for the episodic pain. She did not smoke cigarettes or drink alcohol. Her family history was notable for five other family members with similar complaints. They all experienced a similar early onset, recurrent, and deep aching type of pain mainly in the feet and distal legs, including joints. The pain could occur as frequently as 1–2 times per day. Three of the four affected family members reported relief with NSAIDs.

R. Castoro
Department of Physical Medicine and Rehabilitation, Vanderbilt University Medical Center, Nashville, TN, USA

J. Li
Department of Neurology, Wayne State University School of Medicine and Detroit Medical Center, Detroit, MI, USA

L. Zhou (✉)
Departments of Neurology and Pathology, Boston University Medical Center, Boston, MA, USA
e-mail: lanzhou@bu.edu

L. Zhou et al. (eds.), *A Case-Based Guide to Neuromuscular Pathology*,
https://doi.org/10.1007/978-3-030-25682-1_41

Physical Examination

General examination was unremarkable. Her neurologic examination showed normal mental status, cranial nerve functions, and muscle strength. Her sensation was intact to light touch, pinprick, vibration, and joint position. Her deep tendon reflexes were normal in the upper and lower extremities. Her gait was normal, without appreciable imbalance. All affected and unaffected family members had similar physical examination findings.

Investigations

Her initial rheumatologic workup was positive for a mildly elevated erythrocyte sedimentation rate 32 mm/hr. (0–20 mm/hr), mildly low free T4 0.46 ng/dL (0.61–1.76 ng/dL) and mild anemia with hemoglobin 10.2 gm/dL (11.8–16.0 gm/dL); her laboratory testing was normal for creatinine kinase, free T3, thyroid stimulating hormone, uric acid, vitamin B12 and D. Nerve conduction studies revealed no evidence for a large fiber peripheral neuropathy. Skin biopsy was done to evaluate for possible small fiber sensory neuropathy.

Skin Biopsy Findings

Skin biopsy (Fig. 41.1) showed normal intraepidermal nerve fiber densities (IENFD) at the distal leg, distal thigh, and proximal thigh, with no abnormal morphological changes in the nerve fibers. Thus, there was no evidence to suggest a small fiber sensory neuropathy.

Investigation After Obtaining the Skin Biopsy Diagnosis

Given the history of presentation and a positive family history, the diagnosis of familial episodic pain syndrome (FEPS) was considered. Targeted exome sequencing for common genes associated with FEPS revealed a heterozygous Arg225Cys mutation in the *SCN11A* gene. The same mutation was found in the 5 affected family members but not the 2 unaffected family members. The inheritance pattern is autosomal dominant.

Final Diagnosis

Familial episodic pain syndrome caused by the *SCN11A* Arg225Cys mutation

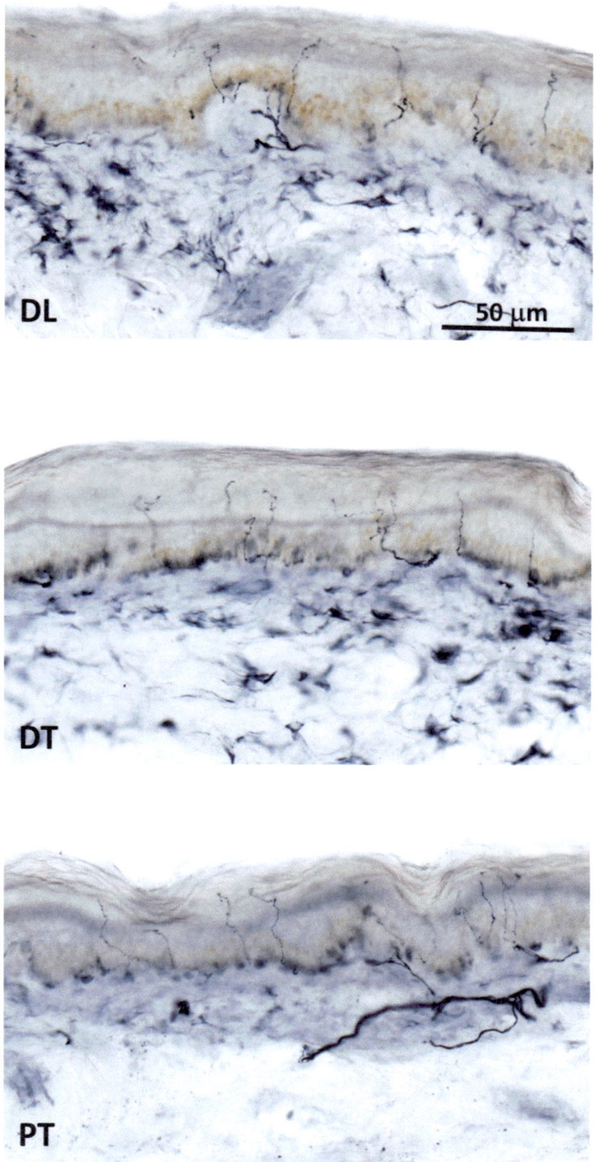

Fig. 41.1 PGP9.5 immunostaining of skin biopsy specimens shows rich innervation of epidermis with normal intraepidermal nerve fiber morphology at the distal leg (DL), distal thigh (DT), and proximal thigh (PT)

Patient Follow-up

The patient had been followed in the clinic for 2 years. She noted partial relief with NSAIDs and was transitioned to Gabapentin. However, she did not get any symptom relief with Gabapentin and switched back to NSAIDs with addition of Acetaminophen which had provided improved relief. She continued to experience pain approximately twice per week, but the intensity was significantly reduced.

Discussion

Human channelopathic pain syndromes have been increasingly recognized by treating neurologists, and the genotype and phenotype spectrums have been continuously expanding [1]. The syndromes can be caused by mutations and abnormal functions of multiple ion channels expressed by nociceptors, including transient receptor potential channel (TRPA1) [2] and voltage-gated sodium channels (Nav1.7-Nav1.9) [3]. Nav1.7, Nav1.8, and Nav1.9 are α-subunit isoforms of the voltage-gated sodium channels that are preferentially expressed in small-diameter dorsal root ganglion (DRG) neurons, trigeminal neurons, and their small peripheral nerve axons [4–7]. Nav1.7, Nav1.8, and Nav1.9 are encoded by the *SCN9A*, *SCN10A*, and *SCN11A* genes, respectively.

Gain-of-function mutations of the *SCN9A* gene have been reported to cause primary erythromelagia [8], paroxysmal extreme pain disorder (PEPD) (previously familial rectal pain syndrome) with episodic perirectal, periorbital and perimandibular deep burning pain [9, 10], and painful small fiber neuropathy [11]. Loss-of-function mutations of the *SCN9A* gene can cause congenital channelopathy-associated insensitivity to pain (CIP) [12]. In a study of 28 patients with skin biopsy-confirmed idiopathic small fiber neuropathy, 8 were found to carry mutations in the *SCN9A* gene with resultant Nav1.7 hyperactivity and DRG hyperexcitability [11]. In a study of 104 patients with predominant painful small fiber neuropathy without *SCN9A* gene mutations, 9 were found to have gain-of-function mutations in the *SCN10A* gene [13]. Gain-of-function mutations in the *SCN11A* gene have also been reported and linked to painful small fiber neuropathy [14, 15], familial episodic pain syndrome (FEPS) [16–18], and congenital inability to feel pain with self-mutilation [19]. In a study of 345 patients with painful neuropathy without *SCN9A* or *SCN10A* gene mutations, 12 had *SCN11A* gene mutations [14].

Familial episodic pain syndromes caused by different mutations in different genes can have different clinical presentations. The FEPS caused by the N855S TRPA1 mutation manifests episodic debilitating upper body pain with normal exam and normal intraepidermal nerve fiber densities in the affected areas [2]. Patients with PEPD caused by the *SCN9A* mutations have early onset autonomic symptoms and episodic excruciating deep burning pain in the rectal, ocular, or jaw areas [10]. The FEPS caused by a mutation in the *SCN10A* gene manifests episodic intense burning pain with reduced intraepidermal nerve fiber densities [13]. The FEPS caused by the *SCN11A* Arg225Cys mutation as seen in our patient and her affected family members mainly presents with episodes of deep aching pain in the feet and distal legs with normal exam and normal intraepdiermal nerve fiber densities [18]. The reason for the different areas of involvement, different qualities of pain, and different changes in intraepidermal nerve fibers in these FEPS is unclear, as all these mutations are found to cause DRG hyperexcitability [2, 13, 17]. It could be due to the potential differences in regional involvement of small-diameter DRG neurons and selective impairment of terminal nerve endings by different mutations. While some mutations with resultant DRG dysfunction cause neurite degeneration due to calcium toxicity, energetic stress, and reactive oxygen species production [20], the others may not.

The neuropathic pain associated with small fiber neuropathy is usually sharp, described as burning, tingling, stabbing, lancinating, or electric shock-like. Dull aching pain often suggests musculoskeletal or joint abnormalities, such as arthritis. The pain in fibromyalgia is also mostly deep aching. Our case illustrates that while *SCN9A-11A* mutations are well known to cause small fiber neuropathy with neuropathic pain and intraepidermal nerve fiber degeneration, some mutations, like *SCN11A* Arg225Cys, may not cause neuropathic pain or intraepidermal nerve fiber degeneration, but cause dull nociceptive pain in distal lower extremities, including joints, which can mimic fibromyalgia. Normal skin biopsy in a patient with pain does not exclude the possibility of a sodium channelopathy, especially when there is a positive family history of the pain disorder. Obtaining a specific genetic diagnosis and understanding pathogenic mechanisms of individual mutations will help develop targeted therapies [3, 21]. It is intriguing that the deep aching pain caused by the *SCN11A* Arg225Cys mutation responds relatively well to NSAIDs [17, 18] but not Gabapentin [18]. The finding suggests an inflammatory component to the pain in this setting.

Pearls

1. Mutations in the TRPA1 ion channel and Nav1.7–1.9 sodium channels can cause various pain syndromes, including paroxysmal extreme pain disorder (familial rectal pain syndrome), primary erythromelagia, painful small fiber neuropathy, and familial episodic pain syndromes.
2. Some pain syndromes associated with channelopathies do not have intraepidermal nerve fiber degeneration. Therefore, normal skin biopsy does not exclude the diagnosis.
3. Nav1.7–1.9 sodium channel gene (*SCN9A-11A*) mutations should be considered in patients with early-onset painful small fiber neuropathy, especially in the presence of a positive family history and absence of other neuropathy etiologies.
4. Patients with episodic pain and a family history of similar symptom should be considered for genetic testing of the genes commonly involved in familial episodic pain syndrome.
5. Familial episodic pain syndrome caused by the *SCN11A* Arg225Cys mutation manifests dull aching pain rather than sharp neuropathic pain in distal lower extremities including joints, which mimics fibromyalgia. The pain responds relatively well to NSAIDs and Acetaminophen but not Gabapentin, which suggests an inflammatory component to the pain. The mutation does not cause detectable intraepidermal nerve fiber degeneration.

References

1. Waxman SG. Channelopathic pain: a growing but still small list of model disorders. Neuron. 2010;66(5):622–4.
2. Kremeyer B, Lopera F, Cox JJ, Momin A, Rugiero F, Marsh S, et al. A gain-of-function mutation in TRPA1 causes familial episodic pain syndrome. Neuron. 2010;66(5):671–80.
3. Hoeijmakers JG, Faber CG, Merkies IS, Waxman SG. Painful peripheral neuropathy and sodium channel mutations. Neurosci Lett. 2015;596:51–9.
4. Dib-Hajj SD, Tyrrell L, Black JA, Waxman SG. NaN, a novel voltage-gated Na channel, is expressed preferentially in peripheral sensory neurons and down-regulated after axotomy. Proc Natl Acad Sci U S A. 1998;95(15):8963–8.
5. Persson AK, Black JA, Gasser A, Cheng X, Fischer TZ, Waxman SG. Sodium-calcium exchanger and multiple sodium channel isoforms in intra-epidermal nerve terminals. Mol Pain. 2010;6:84.
6. Zhao P, Barr TP, Hou Q, Dib-Hajj SD, Black JA, Albrecht PJ, et al. Voltage-gated sodium channel expression in rat and human epidermal keratinocytes: evidence for a role in pain. Pain. 2008;139(1):90–105.
7. Fang X, Djouhri L, Black JA, Dib-Hajj SD, Waxman SG, Lawson SN. The presence and role of the tetrodotoxin-resistant sodium channel Na(v)1.9 (NaN) in nociceptive primary afferent neurons. J Neurosci. 2002;22(17):7425–33.
8. Yang Y, Wang Y, Li S, Xu Z, Li H, Ma L, et al. Mutations in SCN9A, encoding a sodium channel alpha subunit, in patients with primary erythermalgia. J Med Genet. 2004;41(3):171–4.
9. Fertleman CR, Baker MD, Parker KA, Moffatt S, Elmslie FV, Abrahamsen B, et al. SCN9A mutations in paroxysmal extreme pain disorder: allelic variants underlie distinct channel defects and phenotypes. Neuron. 2006;52(5):767–74.
10. Fertleman CR, Ferrie CD, Aicardi J, Bednarek NA, Eeg-Olofsson O, Elmslie FV, et al. Paroxysmal extreme pain disorder (previously familial rectal pain syndrome). Neurology. 2007;69(6):586–95.
11. Faber CG, Hoeijmakers JG, Ahn HS, Cheng X, Han C, Choi JS, et al. Gain of function Nanu1.7 mutations in idiopathic small fiber neuropathy. Ann Neurol. 2012;71(1):26–39.
12. Cox JJ, Reimann F, Nicholas AK, Thornton G, Roberts E, Springell K, et al. An SCN9A channelopathy causes congenital inability to experience pain. Nature. 2006;444(7121):894–8.
13. Faber CG, Lauria G, Merkies IS, Cheng X, Han C, Ahn HS, et al. Gain-of-function Nav1.8 mutations in painful neuropathy. Proc Natl Acad Sci U S A. 2012;109(47):19444–9.
14. Huang J, Han C, Estacion M, Vasylyev D, Hoeijmakers JG, Gerrits MM, et al. Gain-of-function mutations in sodium channel Na(v)1.9 in painful neuropathy. Brain. 2014;137(Pt 6):1627–42.
15. Han C, Yang Y, Te Morsche RH, Drenth JP, Politei JM, Waxman SG, et al. Familial gain-of-function Nav1.9 mutation in a painful channelopathy. J Neurol Neurosurg Psychiatry. 2017;88(3):233–40.
16. Okuda H, Noguchi A, Kobayashi H, Kondo D, Harada KH, Youssefian S, et al. Infantile pain episodes associated with Novel Nav1.9 mutations in familial episodic pain syndrome in Japanese Families. PLoS One. 2016;11(5):e0154827.
17. Zhang XY, Wen J, Yang W, Wang C, Gao L, Zheng LH, et al. Gain-of-function mutations in SCN11A cause familial episodic pain. Am J Hum Genet. 2013;93(5):957–66.
18. Castoro R, Simmons M, Ravi V, Huang D, Lee C, Sergent J, et al. SCN11A Arg225Cys mutation causes nociceptive pain without detectable peripheral nerve pathology. Neurol Genet. 2018;4(4):e255.
19. Leipold E, Liebmann L, Korenke GC, Heinrich T, Giesselmann S, Baets J, et al. A de novo gain-of-function mutation in SCN11A causes loss of pain perception. Nat Genet. 2013;45(11):1399–404.

20. Rolyan H, Liu S, Hoeijmakers JG, Faber CG, Merkies IS, Lauria G, et al. A painful neuropathy-associated Nav1.7 mutant leads to time-dependent degeneration of small-diameter axons associated with intracellular Ca2+ dysregulation and decrease in ATP levels. Mol Pain. 2016;12:174480691667447.
21. de Greef BT, Merkies IS, Geerts M, Faber CG, Hoeijmakers JG. Efficacy, safety, and tolerability of lacosamide in patients with gain-of-function Nav1.7 mutation-related small fiber neuropathy: study protocol of a randomized controlled trial-the LENSS study. Trials. 2016;17(1):306.

Chapter 42
A 35-Year-Old Man with Pain and Numbness in the Left Lateral Thigh

Lan Zhou

History

A 35-year-old Caucasian man presented with pain and numbness in the left lateral thigh and both heels for 6 months. He also reported intermittent low back pain, occasionally shooting towards the bilateral gluteal areas and posterior thighs. He admitted to 60 pounds of weight gain over a period of 2 years. He denied weakness. He denied dry mouth, dry eyes, palpitations, orthostatic dizziness, bowel constipation, or sweating abnormalities. He had a past medical history of asthma. He used albuterol inhaler as needed. Family history was significant for diabetes mellitus. He did not smoke cigarettes, drink alcohol, or abuse illicit drugs.

Physical Examination

The patient was markedly obese with body mass index (BMI) 41.3 kg/m^2. His general examination was otherwise unremarkable. His mental status, cranial nerve functions, motor strength, coordination, and gait were all normal. Pinprick sensation was reduced in the left lateral thigh and both feet. Vibratory sensation, proprioception, and deep tendon reflexes were preserved. There was no spine tenderness.

L. Zhou (✉)
Departments of Neurology and Pathology, Boston University Medical Center, Boston, MA, USA
e-mail: lanzhou@bu.edu

L. Zhou et al. (eds.), *A Case-Based Guide to Neuromuscular Pathology*,
https://doi.org/10.1007/978-3-030-25682-1_42

Investigations

Nerve conduction study (NCS) showed absent lateral femoral cutaneous nerve (LFCN) conduction responses bilaterally but normal sural sensory responses. Needle electromyography (EMG) of selected left distal leg and thigh muscles was normal. Lumbosacral spine MRI showed mild disc bulge at L5/S1. Blood tests revealed borderline diabetes mellitus with HbA1C level 6.1%. ANA, TSH, free T4, B12, and serum immunofixation were unremarkable. Skin biopsy with intraepidermal nerve fiber density (IENFD) evaluation was performed for further evaluation.

Skin Biopsy Findings

3-mm punch skin biopsies showed absent intraepidermal nerve fibers at the left proximal thigh and a normal IENFD at the right proximal thigh (9.3 fibers/mm) (Fig. 42.1). It also showed a borderline reduced IENFD at the left distal leg (4.9 fibers/mm).

Final Diagnosis

1. Left lateral femoral cutaneous neuropathy (meralgia paresthetica)
2. Distal small fiber sensory neuropathy

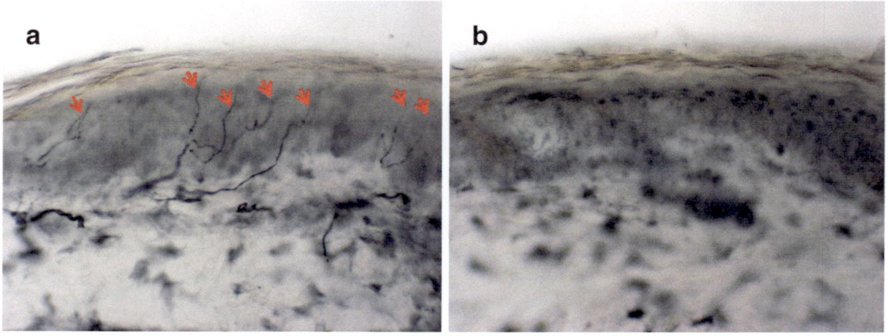

Fig. 42.1 PGP9.5 immunostaining shows normal cutaneous innervation with many intraepidermal nerve fibers (arrows) present at the unaffected right proximal thigh (**a**), but no intraepidermal nerve fibers are seen at the symptomatic left proximal thigh (**b**)

Patient Follow-up

The patient underwent diet control and regular exercise. He also took Gabapentin for pain control. He intentionally lost 40 pounds over 1 year with improvement of his sensory symptoms.

Discussion

Meralgia paresthetica is a focal neuropathy which is caused by compression of the LFCN at the level of the anterior-superior iliac spine or inguinal ligament. The disease can be associated with obesity, diabetes mellitus, wearing tight low cut trousers, and strenuous walking and cycling, among others [1–4]. Patients with meralgia paresthetica commonly present with pain, burning, tingling, and/or numbness in the lateral or anterolateral thigh [5], which can mimic upper lumbar radiculopathy [6, 7]. A reliable and sensitive diagnostic test is needed not only to confirm the diagnosis but also to distinguish it from lumbar radiculopathy. LFCN NCS is often technically challenging due to the high anatomical variability of the nerve and the obesity of patients [1, 4, 8, 9] as seen in our case. Although the symptoms were unilateral in our patient, NCS showed absent LFCN conduction responses bilaterally; therefore, it was non-diagnostic. Using ultrasound-guide surface electrode placement may greatly improve the sensitivity of the test, but it is still suboptimal in evaluating markedly obese patients as the response is difficult to obtain and the interside variability is high [10]. Imaging studies, including ultrasound and magnetic resounance neurography (MRN), may be useful [11–14], but further confirmatory studies are needed and MRN is not widely available.

LFCN arises from the L2 and L3 nerve roots. The nerve specimens derived from neurectomy of patients with chronic meralgia paresthetica showed selective loss of large myelinated fibers with varying degree of intraneural and epineural inflammation [15]. A functional study also suggested small fiber involvement as warm and heat pain sensation thresholds were increased and contact heat-evoked potentials (CHEPs) were reduced in the affected side of 14 patients with meralgia paresthetica as compared with unaffected side and 14 normal controls [16]. Along with the prominent small sensory fiber symptoms and signs in the affected areas of meralgia paresthetica, we studied the diagnostic utility of skin biopsy in this condition, and we found that meralgia paresthetica was indeed associated with focal loss of intraepidermal nerve fibers at the lateral proximal thigh [17]. Therefore, skin biopsy with IENFD evaluation is useful in the diagnosis of this disease. Similar to NCS, skin biopsy can differentiate sensory neuropathy from sensory radiculopathy, as IENFD can be affected by sensory neuropathy but should not be affected by preganglionic root lesions.

Meralgia paresthetica affects anterolateral proximal thigh, and the normal IENFD has been established at the proximal thigh by most cutaneous nerve laboratories. When evaluating meralgia paresthetica, we biopsy bilateral proximal thighs to make a side-to-side comparison and to correlate the IENFD reduction with the side of symptoms and signs. We also biopsy the distal leg to rule out a more generalized peripheral neuropathy as the cause of reduced IENFD at the affected thigh. Our patient did have a distal small fiber neuropathy, which was most likely due to the prediabetes. But the absent IENF at the affected proximal thigh is out of proportion to the borderline reduced IENFD at the distal leg. The absent IENF at the proximal thigh is felt to be due to the meralgia paresthetica rather than related to the distal SFN, and it is unlikely to represent a non-length-dependent SFN given his clinical presentation. The meralgia paresthetica in our patient is mainly caused by the obesity. Prediabetes may also contribute. The key management is weight reduction by lifestyle modification. Pain control is also important. The symptoms of our patient, both pain and numbness, have improved after 1 year of lifestyle modification with reduction of 40 pounds of body weight.

Skin biopsy has been shown useful for assessing focal neuropathies with small fiber degeneration, which include complex regional pain syndrome and diabetic truncal neuropathy in addition to meralgia paresethetica [17–19]. If no normative values are established at the affected sites, the contralateral unaffected sites should also be biopsied for comparison.

Pearls

Clinical Pearls

1. Meralgia paresthetica, a focal neuropathy caused by compression of the lateral femoral cutaneous nerve, is commonly associated with obesity, diabetes mellitus, wearing tight low cut trousers, and strenuous walking and cycling.
2. Patients with meralgia paresthetica commonly present with pain, burning, tingling, and/or numbness in the lateral or anterolateral thigh, which can mimic upper lumbar radiculopathy.
3. LFCN NCS is often technically challenging and non-diagnostic due to the high anatomical variability of the nerve and the obesity of patients.
4. Skin biopsy is useful in assessing meralgia paresthetica and differentiating it from upper lumbar radiculopathy.
5. The management of meralgia paresthetica is to control the underlying causes and to treat the neuropathic pain.

Pathology Pearls

1. Meralgia paresthetic is associated with small fiber degeneration in the affected lateral proximal thigh.
2. When evaluating meralgia paresthetica, bilateral proximal thighs should be biopsied for side-to-side comparison. The distal leg should also be biopsied to rule out a more generalized peripheral neuropathy being the cause of the reduced IENFD at the affected thigh.

References

1. Cheatham SW, Kolber MJ, Salamh PA. Meralgia paresthetica: a review of the literature. Int J Sports Phys Ther. 2013;8(6):883–93.
2. Kho KH, Blijham PJ, Zwarts MJ. Meralgia paresthetica after strenuous exercise. Muscle Nerve. 2005;31(6):761–3.
3. Moucharafieh R, Wehbe J, Maalouf G. Meralgia paresthetica: a result of tight new trendy low cut trousers ('taille basse'). Int J Surg. 2008;6(2):164–8.
4. Parisi TJ, Mandrekar J, Dyck PJ, Klein CJ. Meralgia paresthetica: relation to obesity, advanced age, and diabetes mellitus. Neurology. 2011;77(16):1538–42.
5. Seror P, Seror R. Meralgia paresthetica: clinical and electrophysiological diagnosis in 120 cases. Muscle Nerve. 2006;33(5):650–4.
6. Trummer M, Flaschka G, Unger F, Eustacchio S. Lumbar disc herniation mimicking meralgia paresthetica: case report. Surg Neurol. 2000;54(1):80–1.
7. Yang SN, Kim DH. L1 radiculopathy mimicking meralgia paresthetica: a case report. Muscle Nerve. 2010;41(4):566–8.
8. Mondelli M, Rossi S, Romano C. Body mass index in meralgia paresthetica: a case-control study. Acta Neurol Scand. 2007;116(2):118–23.
9. Moritz T, Prosch H, Berzaczy D, Happak W, Lieba-Samal D, Bernathova M, et al. Common anatomical variation in patients with idiopathic meralgia paresthetica: a high resolution ultrasound case-control study. Pain Physician. 2013;16(3):E287–93.
10. Boon AJ, Bailey PW, Smith J, Sorenson EJ, Harper CM, Hurdle MF. Utility of ultrasound-guided surface electrode placement in lateral femoral cutaneous nerve conduction studies. Muscle Nerve. 2011;44(4):525–30.
11. Aravindakannan T, Wilder-Smith EP. High-resolution ultrasonography in the assessment of meralgia paresthetica. Muscle Nerve. 2012;45(3):434–5.
12. Chhabra A, Del Grande F, Soldatos T, Chalian M, Belzberg AJ, Williams EH, et al. Meralgia paresthetica: 3-Tesla magnetic resonance neurography. Skelet Radiol. 2013;42(6):803–8.
13. Suh DH, Kim DH, Park JW, Park BK. Sonographic and electrophysiologic findings in patients with meralgia paresthetica. Clin Neurophysiol. 2013;124(7):1460–4.
14. Tagliafico A, Padua L, Martinoli C. High-resolution ultrasonography in the assessment of meralgia paresthetica: some clarifications are needed. Muscle Nerve. 2012;45(6):922; author reply
15. Berini SE, Spinner RJ, Jentoft ME, Engelstad JK, Staff NP, Suanprasert N, et al. Chronic meralgia paresthetica and neurectomy: a clinical pathologic study. Neurology. 2014;82(17):1551–5.

16. Schestatsky P, Llado-Carbo E, Casanova-Molla J, Alvarez-Blanco S, Valls-Sole J. Small fibre function in patients with meralgia paresthetica. Pain. 2008;139(2):342–8.
17. Wongmek A, Shin S, Zhou L. Skin biopsy in assessing meralgia paresthetica. Muscle Nerve. 2016;53(4):641–3.
18. Chemali KR, Zhou L. Small fiber degeneration in post-stroke complex regional pain syndrome I. Neurology. 2007;69(3):316–7.
19. Lauria G, McArthur JC, Hauer PE, Griffin JW, Cornblath DR. Neuropathological alterations in diabetic truncal neuropathy: evaluation by skin biopsy. J Neurol Neurosurg Psychiatry. 1998;65(5):762–6.

Index of Cases

Chapter 4: Rhabdomyolysis with normal muscle biopsy
Chapter 5: Antisynthetase Syndrome
Chapter 6: Inclusion body myositis
Chapter 7: Immune-mediated necrotizing myopathy
Chapter 8: Granulomatous myositis
Chapter 9: ANCA-associated vasculitis presenting with severe myalgia
Chapter 10: TB myositis
Chapter 11: Limb girdle muscular dystrophy type 2A
Chapter 12: Myotonic dystrophy type 2
Chapter 13: McArdle disease
Chapter 14: Lipid storage myopathy
Chapter 15: Mitochondrial myopathy
Chapter 16: Late-onset Pompe disease
Chapter 17: Myofibrillar myopathy
Chapter 18: Statin myopathy
Chapter 19: Hydroxychloroquine myopathy
Chapter 20: Myopathy associated with calciphylaxis
Chapter 21: Familial ALS caused by an SOD1 mutation
Chapter 22: Kennedy's disease
Chapter 23: Macrophagic myofasciitis
Chapter 24: Duchenne muscular dystrophy
Chapter 25: Merosin deficient congenital muscular dystrophy
Chapter 26: Central nuclear myopathy
Chapter 27: Nemalin myopathy
Chapter 28: Congenital fiber size variation
Chapter 29: Central core disease
Chapter 30: Pompe Disease
Chapter 31: Spinal muscular atrophy type 1
Chapter 32: Vasculitic neuropathy
Chapter 33: Amyloid neuropathy

L. Zhou et al. (eds.), *A Case-Based Guide to Neuromuscular Pathology*,
https://doi.org/10.1007/978-3-030-25682-1

Index

L. Zhou et al. (eds.), *A Case-Based Guide to Neuromuscular Pathology*,
https://doi.org/10.1007/978-3-030-25682-1

T

MIX
Papier aus verantwortungsvollen Quellen
Paper from responsible sources
FSC® C105338

If you have any concerns about our products,
you can contact us on
ProductSafety@springernature.com

In case Publisher is established outside the EU,
the EU authorized representative is:
Springer Nature Customer Service Center GmbH
Europaplatz 3, 69115 Heidelberg, Germany

Printed by Libri Plureos GmbH
in Hamburg, Germany